E-Health Communities and Online Self-Help Groups:

Applications and Usage

Åsa Smedberg
Stockholm University, Sweden

Medical Information Science
REFERENCE

Managing Director:	Lindsay Johnston
Book Production Manager:	Sean Woznicki
Development Manager:	Joel Gamon
Development Editor:	Myla Harty
Acquisitions Editor:	Erika Carter
Typesetters:	Adrienne Freeland
Print Coordinator:	Jamie Snavely
Cover Design:	Nick Newcomer

Published in the United States of America by
Medical Information Science Reference (an imprint of IGI Global)
701 E. Chocolate Avenue
Hershey PA 17033
Tel: 717-533-8845
Fax: 717-533-8661
E-mail: cust@igi-global.com
Web site: http://www.igi-global.com

Library of Congress Cataloging-in-Publication Data

E-health communities and online self-help groups: applications and usage /
Asa Smedberg, editor.
p. cm.
Includes bibliographical references and index.
ISBN 978-1-60960-866-8 (hardcover) -- ISBN 978-1-60960-868-2 (print & perpetual access) -- ISBN 978-1-60960-867-5 (ebook) 1. Medical informatics. 2. Medicine--Electronic information resources. 3. Self-care, Health. I. Smedberg, Esa.
R858.E227 2012
610.285--dc23

2011020033

British Cataloguing in Publication Data
A Cataloguing in Publication record for this book is available from the British Library.

Editorial Advisory Board

Table of Contents

Foreword vii

Preface ix

Acknowledgment xiv

Chapter 1
Virtual Worlds for Children with Medical Conditions: Experiences for Promoting Positive Youth Development 1
Marina U. Bers, Tufts University, USA
Kathryn A. Cantrell, Tufts University, USA

Chapter 2
An E-Health System for Treatment of Childhood Obesity: The Etiobe Platform 24
Rosa M. Baños, Universidad de Valencia, Spain
Ausiàs Cebolla, Universidad Jaume I, Spain
Elia Oliver, Universidad de Valencia, Spain
Soledad Quero Castellano, Universitat Jaume I, Spain
Cristina Botella, Universidad Jaume I, Spain

Chapter 3
Internet-Based Chronic Disease Self-Management for Youth 36
Jennifer Stinson, The Hospital for Sick Children, Canada
Navreet Gill, The Hospital for Sick Children, Canada

Chapter 4
An E-Health System for Promoting Wellbeing in the Elderly: The Butler System 57
Cristina Botella, Universidad Jaume I, Spain
Rosa M. Baños, Universidad de Valencia, Spain
Ernestina Etchemendy, Universidad de Valencia, Spain
Diana Castilla, Universidad Jaume I, Spain
Azucena García-Palacios, Universidad Jaume I, Spain
Alcañiz Mariano, Universidad Politécnica de Valencia, Spain

Chapter 5
Do Virtual Communities Have an Effect on the Social Network of Cancer Patients? Empirical Insights from Germany ... 72
Jan Marco Leimeister, Universität Kassel, Germany
Karin Janina Schweizer, Microsoft Deutschland GmbH, Germany
Helmut Krcmar, Technische Universität München, Germany

Chapter 6
A Content Analysis of an Online Support Group for Survivors of Sexual Violence ... 85
Jennifer Yeager, University of East London, UK & Waterford Institute of Technology, Ireland

Chapter 7
Blogging: A New Tool for Coping and Accessing Psycho-Social Support for People Living with HIV? ... 106
Cecilia Strand, Uppsala University, Sweden

Chapter 8
Can Stored Data Answer All Questions: A Study of Questions on Eating Disorders ... 121
Jacob Palme, Stockholm University, Sweden

Chapter 9
Dynamic Stress Management: Self-Help through Holistic System Design ... 136
Åsa Smedberg, Stockholm University, Sweden
Hélène Sandmark, Mälardalen University, Sweden

Chapter 10
Living a Healthier Life – Online: On Blending Professional and Experiential Knowledge in Online Self-Help Groups ... 155
Roar Stokken, Norwegian University of Science and Technology, Norway & Sunnmøre Hospital Trust, Norway
Gjermund Eikli, Norwegian Net School, Norway

Chapter 11
The Amazing Impossibilities of Technology: Factors that Inhibit Participation in Skype™ Based Self-Help Groups ... 177
Stein Conradsen, Sunnmøre Hospital Trust, Norway

Chapter 12
E-Health and Digital Inclusion ... 194
Lorna Gibson, University of Dundee, UK
David Sloan, University of Dundee, UK
Wendy Moncur, University of Aberdeen, UK

Chapter 13
Online Health Communities and Health Literacy: Applying a Framework for Understanding Domains of Health Literacy 208
Erin Willis, University of Memphis, USA
Ye Wang, University of Missouri – Kansas City, USA
Shelly Rodgers, Missouri School of Journalism, USA

Chapter 14
Identifying the Essential Design Requirements for Usable E-Health Communities in Mobile Devices 225
Ricardo Mendoza-González, Instituto Tecnológico de Aguascalientes, Mexico
Miguel Vargas Martin, University of Ontario Institute of Technology, Canada
Laura C. Rodríguez-Martínez, Instituto Tecnológico de Aguascalientes, Mexico

Chapter 15
Australian Patient Organizations: Using Digital Technologies to Engage Health Citizen Communities in Health Policy 245
Anni Dugdale, University of Canberra, Australia

Chapter 16
European E-Health Framework: Towards More "Patient-Friendly" Healthcare Services? 262
Korinna Zoi Karamagkioli, Alexandra University Hospital, Greece
Evika Karamagioli, Gov2u, Greece

Chapter 17
Developing Virtual Communities to Support Drug Policy Knowledge Exchange: The Canadian Experience 279
Mowafa Househ, King Saud Bin Abdul Aziz University for Health Sciences, Saudi Arabia
Andre Kushniruk, University of Victoria, Canada
Malcolm Maclure, Harvard University, USA, University of Victoria, Canada & British Columbia Ministry of Health, Canada
Bruce Carleton, University of British Columbia, Canada, Children's and Women's Health Centre of BC, Canada & Child & Family Research Institute, Canada
Denise Cloutier-Fisher, University of Victoria, Canada

About the Contributors 303

Index 312

Foreword

Imagine that you have had excellent health all of your life and you are suddenly diagnosed with cancer. At first you will likely be in a state of shock unable to fully understand how life might change or even end. Gradually you and those around you may start to plan and strategize how to deal with this new reality. Doctors give you information and advise on how to proceed. They answer lots of questions, but sometimes you need more information before you can determine what you really need to know. That's when many of us would turn to the Internet, taking care not to believe everything we read and being careful to warn others to do the same.

The questions that we all need to ask in such situations are which sites should I trust? And what is relevant to me, not just my medical situation, but also my life style? Suddenly, faced with a barrage of strange sounding medical terms, and choices about which drugs or medical procedures to select, we feel scared and alone. In some countries fears about whether costly treatment will be covered by medical insurance add to the trauma. But there is hope. New drugs and procedures are being discovered everyday. But this is not enough; society is waking up to the benefits of e-health and online health support groups.

Like local, face-to-face support communities, their online equivalents enable people, often scattered across the country or even the world, to exchange information and offer support to each other. Such communities are particularly valuable for those who struggle with mobility or have a rare condition that is shared by only a few people. Furthermore, online health communities can be accessed at any time, day or night, which many people find comforting. Perhaps most important of all, they bring together people with similar problems who have a deep understanding of what it is like to have a particular disease.

Other medical problems result when a disease is chronic and requires the patient to stick to a particular routine, for example, a child with an obesity problem or a person with diabetes. In these situations support to manage the health problem on a daily basis is needed and technology can often help here too.

E-Health Communities and Online Self-Help Groups: Applications and Usage edited by Dr. Åsa Smedberg, a Senior Lecturer in the Department of Computer and Systems Sciences at Stockholm University in Sweden provides a diverse selection of chapters written by experts that address many of the important health issues of our age. There are chapters about virtual worlds for children, self-help systems for youths, including those with obesity, and older adults. It has a chapter on the increasingly important topic of health literacy and one on mobile apps for health support, as well as chapters on patient support communities for cancer and other diseases, and many more.

Technology is changing our health systems and empowering patients to understand their own health much better than ever before. Dr. Åsa Smedberg has compiled an impressive "must read" book for anyone interested in E-Health communities and online self-help groups. Each chapter is a valuable resource for patients, practitioners, and researchers interested in how technology can support health care. This book is full of good examples for those wanting to read in depth while also providing an excellent overview of the field.

Jennifer Preece
University of Maryland, USA

Jennifer Preece *is Professor and Dean of the College of Information Studies – Maryland's iSchool - at the University of Maryland. Jenny's teaching and research focuses on the intersection between information, community and technology. She is particularly interested in community participation on- and off-line and social computing. She has researched ways to support empathy online, patterns of online participation and what makes technology-supported communities successful. Jenny is author of over two hundred articles that include refereed journal and conference proceedings and eight books. Her two most recent books are: "Online Communities: Designing Usability, Supporting Sociability" (2000) and a co-authored text entitled "Interaction Design: Beyond Human-Computer Interaction" (1st Ed. 2002; 2nd Ed. 2007). Both books are published by John Wiley & Sons. She is also a regular conference keynote speaker.*

Preface

INTRODUCTION

A traditional community is a place for people who share the same interests and concerns to meet to cooperate and to satisfy each other's needs. E-communities, communities mediated by ICT and the Internet, are used in many areas and for different purposes. Some are open for anyone to join, and some are closed and can only be accessed by an invited group. A common interest and concern for each other is the glue that holds the community together; it should be able to support a sense of togetherness among the community members. It can also be regarded as a virtually social network useful for empathetic support, information sharing, and problem solving.

A certain type of e-communities is used by people who want to discuss health issues with others who share similar health concerns. These e-health communities have become popular arenas for support and sharing of experience, knowledge, and advice among patients and citizens. This group of users has grown rapidly in number and constitutes a large and increasing group on the Internet today. E-health communities are used on a day-to-day basis by people who want to help each other cope with different health conditions and learn together about health-related issues and behaviors. E-health communities create online self-help groups. They exist in many different health areas, from severe physical and mental disorders, such as cancer and depression, to aftercare for patients who are about to return to society, and lifestyle problems such as bad eating and exercising habits, smoking, and stressful lives, that is, lifestyles considered causing health risks to people. There are also self-help systems customized for different age groups, such as children and elderly, and their special conditions and needs.

The growth of e-health communities has contributed to a shift of focus: from healthcare and healthcare givers being the only source of help for most patients, to a situation where patients and citizens take active part in the health and recovery of each other. This has also opened up for patients and citizens to fill a gap: as a group, they can ask for and give support 24 hours a day, 7 days a week. It allows for patients and citizens with health concerns to become both producers and consumers of health information and support. This new active role on the Internet is also called "prosumer," which illustrates the blur between the two previously separate roles. Through the online self-help groups, patients as well as citizens have shown to be more empowered. The Internet and the more available health information and conversations on health issues have even brought empowerment to minority and marginalized groups in the society, such as elderly people. Through the new opportunities, patients can more easily develop confidence to interact effectively with healthcare providers.

The e-health communities help people share experiences, learn together, and provide advice on how to cope with various health problems. In these e-health communities, different types of relationships between participants are developed. There are relationships between people who know each other well, who have access to similar information, common values and approaches, and who provide social and emotional support and self-disclosure reports. There are also relationships characterized by less frequent communication between people who do not know each other well. The latter is also important in order to let the e-health community experience new approaches and opposing ideas.

Although the widespread use of Internet health services and e-health communities has created a lot of new possibilities, they do not automatically lead to certain positive health outcomes or to the public being better informed. It is not given in what ways they affect our health and well-being, and our social or work life. Instead, consequences are highly dependent on contexts. The e-health communities can be utilized in many ways and lead to various social and health outcomes. Community members have different concerns; they communicate on different issues, in different ways, and different community cultures evolve.

In this new world of increased usage of e-health communities, there is a need to discuss different ways of designing and using these systems for communication and learning in groups. There is also a need to systematically evaluate them in terms of learning opportunities, behavioral changes, and impacts on health and well-being.

OBJECTIVE OF THE BOOK

This book offers relevant theoretical frameworks and the latest empirical research findings in the area of e-health communities and online self-help groups. It aims to increase knowledge and understanding of applications and usage of e-health communities for different groups of people who struggle with health disorders, disabilities, lifestyle issues, and other health concerns. The book presents different e-health community settings and aspects, observations of community usage and effects, policy issues, and complementing ways to study and measure effectiveness.

The book addresses health issues that may be of concern to many people. The target audience of this book is researchers and advanced level students in social and health informatics, designers of e-health platforms, and clinical health professionals, such as physicians, dieticians, physiotherapists, and district nurses. It can also be useful for patient interest groups. Moreover, the book provides insights that may support executives concerned with making IT strategies for healthcare.

STRUCTURE OF THE BOOK

The book is organized into five sections. The *first section* is dedicated to e-health communities for different age groups; chapters 1, 2, 3, and 4 are included in this section. This section addresses certain age-related topics for children who are affected by severe illnesses: their relations to peers and siblings, medication, and school work, for example. This section is also concerned with elderly people: their specific needs and concerns, such as changing social lives and the need for continuous mental training. The *second section* of the book, chapters 5, 6, 7, 8, and 9, is concerned with different medical conditions, lifestyle issues, and other health issues. The chapters address e-health communities for people who have been sexually abused, for people with cancer and HIV, with eating disorders and stressful lives. The *third section* of the book includes chapters 10 and 11. The chapters of this section discuss pedagogical and educational aspects of e-health communities. The *fourth section* of the book, chapters 12, 13, and 14, deals with issues related to digital inclusion and usability. The *fifth section* introduces the reader to health policy issues; chapters 15, 16 and 17 address this topic. Below, each chapter is introduced with a few words.

Chapter 1 describes a virtual world for children with critical medical conditions. The chapter guides the reader through two experiences: one with post-transplant pediatric patients and another with pediatric cancer patients. In the first experience, issues of medical adherence and school transition are addressed, and the second experience addresses issues related to sustainable friendship and levels of hope through a virtual summer camp for young patients and their siblings. The virtual world was designed based on a theoretical framework – Positive Technological Development. The designed virtual world offers a range of online activities, such as content creation, collaboration and caring, communication, and community-building. The chapter shows pediatric patients as active and creative participants in the virtual world.

Chapter 2 addresses a great health challenge: treatment of childhood obesity. The chapter discusses how to use e-health technologies to improve treatment adherence, promote mechanisms of self-control in patients, maintain weight loss achievements, and prevent relapses by establishing healthy lifestyles. The chapter presents an e-health system that addresses these weight loss treatment issues. The system consists of three complementary applications: clinical support, home support, and mobile support. The chapter illustrates the system tools, such as a game designed to improve the children's nutrition knowledge, another game to improve their daily behaviors, and devices to record physical habits and physiological responses.

Chapter 3 provides an overview of Internet-based chronic disease self-management treatment programs for children and youth. Promoting self-management for adolescents with chronic diseases requires an understanding of how children with these diseases gradually develop the ability to take the lead from being reliant on parents and caregivers. The chapter defines and describes the theories, processes, and content elements Internet-based self-management programs are based on. It also presents experiences from developing and testing a self-management program for young people with arthritis called "Teens Taking Charge: Managing Arthritis Online." Practical tips for program development and evaluation in this area are discussed.

Chapter 4 addresses how to use ICT for promoting well-being among elderly people. It targets the needs of the elderly population in general, such as the need to break isolation and increase social activities, sustain family companionship, and to ease anxiety. The chapter presents an IT-system in which elderly people, family and friends, and also health professionals, interact. The system has different levels of action: therapeutic, playful, and evaluative. It offers resources that enhance elderly users' social networks, and help them stay in contact with family and friends online, as well as enhance their learning, leisure and training of positive emotions. The platform also allows health practitioners to continuously monitor emotional states of the elderly and offers various clinical resources and therapeutic activities.

Chapter 5 deals with online communities and the social networks of cancer patients. It presents the results of a study of determinants and effects of online communities on the development of social relationships among cancer patients. Determinants for formation of virtual relationships are discussed. Socio-demographical characteristics of patients, type of cancer, Internet usage behavior, and perception of advantages and disadvantages are analyzed. The chapter also outlines some recommendations for patients who use online communities and for providers who administrate them.

Chapter 6 addresses social support as an important coping strategy for survivors of sexual violence. The experience of sexual violence is most traumatic and stressful, and the ones who try to recover from it need social support. The chapter presents the results from a content analysis of an online support group for survivors of sexual violence. The online conversations targeted issues such as appraisal of the situation, the handling of feelings, understanding and sympathy, and guidance to enhance faith in one's abilities. The messages in the studied conversations were categorized according to five different types of support: information support, tangible assistance, esteem support, network support, and emotional support.

Chapter 7 explores blogging as a tool for coping with a lifelong and highly stigmatized disease. The chapter offers insights into the social and health concerns of people living with HIV. It presents results from a study of six HIV-positive individuals' blogs. The blogs are discussed from different perspectives: social interaction, information sharing, self-expression, and social commentary, and illustrative quotes from the blogs are shown.

Chapter 8 challenges the assumption that a small set of stored answers are enough to answer most of the questions in a particular topical area. The chapter presents results from a study of an online service for questions on eating disorders. It offers insights into different types of questions on anorexia nervosa, bulimia nervosa, binge eating disorder and/or obesity, and other or unspecified eating disorders. The results show that the variety of questions is large, and that to provide satisfactory answers, humans are needed.

Chapter 9 addresses holistic system design for online self-help groups. The chapter presents a web-based self-help system for stress management that combines knowledge and experiences of health experts and peers. The system offers research findings, real-life stories, practical exercises and interaction with health experts and peers. The system is based on the active and self-driven participation of people with stress symptoms, and the chapter suggests a model for system evaluation that includes measures related both to the health status of users and to their use of the system, such as patterns of conversations, contents of messages, and the use of systems services.

Chapter 10 addresses blending professional and experiential knowledge in online self-help groups. The chapter offers a theoretical overview of learning processes and self-help groups in a learning context. It also presents and analyzes practical aspects from the course, "Living a healthier life – online," a course that was transformed from face-to-face to online as part of a design-based research project. The chapter argues that online self-help settings need to be facilitated in a firmer manner than face-to-face, and that socialization and overall assignments are two crucial elements in facilitating online self-help initiatives in a learning context.

Chapter 11 addresses motivation and engagement in online self-help groups. Based on theoretical frameworks and practical experiences, the chapter identifies five factors suggested as enablers or constrainers of engagement: synchronicity, identification, specified diagnosis, organizational trust, and accessibility. The chapter applies these five factors to discuss participation in Skype-based self-help groups.

Chapter 12 addresses challenges of digital inclusion. Elderly and disabled people constitute a group of users who can benefit a lot from accessing e-health services and communities, but at the same this group is sensitive to the design of the e-health systems. This is a dilemma that needs further attention. Inclusive design aims to produce solutions available and usable to as many as possible of the target audience. The chapter shows how user-centered and inclusive design is to be used as a basis on which successful e-health systems can be developed and implemented. It also investigates different aspects of online social networks and social connectedness.

Chapter 13 deals with e-health literacy in the context of online health communities. There are different health literacy skills and knowledge needed to understand and communicate effectively about health issues. Not only reading, writing, and communicative skills are needed to function well, but also the ability to critically analyze information, apply information to personal situations, understand health issues as social problems, and recognize cultural differences, for example. The chapter offers a theoretical overview of different health and e-health literacy domains. It also uses the online weight-loss community, the Biggest Loser League, as a case study. A content analysis of the community posts was conducted to examine domains of health literacy.

Chapter 14 addresses design requirements for usable e-health communities in mobile devices. This chapter proposes a set of basic usability requirements specifically oriented to mobile interfaces for blog-based instant messaging e-health communities. The usability requirements are related to interface dimensions, user representation, navigation, adaptability, and turns in online conversations, for example. The chapter also presents an e-health community interface prototype for mobile device based on the proposed requirements.

Chapter 15 addresses the use of digital technologies to engage health citizen communities in health policy. Patient organizations, or citizen health organizations, are engaging with healthcare professionals and government decision-makers in order to advance their interests. The chapter investigates three different models for organizing citizen participation and the role of ICT and the Internet to facilitate and enable engagement on a day-to-day basis. The models are represented by three citizen health organizations; their ways of using ICT and the internet to create practices and e-health communities are examined.

Chapter 16 introduces e-health from a European perspective; it presents insights into the European policy work and discusses drives and barriers towards a Europe with "patient-friendly" healthcare services. The chapter argues that there is a need for political awareness and commitment to take advantage of new technology and to have e-health change the everyday practices of healthcare.

Chapter 17 addresses the development of online communities to support drug policy knowledge exchange and to bridge between academics and policy-makers. It presents results from a study of three drug policy groups and their different virtual knowledge exchange activities. The chapter offers lessons learned regarding the impacts of conferencing technologies on knowledge exchange drug policy groups, and it presents recommendations on how to conduct successful virtual knowledge exchange meetings based on the findings from the studied groups.

Åsa Smedberg
Stockholm University, Sweden

Acknowledgment

I want to thank all contributing authors for making this book possible. Sharing your knowledge and experiences has resulted in a collection of new insights in the field of e-health communities and online self-help groups. Many thanks are also due to Prof. Jacob Palme and Associate Prof. Hélène Sandmark for valuable reviews and advice along the way.

And to the readers – I hope you will find the book enjoyable and useful!

Åsa Smedberg
Stockholm University, Sweden

Chapter 1
Virtual Worlds for Children with Medical Conditions:
Experiences for Promoting Positive Youth Development

Marina U. Bers
Tufts University, USA

Kathryn A. Cantrell
Tufts University, USA

ABSTRACT

This chapter describes an innovative, technology-based intervention for children with critical medical conditions that utilizes the Zora virtual world. Most specifically, the chapter describes two experiences, one with post-transplant pediatric patients and the other with pediatric cancer patients who participated in Zora. The virtual experience was designed to address issues of school transition and medical adherence, while offering psychosocial support in the context of a virtual community of peers. The design of the Zora virtual world is informed by the Positive Technological Development (PTD) framework which was inspired by Positive Youth Development (PYD). In Zora, users can communicate with each other via real-time chat and participate in open-ended guided activities to create a social network of peers. They can also build the personal and public spaces in the virtual city, create interactive characters and write stories for three-dimensional objects.

DOI: 10.4018/978-1-60960-866-8.ch001

SCENARIO

Peter is a 14-year-old boy. He connects to Zora, a virtual city built and inhabited by 11 to 15 year olds. Peter is happy because he feels that the virtual home he created in Zora is almost finished. He put pictures of his favorite things and people, and wrote stories about his family and friends. Peter decides to go around the virtual city. He quickly navigates through Zora's different public spaces: the Transplant Experience House, the Homework Help Cabin, the Medical Center and the Smart Object House. Upon entering the Smart Object House, a virtual doctor welcomes him. "This is clever!" thinks Peter, "I will program a pill box to tell me when to take my medicine!" The Smart Object House is populated by other smart objects and characters created by youth who have experienced a transplant. At first sight, there is an interactive robot that helps you with medical procedures, alarms that sound when you need to fill a prescription, and a teleportation machine that takes you to the beach when one is tired of the hospital. Peter navigates around the three-dimensional space and encounters many different objects. Peter decides to add a pill box to the Smart Object House that sounds an alarm whenever it is time to take his pills. Peter programs the box to say the color of the pill when it sounds so that it's easier to know which to take. He associates the value "organization" to the pillbox and defines it in the Zora Collaborative Values Dictionary as "it is very important to organize your medicine. That way, you can stay healthy after your transplant." As he is about to leave the Smart Object House, he finds a calendar placed by Elena earlier that week. The calendar lists the many medical-related appointments Elena has scheduled that month. He also sees that Elena has used the Zora Values Dictionary to create a new value, "planning", and linked it to the calendar. As Peter is reading Elena's definition of planning, he recalls that he has an appointment in two weeks, and quickly searches for his own calendar to see if it had been written down.

This scenario describes an actual engagement by young people participating in a virtual community for post-transplant pediatric patients with a three-dimensional multi-user environment, called Zora. Zora is a virtual world that provides easy-to-use tools for children to design and program their own virtual city and, in the process, learn about school transition and medical adherence, as well as form peer relationships (Bers, 2001; Bers et al, 2010). Children are put in the role of producers, instead of consumers, of information, knowledge, and habits of mind.

This chapter describes an innovative technology-based intervention for children with critical medical conditions. It presents two case studies that show two potential ways of using a virtual world. The first involved a group of post-transplant youth from two different hospitals, who used Zora from their homes to specifically address issues of medical adherence and school transition in the context of a peer-support network. The second case involved a group of youth with cancer, sickle cell, and healthy siblings participating in a summer camp for children with illnesses and their families. They were introduced to the technology while participating in the face-to-face summer experience and then participated in an intervention that used Zora to sustain the friendships and levels of hope attained during camp, once they were back at home.

This chapter focuses on the virtual curriculum that was designed and implemented within the virtual world while offering psychosocial support in the context of a virtual community of peers. Activities, lead by e-mentors, are designed to foster relationships, teach technological skills, and facilitate the formation of a support network of peers and mentors. The chapter presents both case studies, introduces the Zora technology and the virtual curriculum as well as the theoretical framework upon which it was designed, Positive Technological Development.

INTRODUCTION

As young people discover new ways of using the Internet for social interaction, through social networking sites, multiplayer video games and virtual communities, graphical virtual worlds are emerging as one of the fastest growing on-line environments for youth (Beals & Bers, 2009). For example, the largest virtual world for adults has 13 million registered users, while the largest for children and youth has 90 million users. Furthermore, as of 2008, the Association of Virtual Worlds found that there are over 360 virtual worlds explicitly targeted for this young population (Association of Virtual Worlds, 2008). Within the large presence of virtual worlds, Internet based interventions have been explicitly designed for children facing serious illnesses (Bush & Simonian, 2002). For example, video games (Lieberman, 2001) and virtual reality interventions (Schneider & Workman, 2000), web-based storytelling sites (DeMaso, et al., 1995) and social networking sites (Bush, Huchital, & Simonian, 2002) have been on the rise.

Internet-based psychosocial interventions provide an opportunity to reach children who, due to geographical distance, cannot attend face-to-face meetings. Participation in a peer-based virtual community may engage children in discussion of health related issues, and provides a space to share their needs, feelings and worries. At the same time, a graphical virtual community such as those afforded by virtual worlds, offers different opportunities for participation. Children can choose to express themselves via on-line chat and words, or by drawing and making virtual objects (Bers, 2001). However, when these kinds of psychosocial interventions are put in place, it is not only the technology, but also the social support systems built around the technology and the curriculum mediated by the technology, that can make a difference.

In the past, most young people with a serious medical illness would not survive. Today, advances in medicine make it possible to extend the length of their lives. However, children are trading a life-limiting disease for invasive follow-up interventions and the hardships of medical adherence associated with difficulties in transitioning back to school and socially engaging with peers (Griffin & Elkin, 2001). Frequent clinic visits, medication intake, and dietary and physical exercise restrictions can be disruptive to the patients' academic and social life (Erikson, 1950; Brem et al., 1988; Rodin & Voshart, 1987; Gerson et al., 2004). Therefore it is crucial that help is provided to address the 'medical, psychosocial, educational, and vocational' needs of the patient at various stages of their lives (Blum et al., 1993). Unfortunately, psycho-social services lag behind medical advances, as it is difficult to run effective programs for patients who are geographically dispersed and small in number.

Thus, there is a need to find other vehicles through which to provide the needed supports. This is the driving force at the core of the Zora virtual world project described in this chapter. The first pilot has been running for the last five years with youth transplant recipients aged 11-15 first at Children's Hospital Boston, and then extending it to Tufts Medical Center (Bers, 2009; Bers et al, 2010). The second project was a pilot run for campers aged 13-16 who attended Camp For All in Burton, Texas. The campers, members of the oncology/hematology week at camp, experienced either cancer, a blood disorder, or were siblings (Cantrell & Bers, 2010).

The focus of this chapter is the on-line Zora curriculum used in both interventions, the resulting experiences, and the theoretical framework that informed the development of the virtual curriculum. It is our goal that, by providing a theoretical foundation that presents the key elements for running successful interventions in virtual worlds for children with medical conditions, others might be able to adapt our work to the needs of the specific pediatric populations they serve. While we used the Zora virtual world, other virtual environments that afford similar kinds of experiences might be used.

The chapter will follow the subsequent structure while presenting virtual worlds for children with medical conditions:

1. The Zora Virtual World will introduce the program.
2. Theoretical Background will describe the concepts informing the virtual world.
3. Case Studies will provide two examples of virtual worlds for children with medical conditions
4. Curriculum will describe the e-curriculum utilized within the case studies
5. Future Research Directions will highlight considerations for potential studies.
6. Conclusion will sum up the chapter and explore future research directions.

THE ZORA VIRTUAL WORLD

Zora is a 3D virtual environment that provides easy-to-use authoring tools to create and inhabit a virtual city or summer camp (see Figure 1). Users interact and communicate with each other in real time through a chat system, as well as in asynchronous ways through message boards. Users are graphically represented as avatars. They can populate the virtual world with their own creations by designing 3D graphical objects, interactive characters, personal and public spaces. They can create stories for each of the objects as well as personal or moral values that highlight the special meaning children assign to their objects and characters. Zora provides easy to use authoring tools for young users to create their own objects, but the focus is not only on the aesthetics of 3D objects, but also on the meanings assigned to them. Thus the design elements of Zora are contained within a design framework that encourages users to create stories and values for every object they make in the world, models of identification (such as heroes and villains) for their avatar profiles, and a collective values dictionary for the resulting virtual community.

Upon logging into Zora for the first time, users encounter an initial blank 3D world. Their task is to create the virtual world's public and private spaces and populate the world with interactive objects (e.g., objects that can hold "conversations" with visitors). While using building tools in Zora to construct personally meaning projects, users learn basic computer programming principles as well as gain technological fluency (Barron, Martin, & Roberts, 2006). The underlying assumption is that young people learn best by making, creating, designing and programming their own projects (Papert, 1980; Resnick, Bruckman, & Martin, 1996). Zora allows youth to participate in the virtual community not only by engaging in discussions and arguments, but also by designing and making new objects and new places within the virtual city, to explore psychosocial issues associated with illness. Youth engage in chatting as well as doing, discussing as well as creating, thinking as well as producing (Bers, 2008). The overarching goal of Zora is to provide a safe space for youth to explore issues of identity in hope to promote positive youth development while using technology in positive ways (Bers, 2006; Lerner et al., 2005).

The first version of Zora was developed in 1999 using the Microsoft Virtual Worlds development platform (Bers, 2001b). The current version of Zora used in the studies described in this chapter has been revised and developed using the ActiveWorlds platform (Bers, 2007; Satoh, McVey, Grogan, & Bers, 2006). This platform for developing educational multi-user environments is widely used by educational research projects such as Quest Atlantis (Barab et al., 2005) and River City (Nelson, Ketelhut, Clarke, Bowman, & Dede, 2005). Zora has similarities with the growingly popular Second Life® virtual world (Ondrejka, 2004) in presenting a three dimensional environment for users to develop a virtual community. However, unlike Second Life©, Zora is a

Figure 1. Image of Zora virtual world including chat bar (bottom), navigation screen (middle) and welcome screen (right)

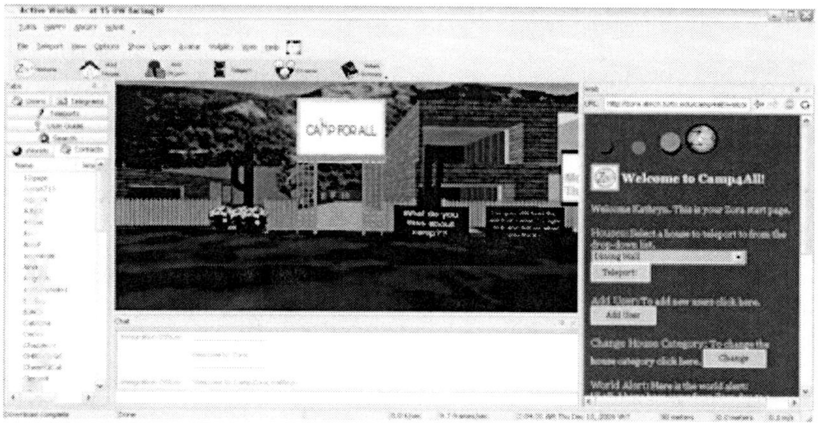

secured and password protected world in which only youth with a particular educational program or intervention, can view and access the world and contribute to it. The design of the Zora virtual world is informed by the Positive Technological Development (PTD) framework. Thus, it supports the implementation of a virtual curriculum that takes advantage of the many features of Zora that are well-aligned with the theoretical model. The next section presents the PTD framework and the theories that informed it.

BACKGROUND

The Positive Technological Development framework (PTD) guides the design of the curriculum implemented in the Zora virtual world. PTD examines the developmental tasks of a child growing up in our digital era, and provides a model for developing and evaluating technology-rich youth programs (Bers, 2008). From a theoretical perspective, PTD is an interdisciplinary approach that integrates ideas from the fields of computer-mediated communication, computer-supported collaborative learning, and constructionist learning with technology, with research in applied development science and positive youth development. In brief, PTD focuses on two related aspects: (1) the design and evaluation of technology-based psycho-educational programs and experiences aimed at helping young people use technology in positive ways, and (2) the trajectory that leads youth to use technology to learn new things, to express themselves in creative ways, to communicate and take care of themselves and others, and to contribute to society, while developing their own sense of identity grounded on personal and moral values.

Two bodies of work have influenced the PTD framework:

Constructionism: Developed by the pioneer in the field of computers and education, Seymour Papert, Constructionism is rooted in Piaget's work and advances the idea that children learn better when they can use computers to create their own meaningful projects by exploring (computational) materials and developing their own (computational) theories. The main tenet is that computers can serve as "objects to think with" when children are given the opportunity and the tools to make their own projects, thus creating their own content. Following Piaget, Constructionism might best be defined as a constructivist philosophy for educational technologies. The claim is that by engaging in the process of creating virtual objects to share and reflect upon, children are more likely to construct internal knowledge, and at the same time, develop technological fluency in a playful way (Kafai & Resnick, 1996). Constructionism has influenced the design of the Zora virtual world by providing an environment, a virtual city, that children can create. They can make their own virtual rooms, their own interactive objects and characters, and write stories and values to define them.

Positive Youth Development (PYD): This research focuses on the dynamic relations between individuals and contexts by emphasizing the strengths and assets of young people, instead of focusing on diminishing or preventing risk-taking behaviors (Lerner et al, 2000; Damon, 2004; King & Furrow, 2004; Larson, 2000; Theokas & Lerner, 2006; Scales, Benson, & Mannes, 2007). The use of the term "positive" connotes the promotion of valued characteristics and activities (i.e., developmental assets) that would lead a young person toward a good developmental trajectory (i.e. development toward improvement of one's self and society). Lerner et al. (2005) frame the various developmental assets into a model of six "C's", competence, confidence, character, connection, caring, and contribution, conceived as pathways to promote thriving and healthy communities. PYD has influenced the design of Zora by including on-line activities that promote the six C's.

PTD borrows the six C's and makes them relevant in our digital world. However, instead of emphasizing only developmental assets, since PTD is about informing interventions, it focuses on positive behaviors supported by the technology and how those behaviors can in turn promote the six C's. For example:

- A sense of *competence* in the technological domain is displayed by the ability to use the computer to *create content* using programming languages or computer applications, to debug projects and problem-solve. Engaging in content creation behaviors promotes, in turn, the development of new concepts and skills.
- A sense of *confidence* in oneself as someone who can act, and learn to act, successfully in a technology-rich world, who knows how to ask for help and who has perseverance over technical difficulties, is further promoted when one uses technology in *creative ways*.
- *Caring*, the willingness to use technology to respond to the others, assumes that people can communicate through the technology. For example, social media promotes new ways of *communication*.
- *Connection*, the capacity to establish and maintain positive bonds and relationships through technology, promotes and supports *collaboration*.
- An orientation to *contribute* to society by using and inventing technologies to solve social problems engages in *community-building*.
- A sense of *character,* a moral compass that guides the use of technology in responsible ways, is built upon having *choice of conduct* in the digital world. In turn, being exposed to choosing our behavior and facing consequences has an impact in the development of character.

Youth programs that are informed by the PTD framework are focused not only on promoting development, but also on choosing technologies and pedagogical approaches that engage children in positive behaviors, such as content creation, creativity, communication, collaboration, community building, and choices of conduct (Bers, in press). The following sections will describe how the virtual curriculum used in the psychosocial interventions with both pediatric cancer and post-transplant patients address each of these aspects.

CASE STUDIES

The PTD theoretical framework and the Zora virtual curriculum were utilized in two different interventions for youth with medical conditions. The next sections will describe each of them by using guidelines identified by previous work as key aspects to consider when developing virtual worlds interventions and educational programs for youth (Bers et al., 2010)

Post-Transplant Pediatric Patients

The goals of the pilot study with post-transplant pediatric patients were:

1. Facilitate peer networking building amongst same age pediatric post-transplant patients.
2. Encourage medical adherence through on-line activities and a virtual environment that foster discussion, sharing of experience and informal content delivery.
3. Support post-transplant patient's psycho-social adjustment to school transition and lifestyle changes by creating a community.

This research project was in collaboration with pediatric psychiatrists and medical staff in the pediatric transplant program at Boston Children's Hospital and the Tufts Floating Hospital for Children and lasted for 12 months. Post-transplant patients were first referred to the project by doctors based on their age (11-15) and health status. Those eligible patients and their families were then contacted and invited to participate in the project. Most participants used Zora from their homes (all over New England, and some other further states in the US) and at times, during hospitalizations (Bers et al., 2007; Bers et al, 2010; Bers et al, 2010a).

Seventy-five patients were originally contacted through phone calls and mailings; 38 verbally agreed to participate and 35 returned the necessary consent and assent forms. Of these 35, we could not provide Internet to 3 due to their remote locations. Thus we worked with a total group of 32. Of the 32 patients, three never logged in into Zora, so our user group was composed of 29 children, however 32 returned questionnaires. Fifty-five percent of the participants were females and the average age at the start of the program was 13.7 years. Participants engaged in weekly online activities for the duration of the study. While they were free to log on at any time, the group activities followed a semi-structured curriculum aimed at sparking conversations about transplant experiences by encouraging them to create virtual spaces such as a Health Museum and a Pharmacy. An example of the e-curriculum is explored in the curriculum section of this chapter.

During the project, each user logged into Zora an average of 60 times and spent an average of 39 hours logged into the program. This represents almost seven hours more online than we had anticipated, as we had planned weekly on-line activities for 32 hours. Users created a total of 4027 objects and made 75 virtual houses. For example, they created a Legislature House where they put recommendations for hospitals to ease the stay of the patients, such as "soft pillows", "beds with comfortable mattress pads on them...especially in the cardiac cathlab, where you have to lay flat for six hours" and suggestions for schools to ease transitions after prolonged hospitalizations, "so kids don't have to tell stories so many times" (Bers et al., 2010).

During the course of the study, three individuals underwent cardiac re-transplantation. Their participation from the hospital both before and after the transplant added an extra dimension to the virtual group discussions. It also provided an opportunity for some of the participants to meet for the first time face to face.

During interviews, users reported positively about their experience with the project, especially about being able to meet other children who had received a transplant as made evident by a feedback from a participant:

I believe that taking part in Zora did give me inspiration. I only had a liver transplant, and I cannot have tunnel vision that there's only me, but there are a multitude of other kids that have gone through similar experiences as myself. They inspired me to help educate others about organ donation, because there are kids like us whose lives have been saved through the gift of organ donation.

Preliminary analysis of the data collected from the questionnaires reveal little change in the participants' medical adherence over the course of the Zora intervention primarily due to the fact that the participants were already exhibiting satisfactory level of adherence prior to participation in the project. However, it became clear that patients with high severity in their illness were the ones who used Zora the most and that participating in Zora helped in ameliorating children's fear of follow-up clinic visits. Based on log analysis and quantitative responses to questionnaires, we have also observed positive impact in terms of peer networking. For example, a social worker described Zora as providing "something that none of [the patient's] Doctors or medical professionals could- a connection to other kids who knew exactly how he was feeling and experience the unpleasant things that go along with transplant each and every day".

The following paragraphs describe specific aspects of the virtual intervention:

Mentoring Model

The facilitator was a child development doctoral student with experience in child health and a clear agenda in terms of the research and learning goals of the project. The facilitator coordinated weekly Zora on-line activities but spent most of her time, helping participants with the technical aspect of the program, from installing it to supporting creative uses. Although the goal was for the facilitator to progressively move towards getting the participants to help each other, this happened very slowly as children were on different schedules (Cantrell, Fischer, Bouzaher, & Bers, 2010). Our mentoring model was composed of a facilitator and several mentors, older teenagers who had had a transplant were identified as potential mentors for the Zora community and were invited to join. For example, when participants discussed on-line their worries about going to college and not having their mothers around to help them to remember to take their medications, we asked one of the mentors, a college student with a transplant, to come on-line to talk about his own experience. The long terms plan is to have the participants, as they become older, to assume the role of mentors.

Diversity

The diversity among this project's participants is found in terms of the type of organ they received, the types of medical situations that lead them to require an organ transplant, the time since transplant, and the severity of their condition. There were 13 participants from the heart transplant program, 3 from liver, and 6 from renal. Diversity is also present based on their location: 12 participants were from Massachusetts, 1 from Florida, 1 from Maine, 3 from New Hampshire, 2 from New York, and 3 from Rhode Island. They all had in common that they underwent the transplant procedure and received post-transplant follow-up treatment at Children's Hospital Boston. Regardless of their original ailment or organ received, they all share the experience of going through organ transplantation and thus were all committed to a life-long regimen of medications and follow-up invasive interventions.

Project Scale

Although 32 post-transplant patients with Internet access signed consent forms, only twenty-one used Zora (logged in more than twice) and half of them participated on a regular basis (N=11).

Although at the beginning of the project, scale was not an issue and children were happy to meet for the first time other post-transplant children, as the project evolved, children wanted to have more participants, as it was difficult to have synchronous activities and conversations. Throughout the study, we had to hold our weekly online meetings at two different times to accommodate different participants' schedules. In addition, the voluntary nature of the project meant that we could not enforce regular attendance. Thus there might be as few as one or two participants attending planned activities. However, participants would be online at other times to work on individual projects. Due to the "constant on" nature of this project, participants were welcomed to sign on at any time; however, our data showed that in many cases, a participant who logs on and finds that only one or two other members are on would sign off. This may be due to the lack of a minimum critical mass to sustain participants' engagement. Other researchers (e.g., Markus, 1987; Preece, 2000) have shared similar experiences for the need to have a minimum critical mass when building a social network or a virtual community. To increase the probability of having a minimum critical mass to sustain a discourse we are increasing the overall user or participant pool by bringing on board a new site, Tufts Floating Hospital for Children.

Types of Contacts with Participants

Besides regular online contact with the regular participants, we have made home visits to a few local participants' homes to gain an understanding of the environment and context in which Zora was being used. We also arranged to meet some patients at the time of their regular hospital's clinical visits or while they were hospitalized for treatment. However, depending on the time since transplant, the frequency of the participants' routine visits to the hospital varied; therefore we could not arrange to meet every participant and their family. For those participants whom we could not visit either at home or at the hospital, interviews were conducted over the phone. In addition, users created a monthly newsletter, *Transplant Times,* which reported on some of the key activities that took place on Zora. The newsletter was printed and mailed to all participants, their families and hospital staff. At the end of the year, we organized a Zora group who would represent the virtual community of transplant patients at the hospital's annual fund raising walk. Five of the participants and their families joined for the walk which gave us, and them, the chance to meet other face-to-face.

Assessment

Data collection included automatically generated logs that provided qualitative and quantitative data of user's online activities, self-report instruments and semi-structured interviews, as well as spontaneous feedback. We collected three sets of data: (1) data pertaining to Zora use and participant feedback through semi-structured face to face or telephone interviews, as well as Zora logs, and home visits to check for fidelity in the way the system was used by the patients and the ways it was intended to be used; (2) data pertaining to the positive development of youth through the use of technology collected through questionnaires; and (3) data about patient's medical adherence and medical history provided by parents, medical staff and children's themselves.

Access Environment

The participants were expected to log online from their computers in their homes. Since not every family had access to a computer suitable for using Zora, we provided computers to three families and also Internet service to one family. During hospitalizations, patients were able to participate from the hospital.

Institutional Context of Usage

Participants were requested to sign a Code of Conduct which outlines some basic rules of Internet behavior (such as not disclosing personal information online) prior to logging into Zora for the first time. This was requested by the hospital IRB to ensure the safety of the participants. The initial items on the Code of Conduct signed by the participants are created by the researchers but once on Zora, we encouraged discussions about appropriate and inappropriate behavior on Zora (such as resolving issues of participants building on top of, or within someone else's "property" without notification). Once consensus was reached as a community, new items were added to the Code in the Zora world. The institutional complexity of hospitals and the interdisciplinarity of this work makes it difficult to be in full control of crafting an innovative educational intervention that, although might not meet the scientific review criteria of the medical field in terms of statistical significance of results, shows clear qualitative signs of having a positive impact

Pediatric Cancer Patients

This pilot study was done with a group of campers at a pediatric campsite called Camp For All in Burton, Texas (Cantrell & Bers, 2010). Zora was introduced to 40 campers with cancer (16), blood disorders (6), and their siblings (18). The four goals for the pilot study were to determine if:

1. Zora could sustain the campers' hopefulness after their week of camp.
2. Zora could sustain the campers' sense of connectedness after their week of camp.
3. Zora could foster positive technological development.
4. Zora could be successfully integrated into pediatric recreation programming.

Zora was utilized as a tool for remaining connected; in addition to this, the program offered an e-curriculum exploring concepts of hopefulness, social connectedness, and positive technological development. Although the virtual world was open for 6 month following the closing of camp, the e-curriculum was administered for 6-weeks. Participants were allowed to access the virtual world 24/7 but the group curricular activities occurred bi-weekly (to accommodate participants' schedules) and lasted an hour. The curriculum is explained further in the curriculum section.

Forty campers signed assent forms and completed the baseline data collection sequence. Twenty-three participants were females and 17 were males. Eighty percent of the participants were returning campers. The ethnicity of the sample was 45% European American, 30% Hispanic American, and 25% African American. Of the 40 who agreed to participate, 26 used Zora as a tool for maintaining contacts and supporting friendships and 10 regularly came online to complete curriculum. The ten individuals who participated the Zora curriculum came online twice a week to discuss issues of hopefulness, social connectedness, and positive technological development.

This Zora virtual world was designed to mirror the actual physical campsite. When it was first constructed, it included all the buildings you would see at camp such as the dining hall and the cabins. Additionally, it contained a virtual lake and areas for the various activities offered at camp such as a ropes course and horses. After introduced to the campers, the participants worked to make the space personalized by adding pictures to the buildings and sharing stories about each of the activities. Ultimately, the virtual camp was designed to look like the physical space but the campers worked to make it reflect the culture.

Overall, the virtual community resembling camp created over 2240 objects, 1788 lines of chat, over 24 stories, 16 values, and 2 interactive characters over the course of 6 months. During the bi-weekly curriculum times, participants worked together to create objects that represented hope, friendship, and camp. For example, campers constructed a Hope Hut, a building that held all their hopeful memories related to illness. One camper who had recently ended treatment for liver cancer created a virtual talking organ: the liver said, "I am hope because I am healthier now." Another camper who had a negative experience with Hurricane Katrina posted this story within the Hope Hut:

Hope is light at the end of the storm like when I lost my house in Hurricane Katrina and that was really hard because I had to move to Texas but now I love it in Texas so it became a blessing!

Campers also constructed buildings that reflected their favorite moments from camp. For example, a Ropes Shack was constructed to hold all the campers' memories from the ropes course. One of the campers explained why the Ropes Shack should be added to the virtual world by saying, "people can go in there when they are down and remember when they were flying and their friends cheered for them."

Data analysis revealed that Zora may contribute to sustaining social connectedness and positive technological development. The mean positive technological development increase (M=2.13, SD=4.55, N=40) demonstrates significance (t=-2.95, p=<.005) and the mean social connectedness increase (M=1.08, SD=2.27, N=40) is also significant (t=-2.99, p<.005). Despite this, there was no significant change in campers' hopefulness after using the program (Cantrell & Bers, 2010). These findings were seen across the population, not within the curriculum cohort; thus, it cannot be confirmed that the curriculum impacted the campers' scores.

Overall campers demonstrated a positive reaction to the program. In interviews, 94% of participants stated that Zora should be used again in the coming summers. Safety was consistently cited as a priority for the population and as a reason for using Zora instead of other online social networking sites; for example, one camper said, "Safety is really important to my parents cause there's lots of crazy people on the Internet and stuff so this will be a way that we can talk and stay in touch but without the dangers."

Mentoring Model

The facilitator was a certified child life specialist with expertise in child development and pediatric psychology. The facilitator was also a former employee of the pediatric camp facility, making communication with the campsite more accessible. Once the campers arrived home, the facilitator spent much of the week on the phone with families as they began installing the program. After most families had installed the program, the facilitator set up weekly meeting times for the participants. Because of scheduling conflicts, the facilitator met campers online twice a week for hour-long sessions that engaged participants in discussions about hopefulness, social connectedness, and positive technological development. The mentoring model was comprised of one facilitator and "camp leaders." The camp leaders were campers that expressed an interest in assisting the facilitator with weekly curricular goals. These campers helped other participants with the technical steps involved in constructing curricular objects within the virtual world.

Diversity

In order to participate in the study, campers were in the age range of 13-17 (the developmental stage the program targets) and receive permission from their camp director (some were omitted by the directors due to behavioral concerns). Of the 120 camp attendees, 45 were eligible for inclusion in the study and 40 assented, resulting in a participation rate of 89%. Forty campers between the ages of 13 and 17 enrolled in the project at Camp For All, 22 from Children's Hospital at Scott and

White (Temple, Texas) and 18 from University of Texas Medical Branch Children's Hospital (Galveston, Texas). Twenty-three participants were females and 17 were males. Eighty percent of participants were returning campers, meaning that they had attended camp before. The ethnicity of the sample was 45% European American, 30% Hispanic American, and 25% African American. Of the participants, 45% were siblings, 40% had been diagnosed with cancer, and 15% were being treated for a blood disorder.

Project Scale

Although 40 campers signed consent forms, only nineteen used Zora and 10 participated weekly, completing the entire curriculum. Interestingly, the 10 campers who came on regularly were not friends at camp; through Zora Camp4All, a new community was created. Additionally, unlike the experience with patients who had received transplants, many campers did come online during non-designated curriculum times. For example, there were two campers who met online every night around midnight and used Zora Camp4All as a chatting tool. Typically, the campers who came online after hours were not members of the 10 who demonstrated consistency within the curriculum.

Types of Contacts with Participants

In addition to the designated curriculum times, the facilitator spent many hours emailing and calling families. Because the participants were located across the country, there was not the ability to visit family homes to aid in technical troubleshooting; instead, all of this had to be completed over the phone. E-mail became the most reliable tool for communicating with the families and updates came nearly daily. In addition to logistical and scheduling emails, the facilitator also updated families on the curricular activities completed online. For the interviews, all were completed over the phone as it was not feasible to schedule face-to-face interviews.

Assessment

Data collection for this study was conducted in two phases. The first phase was at camp, face-to-face while the campers were introduced to the program. The second phase of data collection occurred over the phone after 6-weeks of program usage. Data collection included semi-structured interviews, 3 questionnaires to assess hopefulness (Hind's HSA), social connectedness (Lee's SCS-R) and positive technological development (Bers' PTDQ), and automatically generated logs that provided qualitative and quantitative data of user's online activities. We collected four sets of data: (1) data assessing the affect Zora had on the campers' sense of hopefulness after use; (2) data pertaining to the affect Zora had on the campers' sense of social connectedness after use; (3) data assessing the affect Zora had on the campers' positive technological development after usage; and (4) data assessing the feasibility of incorporating technology in recreational programming.

Access Environment

An installation CD was provided to every participant that assented, so they could take Zora home with them. Additionally, the two participating hospitals installed the program on hospital computers to account for families without computers. During the study, all 40 participants indicated that they had computer access at home. Of the 40 that assented, 36 are recorded as having logged in at least once.

Institutional Context of Usage

Participants were requested to sign a Code of Conduct which outlines some basic rules of Internet behavior (such as not disclosing personal information online) prior to logging into Zora for the first time. The Code of Conduct for this study mirrored many of the ethical codes established at Camp For All. Because Zora was a tool for continuing the camp community, the campsite requested that the code would hold the campers to the same expectations and continue to emphasize inclusivity and compassion. The facilitator also established a strong rapport with the camp director and the hospital staff who were immediately notified if the facilitator became uncomfortable with any online behavior.

THE CURRICULUM

Although both case studies presented above involved two different populations of youth with medical conditions, both followed the PTD framework that guide the design of the program and both used Zora for children to engage in the following activities:

1. *Content creation* by designing a virtual city with personal homes and public spaces, interactive storytellers and objects. The Zora authoring tools foster *competence* in the development of computer literacy and technological fluency.
2. *Creativity* by utilizing different media to express ideas in virtual spaces and solving technical problems. By using the Zora tools in creative ways, children develop a sense of *confidence* in their learning potential.
3. *Collaboration* tools to promote *caring* about others by engaging in shared projects and providing support and guidance to each other in the learning community.
4. *Communication* mechanisms via both synchronous and asynchronous exchanges that promote a sense of *connection* between peers or with adults
5. *Community-building* virtual spaces and tools that enable the formation of a social support network that can bridge, in some cases, to face to face exchanges. This promotes *contribution*, to make a better learning environment, community, and society.
6. *Choice of conduct* by engaging youth in the creation of a collaborative values dictionary that guides actions in the virtual world and the design of narrative-based models of identification, such as heroes and villains, that provoke examination of values. Combined, these Zora features enable users to explore *character traits* and their ethical and moral dimensions while assuming a responsible use of technology in the virtual city.

Next, this chapter will take a closer look at the curriculum within the Zora intervention for post-transplant youth. The following sections describe each of the on-line activities contained within the curriculum that emphasized school transition and medical adherence. Since Zora was explicitly informed by PTD, there is an alignment between the affordances of the technology and the positive behaviors it supports.

Overview

The Zora curriculum was comprised of six objectives that mirrored the six C's of positive technological development. Throughout the virtual meetings, participants were encouraged to complete the objectives within the curriculum. Because the participants came into the project with various technological skill-sets, it was not required that the youth complete the computational knowledge objectives in sequential order or in a certain period of time. Instead, the curriculum followed a loose structure and sequence to encourage and accommodate differentiated levels of instruction and previous expertise. E-mentors, child development students with studies in child life, facilitated the on-line activities and kept track of the youth's progress through the curriculum. When a child came online, e-mentors were able to assist her on an individual basis, knowing the learning objective matched to her progress. Table 1 briefly describes each of the six objectives within the curriculum.

Participation

This section chronicles the six objectives within the curriculum, highlighting the theoretical background informing the prompt given to the child and also providing examples of participation and objects constructed by the youth. Each of the case studies followed the curriculum at their own pace.

Objective 1: Content Creation (Competence)

Construct a Virtual Object That Represents a Struggle You Face While at School

The first objective in the curriculum addresses school transition through the positive technological development term *content creation* and promotes technical proficiency within Zora. Because it was essential that the youth become comfortable with the various elements of the Zora virtual world in order to utilize the technology appropriately and with confidence, this first objective is embedded within the youths' introduction to the program. Participants were encouraged to learn about the technology by constructing their personal homes, decorating it with pictures, and writing stories about their interests. After, they were asked to join the virtual group in the Zora School where the community worked on individual objects representing school-related struggles. During these sessions, participants engaged in conversations that expressed many school transition issues such as strategies for homework completion, concentration struggles, stage fright, and bullying.

Jill was one of the younger participants within the Zora virtual world and had recently received a

Table 1. Curriculum chart

Objective	*Positive Technological Development*	*Positive Youth Development*	*Prompt given to child*	*Relevance*
One	Content Creation	Competence	Construct a virtual object that represents a struggle you face while at school.	Poursanidou (2007) explains how crucial communication with educators and families is. Objective 1 promotes communication about school issues.
Two	Creativity	Confidence	Construct a virtual object that represents a solution to your school struggle.	Objective 2 promotes initiative and problem solving related to school transition.
Three	Collaboration	Caring	Interview another participant about their school struggles and school solutions objects.	Objective 3 promotes awareness of the many school transition concerns (Poursanidou, 2003).
Four	Communication	Connection	Make and program an interactive character that represents someone who has helped you through your transplant experience.	Objective 4 promotes communication about the importance of proper medical care and its continuation through adherence.
Five	Community Building	Contribution	Participate in the virtual scavenger hunt and reflect on the community within Zora. How has it helped you?	Objective 5 encourages reflection on the community comprised of fellow transplant recipients.
Six	Choice of Conduct	Character	Construct an innovative virtual object that will help you manage your medical routine. Add a value for this object and define it.	Objective 6 encourages independent consideration of adherence and creative problem solving related to medical regime. It also promotes adherence responsibility (Shaw et al., 2003).

heart transplant. During a conversation on Zora about school, Jill vocalized a concern about bullies. She explained that there was a reputed group of bullies at her school and was scared that they would antagonize her once she returned from the hospital. Fortunately, her school had recently become aware of the students in question and implemented a "bully awareness" program that taught the student body various ways to prevent bullying. Jill's conversation on Zora motivated her to create a sign that described her fear of bullies. She also built a virtual interactive sign that when clicked on, opened up to a list of ways to prevent bullying. (Figure 2)

Objective 2: Creativity (Confidence)

Construct an Object That Represents a Solution to Your School Struggle

The second objective in the curriculum also focused on promoting technological proficiency within the program. By having the participants utilize the same skills they developed during the first objective, such as object creation, the second objective provided opportunities for the participants to enhance their *confidence* within Zora; they could learn to use new tools within the program to express their *creativity*. During the second objective the facilitators noted a broader range of objects being constructed and an increased level of vocal participation from the youth. The sessions that related to the second objective encouraged participants to consider solutions to their school transition issues, promoting communication, cited as an important aspect of a successful school transition (Poursanidou, 2003; Anthony et al., 2009; Burton et al., 2009). Participants engaged in conversations about how to talk to parents, educators, and healthcare providers about their concerns with school. After construction, the Zora School transformed into a museum of various objects expressing concerns and solutions related to education.

Diane was out of school for five months while she underwent a bone marrow transplant at the age of 13. While the surgery was successful and she has since been in remission, her time away from school was a struggle for her when she returned. During her second week back at school, Diane was asked to give a presentation about the transplant she received. She recalled that the presentation was frightening and that she could barely get any words out because of her stage fright. When asked to program an object that represented a school struggle, Diane immediately expressed how presenting in front of a class made her feel. When she joined us on line for Objective 2, she constructed an object that provided tips for others in Zora on how to get over stage fright. The virtual object she created was a picture of a man

Figure 2. Bully object

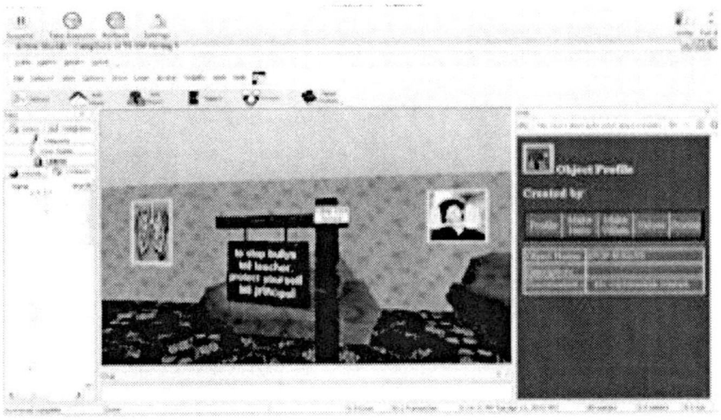

on stage and listed practicing, deep breathing, and talking slowly as tricks for becoming more comfortable in front of the class. (Figure 3)

Objective 3: Collaboration (Caring)

Interview Another Participant about Their School Struggle and School Solution Objects

While a sense of community is promoted within Zora, early on in the experience most of the conversations within the virtual world were initiated by the participating children but directed toward the facilitators. Rarely did participants chat with one another. The third objective was aimed at building a stronger sense of community by promoting *collaboration* between the participants, and enhancing *caring* within the group. For the third objective, participants were asked to interview each other on-line about the school struggle and solution objects they had created. While conducting these interviews, participants were able to learn more about the wide range of topics related to school transition (Poursanidou, 2003). They were also able to start communicating with each other in a direct way, without the need of e-mentor's intervention. Once the dyads had completed the objective, each individual reported to the group what they had discovered, continuing the conversation on a larger scale.

Tanner was one of the older participants in the Zora project. During his time within the virtual world, he often acted as an informal mentor, helping the other participants with the technical elements behind their constructions. During objectives 1 and 2, Tanner expressed having difficulties concentrating in school after his heart transplant. During the group conversation, Tanner was surprised by the response he received from the other participants. His role shifted as the other youth, mostly the younger ones, gave him advice on how to stay awake in class.

Objective 4: Communication (Connection)

Construct and Program an Interactive Character That Represents Someone Who Has Helped You through Your Transplant Experience

The fourth objective extended technical confidence by introducing a new programming skill-set, the programming of an interactive character. Additionally this objective provided an opportunity to enhance *communication*. While the prompt was technically sophisticated, it also asked the participants to think about and share about someone they value. Utilizing *communication* in various forms, this objective promoted *connection*. The interactive character had to be programmed

Figure 3. Stage fright object

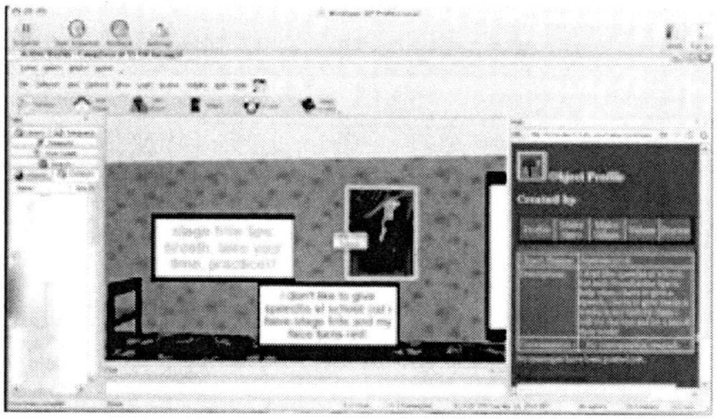

to carry out a dialogue that expressed how the individual was helpful. Participants were able to place the character wherever they liked within the world. After multiple participants had built their characters, the group toured the world, searching for one another's characters and engaging in conversations with them.

Mary was 10 when she had her lung transplant. During the experience, her parents used the metaphor of a butterfly to emphasize how much healthier she would feel after her transformation. Since that time, the butterfly has turned into her favorite image. When giving the prompt for the fourth objective, facilitators expected to see characters inspired by parents, doctors, and child life specialists. Instead, Mary, the first participant to complete the objective, constructed a butterfly named Flutter. When asked how the character helped her through her transplant experience, Mary's answer was simple: Flutter means hope. (Figure 4)

Objective 5: Community-Building (Contribution)

Follow the Scavenger Hunt and Reflect on the Community within Zora: How Has it Helped You?

The fifth objective was designed to promote reflection about time spent on Zora. Recalling how the group had developed throughout the project promoted further *community-building*. Likewise, the group format of the scavenger hunt promoted *contribution* and collaboration. Together, the group chatted about how each participant had contributed to the Zora family. The scavenger hunt was a collection of riddles throughout the virtual world asking the participants to leave behind an object at each stop. After the objective's completion, there were dozens of objects throughout the virtual world reflective of the Zora community. This objective, like many of the others, worked to promote communication and expression within the participants; in this manner, the youth gained skills that could later be accessed at school and at the hospital.

The last sign on the scavenger read, "can everyone please build an object that represents what Zora means to you?" One of our most loyal participants, Johnny, had a difficult time throughout the program initiating conversation with the other participants and coming out of his shell. In fact, most of his chat had been directed toward the facilitators. During his time with the program, he frequently voiced how difficult it had been for him to make friends since his heart transplant. He had found that he couldn't relate to his peers after going through so many health challenges. To the facilitators' surprise, the object he chose to build at the end of the scavenger hunt was a dedication to the friends he had made on Zora. The object's description said, "Zora is about friendship." (Figure 5)

Objective 6: Choice of Conduct (Character)

Construct an Innovative Object That Will Help You Manage Your Medical Routine: Add a Value and Indicate if it's a Hero or a Villain

The last objective of the project addressed the topic of medical adherence by asking participants to construct an innovative virtual object to assist with their medical routine. The prompt asked the youth to categorize the object as either a hero or a villain; also, they were encouraged to give the object a value that represented how it was constructive. This examination of values, provoked by the participant's *choice of conduct*, promoted *character*. In the Zora Smart Shop, participants were asked to gather and discuss innovative objects that aid in managing medical routines. During the conversation, facilitators promoted simple strategies for adherence; likewise, the group discussed the long-term responsibilities of adherence including adapting a medical regime to college-life (Shaw et al., 2003). Participants recalled pill-boxes, calendars, and phones with

Figure 4. "Flutter" interactive character

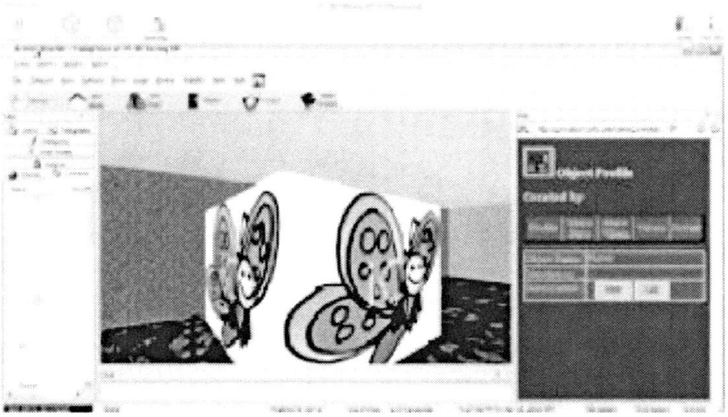

alarms. Facilitators then asked the participants to create their own innovative, futuristic object to help with medical adherence; there were no limits to their creation.

During the sixth objective, creations ranged from robots to time machines to virtual alarms. One participant, Dan, decided to be more literal with his response to the prompt. "My innovative object that helps me is my new kidney," Dan explained during the conversation. While other participants were constructing machines, Dan built in the virtual world the kidney he had recently received. Dan explained, "My kidney helps me remember why I have to take my medicine because it keeps my body going." (Figure 6)

FUTURE RESEARCH DIRECTIONS

The facilitation of psychosocial programming through virtual communities can be a challenge. In order to maintain the virtual world, collaboration between healthcare professionals, families, researchers, and the youth must be consistent and frequent. Due to this limitation, the virtual format for psychosocial curriculum can seem less than feasible; despite this, both case studies demonstrate that there is a population of youth embracing the technology. Additionally, the portability of the format provides an additional outlet for educating youth when distance and medical isolation are factors.

Figure 5. Friendship object

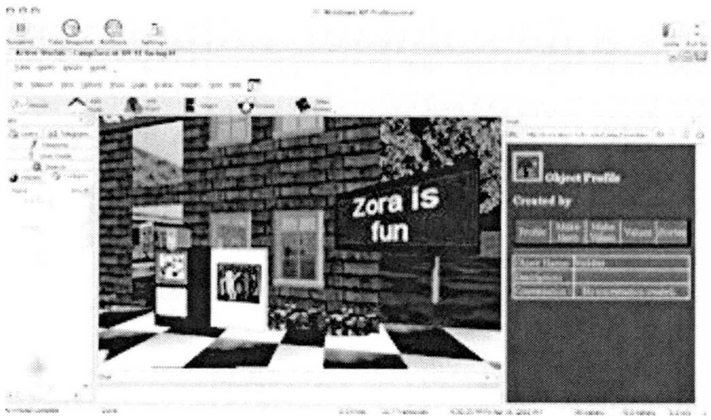

Figure 6. Innovative object

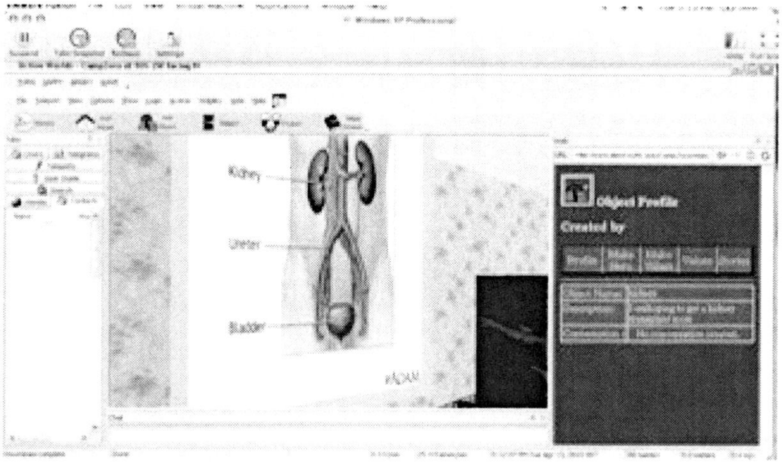

The case study chronicling the program for post-transplant youth saw about 11 devoted participants. Similarly, the program for youth with cancer had 10 participants who religiously contributed to the curricular activities. This rate, approximately 25% of the assenting population, may seem small; despite this, those that did consistently use the program excelled in the virtual world, devoting hours to constructing objects and personal cabins. For many youth, this alternative form of socialization may be more comforting than face-to-face conversation. Additionally, the ability to not just chat but also construct objects together might be more appealing for some youth. For these populations, the virtual form of intervention may be ideal in the face of illness.

Considering these factors, more strides need to be made in the field of technologically based interventions. The case studies presented in the chapter involve a small sample of participants and both were conducted over the span of a year. Increasing the sample size and maintaining the project for an extended amount of time would not only validate data analysis but also provide an example of how much work is required to keep a virtual intervention running continuously.

In addition to larger sample sizes and longer timeframes, virtual interventions for youth with illnesses need a strong advocate within healthcare. Conducting these projects from within hospital walls provides immediate access to participants and a consistent face behind the technology. Knowing that the tool would be a strong resource in programming for youth with chronic illnesses, interdisciplinary collaboration with the clinical teams caring for the participants is imperative.

CONCLUSION

This chapter conveys the prevalence of virtual worlds in the lives of young people and presents two case studies of programs that used the Zora virtual world with children with medical conditions. Zora was designed and implemented to be used by researchers and practitioners developing psycho-educational interventions. However, in order to have successful experiences, the virtual world by itself is not enough. It is important to have a theoretical framework, in this case Positive Technological Development, that guides the design of the technology, the development of the virtual curriculum, the type of participation, mentoring approach and activities to happen online. While the projects presented in these case studies engage two different populations, both were strongly designed upon the PTD framework.

The curriculum within the Zora virtual community acted as the structure behind the technological intervention and was designed to promote positive adaptation to school transition, medical adherence and a sense of hopefulness in the context of a community of peers. The curriculum's skeleton was the six C's of positive technological development, the theoretical framework that simultaneously informs community growth and technological skill development. While technology continues to develop, more clinicians might have the opportunity to facilitate interventions online. Because these population's experience the chronic stress of illness and the risk factors associated with it, a foundation of accountability for online curriculum is needed to maintain safety and promote success in this setting.

We live in a society where concepts of self and community are constantly changing. This context makes it challenging for young people to construct a sense of self and grow into positive contributors to civil society. This becomes even more challenging for youth suffering from a severe medical condition that requires invasive medical interventions. Today, the current advances in medicine make it possible not only to extend their length of life, but also their quality. However, life style changes and compliance to demanding medication regiments and dietary restrictions are needed. As shown in this chapter, new technologies, such as virtual worlds can help young patients to tackle this challenge by integrating already existing face-to-face psycho-educational programs with virtual environment and by allowing them to participate in novel virtual interventions.

ACKNOWLEDGMENT

We thank Clement Chau, Laura Beals, Amy Fischer, and Keiko Satoh, from the DevTech research group at Tufts University, as well as our collaborators at Children Hospital Boston, Tufts Floating Hospital for Children, and Camp For All. We also thank the National Science Foundation for support of this research through an NSF Career grant # IIS-0447166 and the Deborah Munroe Noonan Memorial Research Fund. Any opinions, findings, and conclusions or recommendations expressed in this chapter are those of the authors and do not necessarily reflect the views of the National Science Foundation.

REFERENCES

Barab, S. A., Thomas, M., Dodge, T., Carteaux, R., & Tuzun, H. (2005). Making learning fun: Quest Atlantis, a game without guns. *Educational Technology Research and Development*, *53*(1), 86–108. doi:10.1007/BF02504859

Beals, L., & Bers, M. U. (2008). A developmental lens for designing virtual worlds for children and youth. *International Journal of Learning and Media*, *1*(1), 51–65. doi:10.1162/ijlm.2009.0001

Berquist, R. K., Berquist, W. E., Esquivel, C. O., Cox, K. L., Wayman, K. I., & Litt, I. F. (2008). Non-adherence to post-transplant care: Prevalence, risk factors and outcomes in adolescent liver transplant recipients. *Pediatric Transplantation*, *12*(2), 192–200. doi:10.1111/j.1399-3046.2007.00809.x

Bers, M., Beals, L., Chau, C., Satoh, K., Blume, B., DeMaso, D., & Gonzalez-Heydrich, J. (2010). Use of a virtual community as a psychosocial support system in pediatric transplantation. *Pediatric Transplantation*, *14*, 261–267. doi:10.1111/j.1399-3046.2010.01271.x

Bers, M. U. (2001). Identity construction environments: Developing personal and moral values through the design of a virtual city. *Journal of the Learning Sciences*, *10*, 365–415. doi:10.1207/S15327809JLS1004new_1

Bers, M. U. (2006). The role of new technologies to foster positive youth development. [Mahwah, NJ: Lawrence Erlbaum Associates.]. *Applied Developmental Science*, *10*(4), 200–219. doi:10.1207/s1532480xads1004_4

Bers, M. U. (2007). Positive technological development: Working with computers, children, and the Internet. *MassPsych, 51*(1), 5-7, 18-19.

Bers, M. U. (2008). Civic engagement and the internet: Developing technologically-rich educational programs to promote civic participation online and offline. In Bennett, L. (Ed.), *Volume on digital media and civic engagement* (pp. 139–160). Cambridge, MA: MIT Press.

Bers, M. U. (2009). New media for new organs: A virtual community for pediatric post- transplant patients. *Convergence (London)*, *15*(4), 462–469. doi:10.1177/1354856509342344

Blum, R., Garell, D., & Hadgman, C. (1993). Transition from child-centered to adult health- care systems for adolescents with chronic conditions. A position paper of the Society for Adolescent Medicine. *The Journal of Adolescent Health*, *14*, 570–576. doi:10.1016/1054-139X(93)90143-D

Brem, A., Brem, F., McGrath, M., & Spirito, A. (1988). Psychosocial characteristics and coping skills in children maintained on chronic dialysis. *Pediatric Nephrology (Berlin, Germany)*, *2*(4), 460–465. doi:10.1007/BF00853442

Bunzel, B., & Laederach-Hofmann, K. (2000). Solid organ transplantation: Are there predictors for post transplant noncompliance? A literature overview. *Transplantation*, *70*, 711–716. doi:10.1097/00007890-200009150-00001

Burton, J. H., Marshall, J. M., Munro, P., Moule, W., Snell, G. I., & Westall, G. P. (2009). Rehabilitation and transition after lung transplantation in children. *Transplantation Proceedings*, *41*, 296–299. doi:10.1016/j.transproceed.2008.10.047

Bush, J., Huchital, J., & Simonian, S. (2002). An introduction to program and research initiatives of the Starbright foundation. *Children's Health Care*, *31*(1), 1–10. doi:10.1207/S15326888CHC3101_1

Bush, J., & Simonian, S. (2002). Program and research initiatives of the Starbright foundation. *Children's Health Care*, *31*(1), 1–10. doi:10.1207/S15326888CHC3101_1

Cantrell, K., & Bers, M. (2010). Zora Camp4All: A virtual community to augment the hopefulness of pediatric camping. *Child Life Focus, 28*(3).

Cantrell, K., Fischer, A., Bouzaher, A., & Bers, M. (2010). The role of e-mentorship in a virtual world for youth transplant recipients. *Journal of Pediatric Oncology Nursing*, *27*(6), 344–355. doi:10.1177/1043454210372617

Damon, W. (2004). What is positive youth development? *The Annals of the American Academy of Political and Social Science*, *591*(1), 13–24. doi:10.1177/0002716203260092

DeMaso, D., Twente, A., Spratt, E., & O'Brien, P. (1995). The impact of psychological functioning, medical severity, and family functioning in pediatric heart transplantation. *The Journal of Heart and Lung Transplantation*, *14*, 1102–1108.

Erikson, E. (1950). *Childhood and society*. New York, NY: W.W. Norton.

Gerson, A., Furth, S., Neu, A., & Fivush, B. (2004). Assessing associations between medication adherence and potentially modifiable psychosocial variables in pediatric kidney transplant recipients and their families. *Pediatric Transplantation*, *8*, 543–550. doi:10.1111/j.1399-3046.2004.00215.x

Griffin, K. J., & Elkin, T. D. (2001). Non-adherence in pediatric transplantation: A review of the existing literature. *Pediatric Transplantation*, *4*, 246–249. doi:10.1034/j.1399-3046.2001.005004246.x

Kafai, Y., & Resnick, M. (Eds.). (1996). *Constructionism in practice: Designing, thinking, and learning in a digital world.* Mahwah, NJ: Lawrence Erlbaum.

King, P. E., & Furrow, J. L. (2004). Religion as a resource for positive youth development: Religion, social capital, and moral outcomes. *Developmental Psychology*, *40*, 703–714. doi:10.1037/0012-1649.40.5.703

Larson, R. W. (2000). Toward a psychology of positive youth development. *The American Psychologist*, *55*, 170–183. doi:10.1037/0003-066X.55.1.170

Lerner, R., Fischer, C., & Weinberg, R. (2000). Toward a science for and of the people: Promoting civil society through the application of developmental science. *Child Development*, *71*, 11–20. doi:10.1111/1467-8624.00113

Lerner, R., Lerner, J., Almerigi, J., Theokas, C., Phelps, E., & Gestsdottir, S. (2005). Positive youth development, participation in community youth development programs, and community contributions of fifth-grade adolescents: Findings from the first wave of the 4-H study of positive youth development. *The Journal of Early Adolescence*, *25*(1), 17–71. doi:10.1177/0272431604272461

Lieberman, D. A. (2001). Management of chronic pediatric diseases with interactive health games: Theory and research findings. *The Journal of Ambulatory Care Management*, *24*(1), 26–38.

Nelson, B., Ketelhut, D. J., Clarke, J., Bowman, C., & Dede, C. (2005). Design-based research strategies for developing a scientific inquiry curriculum in a multi-user virtual environment. *Educational Technology*, *45*(1), 21–27.

Papert, S. (1980). *Mindstorms: Children, computers and powerful ideas*. New York, NY: Basic Books.

Penkower, L., Dew, M. A., Ellis, D., Sereika, S. M., Kitutu, J. M., & Sharpiro, R. (2003). Psychological distress and adherence to the medical regimen among adolescent renal transplant recipients. *American Journal of Transplantation*, *3*, 1418–1425. doi:10.1046/j.1600-6135.2003.00226.x

Poursanidou, K., Garner, P., Watson, A., & Stephenson, R. (2003). Difficulties and support at school for children following renal transplantation: A case study. *Support for Learning*, *18*(4), 170–176. doi:10.1046/j.0268-2141.2003.00303.x

Preece, J. (2000). *Online communities: Designing usability, supporting sociability*. Chichester, UK: Wiley.

Resnick, M., Bruckman, A., & Martin, F. (1996). Pianos not stereos: Creating computational construction kits. *Interaction*, *3*(5), 40–50. doi:10.1145/234757.234762

Rodin, G., & Voshart, K. (1987). Depressive symptoms and functional impairment in the medically ill. *General Hospital Psychiatry*, *9*(4), 251–258. doi:10.1016/0163-8343(87)90080-6

Satoh, K., McVey, M., Grogan, D., & Bers, M. (2006). *Zora: Implementing virtual communities of learning and care (VCLC)*. Presentation at the New Media Consortium's, Regional Conference at San Antonio TX.

Scales, P., Benson, P., & Mannes, M. (2006). The contribution to adolescent well-being made by nonfamily adults: An examination of developmental assets as contexts and processes. *Journal of Community Psychology*, *34*, 401–413. doi:10.1002/jcop.20106

Schneider, S. M., & Workman, M. L. (2000). Virtual reality as a distraction intervention for older children receiving chemotherapy. *Pediatric Nursing*, *26*, 593.

Shaw, R. J., Palmer, L., Blasey, C., & Sarwal, M. (2003). A typology of non-adherence in pediatric renal transplant recipients. *Pediatric Transplantation*, *7*, 489–493. doi:10.1046/j.1397-3142.2003.00117.x

Shaw, S. R., & McCabe, P. C. (2008). Hospital-to-school transition for children with chronic illness: meeting the new challenges of an evolving health care system. *Psychology in the Schools*, *45*(1), 74–87. doi:10.1002/pits.20280

Shemesh, A., Lurie, S., & Stuber, M. (2000). A pilot study of posttraumatic stress and non- adherence in pediatric liver transplant recipients. *Pediatrics*, *105*, 1–7. doi:10.1542/peds.105.2.e29

Stilley, C. S., Lawrence, K., Bender, A., Olshansky, E., Webber, S. A., & Dew, M. A. (2006). Maturity and adherence in adolescent and young adult heart recipients. *Pediatric Transplantation*, *10*, 323–330. doi:10.1111/j.1399-3046.2005.00473.x

Theokas, C., & Lerner, R. (2006). Promoting positive development in adolescence: The role of ecological assets in families, schools, and neighborhoods. *Applied Developmental Science*, *10*(2), 61–74. doi:10.1207/s1532480xads1002_2

ADDITIONAL READING

Bennett, W. L. (Ed.). (2008). *Civic Life Online: Learning how digital media can engage youth*. Cambridge, MA: The MIT Press.

Ching, C. C., & Foley, B. J. (Eds.). (2009). *Technology, Learning, and Identity: Research on the Development and Exploration of Selves in a Digital World*. Cambridge University Press.

Khine, M., & Saleh, I. (Eds.). (2010). *New Science of Learning: Cognition, Computers, and Collaboration in Education*. New York: Springer Publishing Company.

Papert, S. (1980). *Mondstorms: children, computers and powerful ideas*. New York: Basic Books.

KEY TERMS AND DEFINITIONS

Constructionism: Learning theory which claims that learning can happen most effectively when people are also active in making tangible objects in the real world.

E-Curriculum: Curriculum designed and facilitated virtually.

Positive Youth Development (PYD): Summarizes the intentional efforts of other youth, adults, communities, government agencies, and schools to provide opportunities for youth to enhance their strengths, promoting positive development.

Positive Technological Development (PTD): A research model that details the overall impact of a technology on youth and their development.

Chapter 2
An E-Health System for Treatment of Childhood Obesity:
The Etiobe Platform

Rosa M. Baños
Universidad de Valencia, Spain

Ausiàs Cebolla
Universidad Jaume I, Spain

Elia Oliver
Universidad de Valencia, Spain

Soledad Quero Castellano
Universidad Jaume I, Spain

Cristina Botella
Universidad Jaume I, Spain

ABSTRACT

Obesity is one of the greatest public health challenges of the 21st century and the most prevalent health problem among children in Europe. Treatment is complex due to the multiple causes of obesity that include many dimensions of children's lives, such as nutritional habits, physical activity, and lifestyle. E-health technologies can be useful in this area; they may improve health care delivery and acceptability, facilitate the provision of interventions to wider populations, and improve treatment efficacy by taking advantage of new technologies such as the Internet and mobile technologies. The objective of this chapter is to describe an e-health platform called ETIOBE. It comprises three complementary applications connected in real time that support different components of weight loss treatment: the Clinical Support System (CSS), the Home Support System (HSS), and the Mobile Support System (MSS). It was designed to treat childhood obesity by improving treatment adherence, promoting the mechanisms of self-control in patients, obtaining the maintenance of patients' achievements (reducing body weight), and preventing relapses by establishing healthy life habits.

DOI: 10.4018/978-1-60960-866-8.ch002

INTRODUCTION

Childhood obesity is one of the greatest public health challenges of the 21st century (Branca, Nikogosian, & Lobstein, T., 2007). In fact, it is the most prevalent health problem among children in Europe. The prevalence of obesity has tripled in many countries in the European Region since the 1980s, and now spans from 9% in the Netherlands to 30% in Greece (IOTF, 2007). The children obesity global data in Europe are nearly around 20% of the total, and the numbers of those affected continue to rise at an alarming rate to "epidemic" status (EASO, 2002). Moreover, general obesity treatment and associated health problems such as medical illness (diabetes, hypertension, etc.) and psychological problems (low self-esteem, body dissatisfaction, etc.) have a significant economic impact. In the European Union, obesity is already responsible for 2-7% of health costs (Branca, Nikogosian, & Lobstein, T., 2007).

The rapid and significant increase in the prevalence of obesity indicates that, although there may be some genetic factors, the main causes are environmental. According to the European Association of Obesity (EASO, 2002), the causes of this epidemic are basically twofold: (a) an increase in consumption of energy-dense beverages and foods (foods high in fat and sugar); this promotes excessive calorie consumption and drives a culture of continuous snacking and omnipresent, leading to "passive over-consumption" of energy, and (b) developments that restrict opportunities for physical activity, creating an almost universal sedentary state. Because causality involves many dimensions of children's lives such as nutritional habits, physical activity, and lifestyle, treatment of this problem needs to include not only medical factors, but also

As the International Obesity TaskForce warns, governments should address childhood obesity by improving the evidence base for treatments (EASO, 2003). A growing number of children in western countries need more effective therapeutic management to control their obesity and to reduce their risks. Furthermore, treatment in early years is crucial because child obesity is a powerful predictor of adult obesity (Guo, Wu, Chumlea & Roche, 2002). This problem is overwhelming the capacities of European public health systems to the point where many children in need do not receive effective treatments or prevention tools in their struggles against obesity.

Children in western cultures are living in an environment that encourages the overconsumption of energy-dense foods. The main objective of the treatment and prevention of obesity is to protect children from the "obesogenic environment" (including factors that tend to make people fat) that surrounds them. However, such strategies are difficult to apply in a clinical context wherein professionals must manage many patients daily. E-health technologies are being proposed as one solution to this growing problem.

BACKGROUND

E-health technologies constitute an innovative approach to improving health service delivery and acceptability (Stinson, Wilson, Gill, Yamada, & Holt, 2009). They facilitate the provision of interventions to wider populations and improve treatment efficacy by utilizing new technologies, such as the Internet and mobile technologies. It has been suggested that e-health interventions make health-related goals more attainable because they (a) break treatment goals into smaller, more manageable pieces, (b) automatically assess success, and (c) modify previously attained goals in response to program success (Norman et al., 2007). The use of e-health technologies in children can be even more powerful than in adults; because most children are proficient in using the Internet and mobile devices for entertainment, e-mail, chat and instant messaging, they show high levels of acceptability of their usage in treatment. Furthermore, one of the clear benefits of Information and

Communication Technologies (ICTs) is that they can provide immediate feedback to users and thus can help to remind them of tasks to be performed every day (such as exercising and eating well), reinforcing them immediately. Therefore, new ICTs may help improve treatment for childhood obesity by providing continuingly supportive mechanisms that increase motivation and alert patients to their problems, providing incentives while strengthening children in a social environment that may not favor new healthy habits.

E-HEALTH ON OBESITY

E-Health Platforms in the Treatment of Obesity

There is already evidence that the Internet can be a helpful tool in treating obesity. Tate, Jackovony & Wing (2003, 2006) have shown the effectiveness of Cognitive-Behavioral Treatment (CBT) for weight loss applied through the Internet, and they found that the treatment program increased its effectiveness when paired with advice applied via email by a therapist.

Furthermore, Harvey-Berino et al. (2002) compared an Internet-based program with two programs including different levels of face-to-face contact (frequent and infrequent) to maintain weight loss. Although the results showed that both of the face-to-face groups obtained better results than the Internet-based group, differences between the Internet group and the infrequent contact face-to-face group were minimal.

Finally, Williamson et al. (2005) evaluated the effectiveness of an Internet-based program for lifestyle modification in obese adolescents and their obese biological parents. Results showed that adolescents lost more body fat, parents lost more weight, and all reduced their intake of dietary fat compared to the group following the control condition program (a passive non-interactive educational program that was also Internet-based).

E-Health Applications for Children's Weight Loss Treatment

In contrast to the body of research on adult populations, evidence-based interactive e-health applications for children are scarce (Ahern, Phalen, Le & Goldman., 2007). Only a few published studies to date focus on methods for changing physical activity, sedentary behaviors, and nutritional patterns to manage weight in children. Baranowski et al. (2003) evaluated a computer game that was successful in increasing children's consumption of fruits and vegetables in the experimental group. Casazza and Ciccazzo (2007) found that, compared to both the control group and to students who received traditionally-based education, students who utilized a computer-based nutrition and physical activity program increased their physical activity and nutrition knowledge base and reduced their meal-skipping. Saelens et al. (2002) analyzed a weight management program that combined a computer-based behavioral assessment with a single session of weight counseling by a by a physician, with all further contact provided by telephone and mail. Results showed improving body mass index (BMI) scores in a group of overweight research subjects. Patrick et al. (2006) found that a one-year intervention that combined computer-assisted behavioral assessment and action planning with health provider counseling as well as mail and telephone contact improved patients' physical activity levels and food habits.

For the treatment of childhood obesity, ICTs have been used mainly as a communication tool in the clinician-patient relationship and for transmitting nutritional knowledge and physical activity information. Although e-health platforms have been developed which focus on individual components of obesity treatment (Ahern et al., 2007), there are no existing studies about the effectiveness of ICT platforms for comprehensive weight loss treatment. ETIOBE is an e-health platform designed to achieve this goal. This chapter will describe this system's method for treating and preventing childhood obesity.

THE ETIOBE PLATFORM

The ETIOBE platform is an e-therapy system whose objectives are to improve treatment adherence and to promote patients' self-control, to maintain weight loss achievements and to prevent relapses through the establishment of healthy life habits.

The e-health ETIOBE platform comprises three complementary applications that support different components of weight loss treatment: the *Clinical Support System* (CSS), the *Home Support System* (HSS), and the *Mobile Support System (MSS).*

Clinical Support System (CSS)

This application is used by clinicians to incorporate medical and psychological data into a patient's profile. This tool has been designed according to clinicians' recommendations, and it has been validated in a usability study which found it intuitive and easy to use (Baños, Cebolla, Zaragoza, Botella, Alcañiz, et al., 2009). CSS allows clinicians to design and adapt guidelines for assessment and intervention (e.g., sedentary lifestyle reduction, healthy food habits establishment, etc.) to suit the needs of individual clients while allowing flexibility depending upon their progress (See Figure 1).

CSS incorporates psychological questionnaires with medical data. Questionnaires and responses are computerized, and results are accessible and incorporated immediately into children's profiles (children can also respond to the questions through the HSS). Medical data are gathered and entered by clinicians and the results are automatically compared with normative data. Furthermore, the system includes several alerts: if a child is shown to be at risk physically or psychologically, the system notifies the appropriate medical professional. For example, if ETIOBE detects high scores in medical variables such as blood sugar or cholesterol or psychological markers for concern such as depression or anxiety, the system

Figure 1. The clinical support system (CSS)

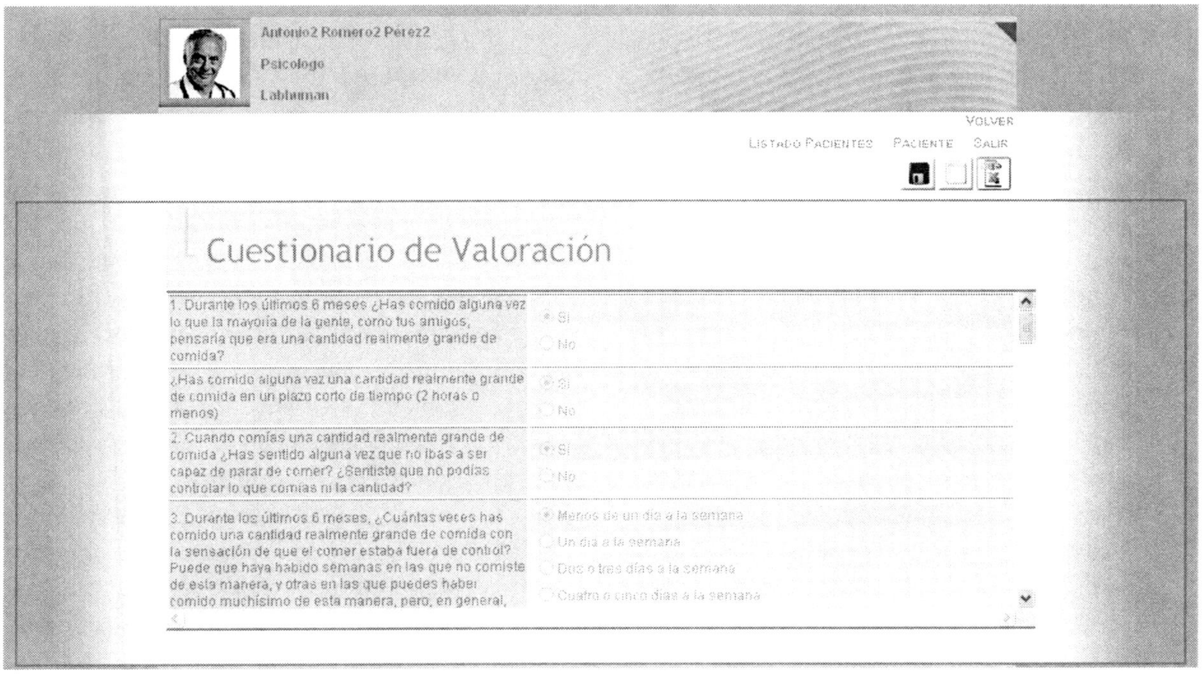

sends an alert to the clinician indicating the specific risk level for that patient.

CSS also gives clinicians the ability to adapt the intervention program to each patient and to customize the program according to the patient's progress. Therapists can monitor children's development in real time, encouraging their adherence to their treatment (food habit changes, home tasks, physical exercise, etc.) through feedback given in the other two platforms (HSS and MSS). This information allows the treatment to be customized to the specific characteristics of the children in each phase, thereby improving their motivation and adherence to the treatment. In addition, clinicians can assess and treat the children without a face-to-face interview, avoiding removals and delays in the intervention. In this manner clinicians can also provide feedback and all the information that they consider necessary for proper intervention.

Home Support System (HSS): The ETIOBE Mates

This application is called "The ETIOBE mates", and is used by patients at home on a computer connected to the Internet (see Figure 2). This platform allows children to contact the therapist and access tasks and activities (questionnaires, registers, games, etc.) set by the clinician. The HSS also includes various activities designed to increase children's nutrition literacy in an entertaining way. The HSS has several components:

- **Cooking:** A section of the website that includes healthy recipes and how to make them.
- **Feeding:** Here children can find interactive pages with nutritional knowledge: the food pyramid, the components of food, medical consequences of unhealthy living, etc.
- **Moving:** This section includes information about physical activity and healthy lifestyles. It includes a physical activity pyramid that is similar to the food pyramid but describes activities that should be done most frequently in order to maintain health.

The HSS allows children to design a virtual agent, or avatar, who guides them and recommends the tasks the clinician has proposed. This avatar also provides children with "rewards". Children acquire points for completing the prescribed tasks, which allows them to progress from beginner to expert ranks. Patients can see how many points they are acquiring by completing the tasks through playing serious games, filling out self-registers, and other activities. All results and data are sent to the *CSS* in real time, allowing the clinician to monitor the children's status and adherence to the tasks.

The HSS also includes several serious games which are presented by different characters. "Serious game" refers to a software application developed with informatics technology and game design principles used for educational, persuasive or health purposes (Baños, Cebolla, Etchemendy et al., 2009). These games combine learning and play, making the process of learning new concepts and skills more attractive for children. Thus, this format is expected to increase children's learning of new information. The research literature shows that computer games are effective tools in psychological skills training and educative learning, accelerating the learning process and improving motivation levels (Garris, Ahlers & Driskell, 2002). Other advantages of this educative tool include its appeal to children who are already conversant in Internet and computer game formats, its entertainment value which makes learning fun, and its adaptability (it can be controlled by the clinician and the targets can be modified according to the objectives). (See Figure 3).

The three games developed thus far include:

The Healthy Plate: This game was designed for young children as an introduction to nutritional knowledge. The objective is to teach the categories

Figure 2. The home support system (HSS)

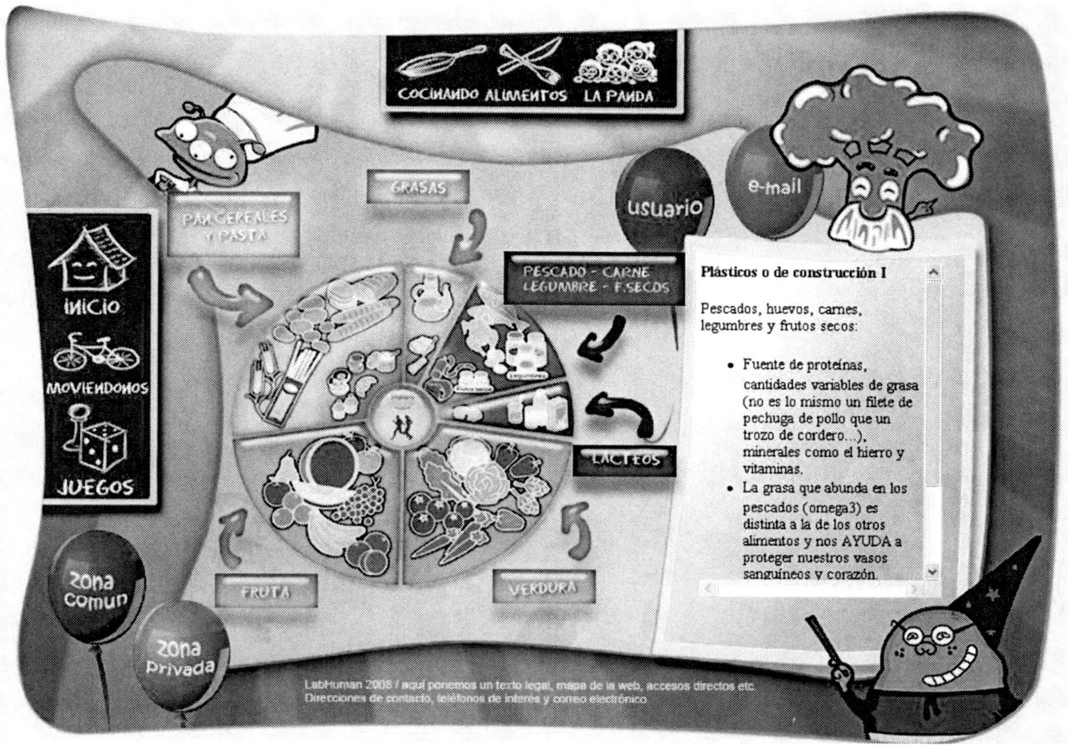

of the food pyramid. The user has to sort different foods into the correct categories in the pyramid and select the food properties. For example, potatoes belong in the category of "vegetable".

The Memory Game: This game is designed to help children learn nutrition trivia, and is based on a classical memory game for children. Different cards with pictures of food are presented one by one. The user has to find matching pairs of foods in the panel. When the pair is found, the user then has to answer a multiple choice question about this food's specific characteristics. The player receives points if the question is answered correctly.

SuperETIOBE: This game is designed to show how some daily behaviors can easily be altered for a healthier life. It consists of graphic adventures wherein the child has to help a detective, called "SuperETIOBE", solve cases of children who have imbalanced food habits or sedentary lifestyles. In each case, the game presents a character and the daily difficulties that prevent a healthy lifestyle; each case must be resolved in a limited time. For example, one boy character always watches TV when he gets home. The players must choose the best methods for improving his physical activity or food habits.

Mobile Support System (MSS)

The MSS is composed of a self-register system and a therapy intelligent network (TIN). The self-register is made with software developed to run with a Personal Digital Assistant (PDA). The objective of this software is to record children's dietary and physical activity habits.

Traditionally, self-register techniques are used to evaluate behaviors in a natural setting (e.g. home or school) and are considered important tools for both the assessment and treatment phases of weight loss treatment. The information obtained

Figure 3. Game image from HSS

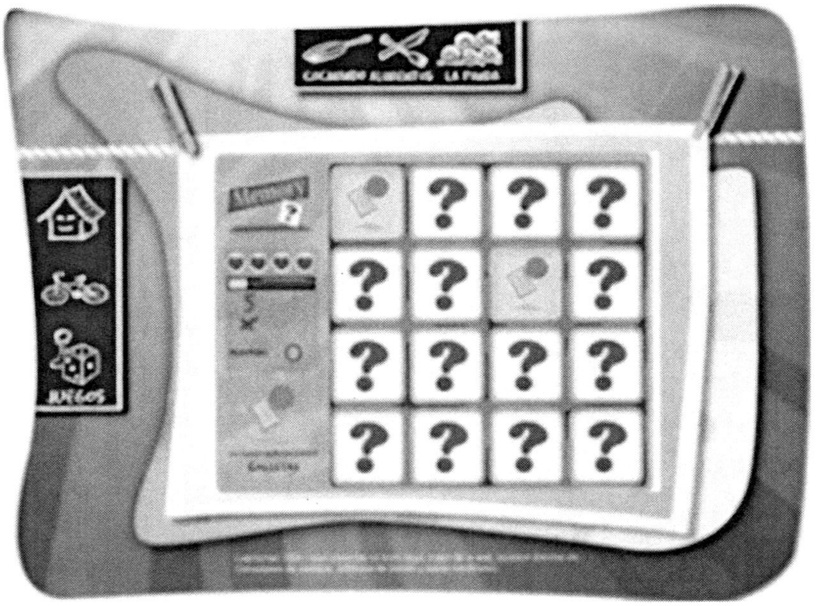

by them allows clinician to identify behavioral cues and the thoughts and emotions associated with these behaviors. Traditionally, these registers are completed with pencil and paper. However, such analog registers have several limitations, including inconvenience, difficulty with recording information in real time (Burke et al, 2008), and poor rates of adherence to the treatment (Baker & Kirschenbaum, 1993; Germann, Kirschenbaum, & Rich, 2007), which worsen over time (Burke et al, 2005). These limitations are significant, because the frequency of dietary self-monitoring during weight loss treatments has been found to be a reliable predictor of success (Streit, Stevens, Stevens & Rossner, 1991).

Research has indicated that the use of a PDA improves the frequency of dietary self-monitoring (Stone et al., 2002; Yon et al., 2007; Lee & Bakken, 2007), adherence to treatments (Beasley et al., 2008), as well as levels of acceptability (Fowles & Gentry, 2008) over paper diary systems.

The electronic self-register included in ETIOBE allows children to register information about the food eaten (amount, order, food name, time and place injested), thoughts and emotions previous to and after eating, and physical activities. For more detailed information about the PDA self-register system see Baños, Cebolla, Zaragoza, Botella, & Alcañiz, (2009) (See Figure 4). This information is transmitted to the clinician in real time through the Internet.

The MSS also includes a therapy intelligent network (tin). It is an open platform that captures information in real time by means of a sensor network focused on the patient. The tin is incorporated into a shirt (developed by the i3bh institute and nuubo). Physiological and activity parameters are acquired from "smart fabrics" that the child wears in regular daily life. The tin shirt includes an accelerometer and heart signal receptor linked to a mobile device with internal geoposition signals to record physical habits and physiological responses in the mss. In order to develop this module, a study is being conducted to analyze the different options to determine bodily position, physical activity, and power consumption without disturbing the daily activity of the patient. Signals acquired by the tin-shirt

Figure 4. The Mobile Support System (MSS)

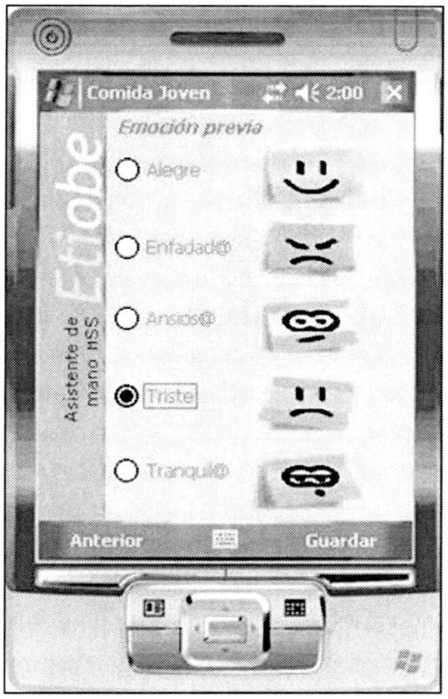

will be uploaded to the css for processing and evaluation. Once processed, the information will be delivered to the clinician and can be used to create a suitable profile of the movement habits of the patients as well as their physiological and health status. This information will also be used to monitor the progress of the patients, including adherence level and difficulties.

FUTURE RESEARCH DIRECTIONS

The development of the ETIOBE platform has been a significant undertaking. First, functional specifications of each application were defined, taking into account the needs of the different users (clinicians, psychologists, and children). Next, the three applications were independently developed and validated; various studies on them were then conducted. For the CSS application, usability and acceptability by clinicians were accessed (Baños, Cebolla, Zaragoza, et al., 2009). The clinicians specialized in obesity treatment (psychologist and medics) received a password to get inside the web and navigate during 30 minutes, after that they answered a questionnaire asking about suitability of the tool, things to improve or to change, and acceptability. Results showed good levels of acceptability and usability (Baños, Cebolla, Zaragoza, et al., 2009). For the HSS, the games were tested for acceptability, user-friendliness, and efficacy of the games platform to learn nutritional knowledge in a children sample (Baños, Cebolla, Etchemendy, et al., 2009). Children's nutritional knowledge was measured, and then participants were randomized into two groups, traditional and Etiobe conditions. In the traditional condition, participants received a pamphlet that they had to study during 2 weeks; in the Etiobe condition, participants received password to get into HSS application and play the games. Results indicated that the group which got inside Etiobe learnt more nutritional knowledge (Cebolla et al., 2010). For the MSS, acceptability of the PDA as a self-register technique is currently being studied; the objective is to compare the traditional self-register method (paper-pencil) with a PDA self-register method in acceptability, efficacy or suitability. Once the three applications are validated, the next step will be a controlled study in which the three applications will be used as a whole system to support a childhood weight loss treatment. This controlled study will compare the efficacy and efficiency of the e-health platform with a traditional cognitive-behavioural treatment.

The ETIOBE design will continue beyond the controlled study. With the objectives of making the HSS more appealing to children and increasing the frequency with which they learn about nutrition, more serious games are needed. Our medium-term objective is to generate several serious games focusing on each of the main abilities involved in the treatment of childhood weight loss, such as self-control, physical activity, and self-esteem. The existing serious games focus solely on nutritional knowledge; however, games focusing on other components of weight loss are needed. Interestingly, physical activity is increasingly being promoted using new generation active computer and video console games, called exergaming (Daley, 2000). These games provide an interesting opportunity to convert what has traditionally been a sedentary activity into one that requires children to be physically active. Evidence has shown that exergaming engages children in low-intensity exercise (Daley, 2000) and can be a suitable tool for childhood weight loss treatment. In fact, research has shown that some exergames are a useful tool in weight loss therapy (Graff, Pratt, Hester, & Short, 2009).

Another component that should be incorporated into the HSS is a section addressing the children's parents, since family is a crucial factor in childhood obesity treatment. In the future, HSS will also include information for parents on where they can receive suitable guidelines on how to help their children change their habits and modify their lifestyles.

CONCLUSION

The use of ICTs in childhood obesity treatment can be effective in preventing increasing treatment adherence, according to user characteristics. The most important guidelines and international associations recommend further research on treatments for childhood obesity and development of more efficient weight loss treatments. E-health technologies such as the ETIOBE system can help achieve this goal and improve the efficacy of the treatments. It is expected that they will improve children's adherence to weight loss treatments due to several factors, such as better user acceptability of the technologies, treatment goal flexibility, and continued monitoring of patient progress. According to Cushing and Steel (2010), technology has been and will continue to become an ever-increasing part of children's lives. Therefore, intervention programs aimed at changing young people's health behaviors may have far greater reach and be much more effective if delivered via the channels that children and teenagers prefer and in the forms that they recognize and will use.

One of the biggest challenges for obesity treatments is helping patients maintain weight loss over time. To address this, e-health platforms help clinicians work with patients even when they are far away or after the treatment session has finished. ICTs may improve adherence and greater motivation for treatment, helping children maintain their daily therapeutic requirements while supervised and monitored. Thus, ICTs can provide information and resources to enable children to counter the influences of the "obesogenic environment" that surrounds them, resulting in medium- and long-term maintenance of healthy body weight.

Childhood obesity prevention and treatment are complex and difficult problems, and development of novel tools is critical to achieving effective intervention. E-health technologies have the potential to improve treatments for obesity, providing national health services with an increased ability to reach everyone in need of personalized weight loss therapy.

ACKNOWLEDGMENT

CIBERobn is an initiative of ISCIII. This research has been made possible, in part, by the support of Ministerio de Ciencia e Innovación (Plan Nacional de Investigación Científica, Desarrollo e Innovación Tecnológica 2008-2011), in the project (PSI2008-04392/PSIC), and the Excellence Research Program PROMETEO (Generalitat Valenciana. Conselleria de Educación; 2008/157).

REFERENCES

Ahern, D. K., Phalen, J. M., Le, L. X., & Goldman, R. E. (2007). *Childhood obesity prevention and reduction: Role of eHealth. Exploring the role of technology can play in reducing the incidence and prevalence of childhood obesity*. Health E-Technologies Inititative. Retrieved April 15, 2010, from www.hetinitiative.org

Baker, R., & Kirschenbaum, D. (1993). Self-monitoring may be necessary for successful weight control. *Behavior Therapy*, *24*, 377–394. doi:10.1016/S0005-7894(05)80212-6

Baños, R., Botella, C., Frías, A., Alcañiz, M., Cebolla, A., & Etxemendy, E. ... Andreu S. (2008). *The ETIOBE Project: A supporting system for childhood obesity*. Cybertherapy 13th Conference: Changing the face of healthcare. San Diego, California.

Baños, R., Cebolla, A., Etchemendy, E., Rasal, P., Botella, C., & Alcañiz, M. ... Frias, A. (2009). *Serious game platform for nutritional education: Memory game acceptability and playability results*. 2nd European Conference on Games Based Learning. Graz, Austria.

Baños, R., Cebolla, A., Frías, A., Etchemendy, E., Botella, C., Garcia-Palacios, A., & Alcañiz, A. (2009). *The Etiobe Mates: A serious game platform to improve the learning of nutritional knowledge in children*. Frontiers in Neuroengineering. 14th Annual Cybertherapy & Cyberpsychology Conference.

Baños, R., Cebolla, A., Zaragoza, I., Botella, C., & Alcañiz, M. (2009). Electronic PDA dietary and physical activity registers in a weight loss treatment program for children: A description of the ETIOBE personal digital assistant system. *Journal of Cybertherapy and Rehabilitation*, *3*, 235–241.

Baños, R., Cebolla, A., Zaragoza, I., Botella, C., Alcañiz, M., & Jiménez, S. ... Alvarez Pitti, J. (2009). *Usability study of the clinic support system of ETIOBE platform*. III Symposium CIBEROBN Fisiopatología de la Obesidad y la Nutrición. La Toja (A Coruña).

Baranowsky, T., Baranowsky, J., Cullen, K. W., Marsh, T., Islam, N., & Zakeri, I. (2003). Squire's quest: Dietary evaluation of a multimedia game. *American Journal of Preventive Medicine*, *24*, 52–61.

Beasley, M., Riley, W. T., Davis, A., & Singh, J. (2008). Evaluation of a PDA-based dietary assessment and intervention program: A randomized controlled trial. *Journal of the American College of Nutrition*, *27*, 380–386.

Branca, F., Nikogosian, H., & Lobstein, T. (2007). *World Health Organization: The challenge of obesity in the WHO European region and the strategies for response*. Retrieved February 2, 2010, from http://www.euro.who.int/ en/home

Burke, L. E., Choo, J., Music, E., Warziski, M., Styn, M. A., Kim, Y., & Sevick, M. A. (2005). PREFER study: A randomized clinical trial testing treatment preference and two dietary options in behavioral weight management: Rationale, design and baseline characteristics. *Contemporary Clinical Trials*, *27*, 34–48. doi:10.1016/j.cct.2005.08.002

Burke, L. E., Sereika, S. M., Music, E., Warziski, M., Styn, M. A., & Stone, A. (2008). Using instrumented paper diaries to document self-monitoring patterns in weight-loss. *Contemporary Clinical Trials*, *29*, 182–193. doi:10.1016/j.cct.2007.07.004

Casazza, K., & Ciccazzo, M. (2007). The method of delivery of nutrition and physical activity information may play a role in eliciting behavior changes in adolescents. *Eating Behaviors*, *8*, 73–82. doi:10.1016/j.eatbeh.2006.01.007

Cebolla, A., Baños, R., Oliver, E., Etchemendy, E., Botella, C., & García-Palacios, A. ... Alcañiz, M. (2010). "La panda Etiobe": Utilidad de una plataforma de juegos serios para el aprendizaje de conocimientos nutricionales en población infantil. Paper presented in SEAS Congress. Valencia, Spain.

Daley, A. (2009). Can exergaming contribute to improving physical activity and health outcomes in children? *Pediatrics*, *124*, 763–771. doi:10.1542/peds.2008-2357

European Association for the Study of Obesity. (2002). *Obesity in Europe: The case for action* (on line). Retrieved April 5, 2008, from www.iotf.org

Fowles, E. R., & Gentri, B. (2008). The feasibility of personal digital assistants (PDAs) to collect dietary intake data in low-income pregnant women. *Journal of Nutrition Education and Behavior*, *40*, 374–377. doi:10.1016/j.jneb.2007.08.015

Garris, R., Ahlers, R., & Driskell, J. (2002). Games, motivation and learning: A research and practice model. *Simulation & Gaming*, *33*, 441–467. doi:10.1177/1046878102238607

Germann, J. N., Kirschenbaum, D. S., & Rich, B. H. (2007). Child and parental self-monitoring as determinants of success in the treatment of morbid obesity in low-income minority children. *Journal of Pediatric Psychology*, *32*, 111–121. doi:10.1093/jpepsy/jsl007

Graf, D. L., Pratt, L. V., Hester, C. N., & Short, K. (2009). Playing active games increases energy expenditure in children. *Pediatrics*, *124*, 534–540. doi:10.1542/peds.2008-2851

Guo, S. S., Wu, W., Chumlea, W. C., & Roche, A. F. (2002). Predicting overweight and obesity in adulthood from body mass index values in childhood and adolescence. *The American Journal of Clinical Nutrition*, *76*, 653–658.

Harvey-Berino, J., Pintauro, S. J., & Gold, E. C. (2002). The feasibility of using internet support for the maintenance of weight loss. *Behavior Modification*, *26*, 103–116. doi:10.1177/0145445502026001006

International Association for the Study of Obesity. (2007). *Childhood and adolescent overweight in Europe*. Retrieved May 15, 2010, from http://www.iotf.org/database/ Childhoodandadolescentover weightineurope.htm

Kirschenbaum, D. S., Germann, J. N., & Rich, B. H. (2005). Treatment of morbid obesity in low-income adolescents: Effects of parental self-monitoring. *Obesity Research*, *9*, 1527–1529. doi:10.1038/oby.2005.187

Lee, N. J., & Bakken, S. (2007). Development of a prototype personal digital assistant-decision support system for the management of adult obesity. *International Journal of Medical Informatics*, *76*, 281–292. doi:10.1016/j.ijmedinf.2007.05.009

Norman, G. J., Zabinski, M. F., Adams, M. A., Rosenberg, D. E., Yaroch, A. L., & Atienza, A. A. (2007). A review of eHealth interventions for physical activity and dietary behavior change. *American Journal of Preventive Medicine*, *33*, 336–345. doi:10.1016/j.amepre.2007.05.007

Patrick, K., Calfas, K. J., Norman, G. J., Zabinski, M. F., Sallis, J. F., Rupp, J., & Covin, J. (2006). A randomized controlled trial of a primary care and home based intervention for physical activity and nutritiobehaviors: PACE+ for adolescents. *Archives of Pediatrics & Adolescent Medicine*, *160*, 128–136. doi:10.1001/archpedi.160.2.128

Saelens, B. E., Sallis, J., Wilfleym, D., Patrick, K., Cella, J., & Buchta, R. (2002). A randomized trial of a multicomponential behavioral weight control treatment initiated in primary care versus typical care for overweight adolescents. *Obesity Research*, *10*, 22–32. doi:10.1038/oby.2002.4

Stinson, J., Wilson, R., Gill, N., Yamada, J., & Holt, J. (2009). A systematic review of internet-based self-management interventions for youth with health conditions. *Journal of Pediatric Psychology, 34*, 495–510. doi:10.1093/jpepsy/jsn115

Stone, A. A., Shiffman, S., Schwartz, J. E., Broderick, J. E., & Hufford, M. R. (2002). Patient non-compliance with paper diaries. *British Medical Journal, 324*, 1193–1194. doi:10.1136/bmj.324.7347.1193

Streit, K. J., Stevens, N. H., Stevens, V. J., & Rossner, J. (1991). Food records: A predictor and modification of weight change in a long-term weight loss program. *Journal of the American Dietetic Association, 91*, 13–216.

Tate, D., Jackvony, E., & Wing, R. (2003). Effects of Internet behavioral counseling on weight loss in adults at risk for Type 2 Diabetes. *Journal of the American Medical Association, 289*, 1833–1836. doi:10.1001/jama.289.14.1833

Tate, D. F., Jackvony, E. H., & Wing, R. R. (2006). A randomized trial comparing human e-mail counseling, computer-automated tailored counseling, and no counseling in an Internet weight loss program. *Archives of Internal Medicine, 166*, 1620–1625. doi:10.1001/archinte.166.15.1620

Williamson, D. A., Walden, H. M., White, M. A., York-Crowe, E., Newton, R. L., & Alfonso, A. (2006). Two-year randomized controlled trial for weight loss in African-American girls. *Obesity Research, 14*, 1231–1243. doi:10.1038/oby.2006.140

Yon, B. A., Johnson, R. K., Harvey-Berino, J., Gold, B. C., & Howard, A. B. (2007). Personal digital assistants are comparable to traditional dietary self-monitoring during a weight loss program. *Journal of Behavioral Medicine, 30*, 165–175. doi:10.1007/s10865-006-9092-1

KEY TERMS AND DEFINITIONS

Adherence Treatment: It refers to how closely patient follow a prescribed treatment, and includes his/her willingness to start treatment and his/her ability to do the tasks and recommendations suggested by the therapist.

Childhood Obesity: A medical condition in which excess body fat negatively affects child's health and wellbeing.

E-Health: The use of emerging interactive Information and Communication Technologies (i.e., Internet, interactive TV, interactive voice response systems, kiosks, internet-enabled cell phones and personal digital assistants [PDAs], CD-ROMs, DVDs) to facilitate access to healthcare and to enable health improvement and health care services.

Internet Based Intervention: Intervention which uses Internet to deliver treatment programs with the objective to improve treatment efficiency.

Obesogenic Environment: An environment that encourages the overconsumption of energy-dense foods and promotes gaining weight.

Serious Games: Software applications developed with informatics technology and game design principles used for educational, persuasive or health purposes.

Weight Loss Treatment: Medical and psychological interventions designed to reduce the excess of body fat and improve the general health of obese patients. It usually includes changes in lifestyle, exercise, dieting, and, in some cases, weight loss medicines or weight loss surgery.

Chapter 3
Internet-Based Chronic Disease Self-Management for Youth

Jennifer Stinson
The Hospital for Sick Children, Canada

Navreet Gill
The Hospital for Sick Children, Canada

ABSTRACT

Chronic health conditions in children and youth are important health problems that seriously affect all aspects of their everyday lives. There is growing recognition of the need to promote disease self-management in youth with chronic health conditions. While there is evidence of the effectiveness of self-management programs to improve health outcomes in pediatric chronic illnesses, there are barriers to youth receiving these services. Internet-based programs offer an innovative approach to improve the availability, accessibility, and acceptability of these programs. This chapter provides an overview of Internet-based chronic disease self-management treatment programs for children and youth. It defines and describes the underlying theories, processes, and content elements of Internet-based self-management programs. Practical tips for program development and evaluation in terms of improved health outcomes are also discussed based on the authors' experience with developing the "Teens Taking Charge: Managing Arthritis Online" self-management program for adolescents with arthritis. Future directions for theory, research, and clinical practice are also described.

INTRODUCTION

Despite the focus on chronic disease self-management in adults; little attention has been directed to promoting disease self-management in children and youth with chronic health conditions. It is estimated that 10-15% of children and adolescents have significant ongoing health care needs related to chronic health conditions that will persist into adulthood (van der Lee, Mokkink, Grootenhuis, Heymans, & Offringa, 2007). Childhood chronic illness can negatively impact all aspects of health-related quality of life and also have a significant

DOI: 10.4018/978-1-60960-866-8.ch003

economic impact on the health care system and families (Barlow & Ellard, 2006; Bernatasky et al., 2007; Newacheck, Inkelas, & Kim, 2004; Shaw, Southwood, Duffy, & McDonough, 2006; Turkel & Pao, 2007). Disease course can be unpredictable and children commonly experience a myriad of symptoms that restrict physical and social interactions (Barlow & Ellard, 2006; Shaw et al., 2006; Turkel & Pao, 2007). Disease management is often complex, involving multiple therapies over long periods of time that require frequent monitoring. In the absence of cure, improving health-related quality of life through better disease self-management becomes critical (Phelps, 2006). While there is evidence of the effectiveness of self-management programs improving health outcomes in children (e.g., asthma and diabetes), many youth with chronic health conditions do not receive comprehensive disease education with self-management strategies and meaningful social support (Barlow & Ellard, 2006; Barlow, Shaw, & Southwood, 1998; Smith et al., 2005). The Internet is a widely available, affordable, and interactive medium that is well suited to teaching disease self-management skills and can easily address barriers such as inaccessibility and unavailability. From a public health perspective, there is much potential for self-administered treatments to improve the health of children who suffer from chronic illnesses but are unable to access services.

BACKGROUND

Self-management can be defined as "the individual's ability to manage the symptoms, treatment, physical and psychological consequences, and life style changes inherent in living with a chronic illness" (Barlow, Wright, Sheasby, Turner, & Hainsworth, 2002, pp.178). It is a dynamic and continuous process of self-regulation that encompasses the ability to monitor one's health condition and to carry out the cognitive, behavioural and emotional responses necessary to maintain a satisfactory quality of life (Barlow et al, 2002). The daily tasks requiring self-management are three-fold: (1) taking care of one's overall health (e.g., healthy eating, being physically active, relaxing and reducing stress, and being knowledgeable about one's condition, treatments and medications, etc.); (2) carrying on with normal activities and roles in life (e.g., maintaining healthy social relationships and staying involved in home, social, and school/work activities) and; (3) managing the emotional changes that are inherent in the chronic illness experience such as anger, fear, frustration, low mood, etc. (Lorig & Holman, 2003; McGillion LeFort, & Stinson, 2008). To successfully manage these tasks, individuals with chronic health conditions need a set of core self-management skills which include: problem-solving skills; decision-making skills; how to find, evaluate and utilize appropriate resources; how to work effectively in partnership with health care providers and; how to take action to change behavior (McGillion et al., 2008).

Traditional patient education provides information and teaches technical skills about how to manage the chronic condition itself. By contrast, self-management education is broader in scope emphasizing problem solving, action planning for behavior change, and confidence building to enable people to better deal with everyday problems that result from chronic conditions (McGillion et al., 2008). In other words, self-management education helps people with a chronic condition better manage their lives. Self-management interventions typically encompass information-based material and cognitive-behavioural strategies designed to increase participants' knowledge, self-efficacy and use of self-management behaviors (see Table 1 for elements of a self-management program for youth). Self-management interventions also involve a collaborative partnership between patients and their health care providers to support at-home management of their disease.

Studies in both adult and paediatric chronic illness have shown that comprehensive interactive

Table 1. Elements of a self-management program for children and youth

Elements	Sub-elements
Disease-specific information	• Pathophysiology • Causes • Symptoms • Determining a diagnosis • Subtypes • Complications • Prognosis
Symptom management	• Medication information (e.g., purpose, side effects) • Cognitive-behavioural strategies (e.g., imagery, distraction, relaxation) • Other types of care (e.g., surgery, exercise, physiotherapy)
Communication	• Communicating with physicians, teachers, and peers • Advocating
Healthy Living	• Exercise and staying active • Nutrition • Sexuality • Body Image and self-esteem • Recreational drugs • Smoking • Alcohol use
Social Support	• Family support • Peer support • Support from teachers • Support from health care professionals
Transition to Adulthood	• Care provision in adult health care centres • Higher education • Career planning
Other	• Goal-setting • Other resources

face-to-face self-management interventions lead to symptom reduction and improved quality of life compared with care that is strictly medically focused (Barlow & Ellard, 2006; Eccleston, Morley, Williams, Yorke, & Mastroyannopoulou, 2002; Superio-Cabuslay, Ward, & Lorig, 1996; Walco, Sterling, Conte, & Engel, 1999). For example, Barlow and colleagues (2002) conducted a systematic review of 145 studies of self-management interventions for individuals (children and adults) with 28 different chronic health conditions. Self-management interventions were found to improve knowledge, performance of self-management behaviours (e.g., exercise, relaxation, energy conservation, and stress reduction), and various aspects of physical and emotional functioning such as exercise capacity and mood compared to standard care or no intervention. The self-management interventions were: (a) delivered within either clinical or home environments; (b) facilitated by health care professionals or lay tutors with chronic conditions and; (c) either group-based with 6-12 participants, individualized, or a combination of both, each of which was equally effective. Regardless of format, most programs utilize a multi-component approach, offering an array of self-management techniques that participants can rehearse and incorporate into their day-to-day lives. They also found that the majority of self-management programs to date are designed for adult patients.

Promoting chronic disease self-management in youth requires an understanding of how children with chronic health conditions gradually develop these skills within a shared management model of care. A shared management model has been proposed as a framework to help young children move from a stage where their parents manage all aspects of their chronic illness with support from the health care team (shared management), to one where the youth and or young adult ultimately assumes the management role (self-management) (Gall, Kingsnorth, & Healy, 2006; Kieckhefer & Trahms, 2000).

In younger years, activities necessary to manage chronic illness are shared by the child and family with support from health care professionals (Gall et al., 2006; Kieckhefer & Trahms, 2000). In a shared management model, parents may influence their child's developing self-efficacy by (a) provision of support and encouragement and; (b) assisting children to interpret disease specific education and strategies to manage their chronic health condition depending on their developmental readiness. In addition, engaging children at this age may help them to become knowledgeable and capable participants in their own care as they move into the adolescent period where they will be expected to take more control over managing their chronic condition (self-management) (Gall et al., 2006; Kieckhefer & Trahms, 2000). For these reasons, it is important to develop programs to make it easier for school-age children with chronic conditions and their parents to jointly manage their disease.

As children mature, they are expected to assume increasing responsibility for disease management concomitant with their growing independence and autonomy (Sawyer & Aroni, 2005). However, adolescents' acceptance of and ability to implement this increasing responsibility is not always optimal, thereby often reducing the potential benefits of treatment and adversely impacting health-related quality of life (April, Feldman, Platt, & Duffy, 2006; Rapoff, 2002). Promoting self-management amongst adolescents with chronic illnesses can improve health outcomes (symptom reduction) and ultimately can facilitate transition into the adult health care system (Barlow et al., 2002; Phelps, 2006).

NEED FOR NEW MODELS OF SELF-MANAGEMENT FOR CHILDREN AND YOUTH

Issues, Controversies, Problems

Many school-age children and adolescents with chronic health conditions do not receive comprehensive disease self-management education due to: (1) difficulty accessing these services because of limited services available in many geographic areas (including the rural and remote regions, language barriers, and long-wait times); (2) limited availability of trained professionals such as nurses and psychologists especially in rural and remote areas and; (3) costs including time off school and work for youth and their parents associated with these therapies (Barlow, Shaw, & Harrison, 1999; Elgar & McGrath, 2003; Lineker, Badley, & Dalby, 1996; Newacheck et al., 2004). Moreover, existing self-management therapies for childhood chronic illnesses have been reported to be: (1) limited in scope; (2) directed at parents rather than school-age children and or adolescents; (3) delivered in individual or group sessions in specialty clinics by highly trained personnel and; (4) not suitable for wide-spread distribution in community and home-based settings (Barlow et al., 1999; Barlow & Ellard, 2004). With emerging interactive and communication technologies (e-health), especially the Internet, new media for the delivery of health interventions are now available (Ritterband et al., 2003). The Internet has emerged as one of the top health information resources and modes of social communication for youth and is, therefore, ideally suited to the provision of online health care services (Gray, Klein, Noyce, Sesselberg, & Cantrill, 2005; Rainie, 2010). Internet self-management interventions are a promising method for improving the accessibility and availability of self-management interventions and social supports for youth with chronic diseases.

The Internet provides patients, families, and health care professionals with unparalleled opportunities to: (a) learn, inform and communicate with one another; (b) receive meaningful social support; (c) fulfill the rising demand for expedient access to evidence-based health information and; (d) achieve greater involvement in health care decision-making (Drotar et al., 2006; Griffiths, Lindenmeyer, Powell, Lowe, & Thorogood, 2006). Access to online health interventions eliminates geographic constraints, allows for anonymity, and provides 24-hour access to disease-related information and self-management strategies that may help patients feel more in control of managing their chronic condition and minimize feelings of isolation. Other advantages include: (a) a secure server which can deliver, customize and record homework sessions, and provide individuals with opportunities to communicate with their health care team and their peers; (b) private access to information at any time, increasing treatment convenience as well as helping decrease costs; (c) a range of self-management modules, which enables individuals to personalize their treatment by selecting the modules that are most relevant to them or those they wish to explore in greater depth and; (d) a mode of communication – the computer - that is highly appealing to children and youth.

Internet-based interventions are treatments that are usually based on effective face-to-face interventions that are transformed for delivery via the Internet with the goal of improved health outcomes (symptom reduction and improved health status or health-related quality of life). There are three broad types of Internet-based interventions: (1) education interventions (tend to be static sites that are relatively therapeutically inactive); (2) self-guided therapeutic interventions and; (3) human-supported therapeutic interventions (Barak, Klein, & Proudfoot, 2009). Internet-based self-management programs are therapeutic interventions that are highly structured, self-guided or partly self-guided (i.e., minimal therapist support through regular brief telephone and or email contact), tailored to the user's needs, and interactive (Ritterband et al., 2003). While this is a burgeoning field, the Internet remains a relatively new medium for delivery of health care. Formal evaluations of the impact of Internet health interventions on health outcomes, level of resource utilization and user satisfaction have lagged far behind their development (Danaher & Steeley, 2009; Nguyen, Carrieri-Kohlman, Ranki, Slaughter, & Stulbarg, 2004).

Theoretical Frameworks for Internet Self-Management Programs

Like face-to-face self-management programs, Internet self-management interventions aim to produce cognitive and behavioral change to impact patient behavior and reduce unwanted symptoms and improve quality of life. A critical feature of successful self-management education programs is a firm grounding in social, cognitive and/or behavioural theories, targeting individuals' (a) confidence to achieve optimal functioning; (b) acceptance of their chronic illness-induced limitations and; (c) adaptive ways of thinking, feeling and behaving (Barlow et al., 2002; McGillion et al., 2008). Researchers have postulated that enhanced self-efficacy (a person's belief in their capacity to carry out a specific action) and empowerment (process whereby an individual gains control over their own lives) are key mediators in effective self-management programs (Marks, Allegrante, & Lorig, 2005a; Marks, Allegrante, & Lorig, 2005b).

Murray and colleagues (2005) have postulated a pathway for change whereby interactive health communication applications (primarily Internet-based programs) are hypothesized to work by combining information with peer, decision-making, and behavioural change supports to allow internalization and interpretation of the information by the user. A combination of enhanced self-efficacy with motivation and knowledge enables users to change their health behaviours leading to changes in clinical outcomes.

Ritterband and colleagues (2009) have built upon this postulated pathway of change by including characteristics of the end-users (i.e., demographic, disease, cognitive and physiological factors; personality traits; beliefs and attitudes; self-efficacy and skills), the environment and the web-based program. The model purports that program users are influenced by environmental factors (i.e., family, friends, significant others, employers/school, health care system, community and societal influences) which affect website use and adherence. Website use and adherence is also influenced by the type of support provided (e.g., email, phone, face-to-face) and characteristics of the website (e.g., appearance, behavioral prescriptions [e.g., contracts, prompts], content, burden [e.g., difficulty of use, length], delivery [e.g., animations, audio, illustrations, text, testimonials], message [e.g., source and style], participation [e.g., interaction, reinforcement, testing] and assessment [e.g., personalized or tailoring]). Website use leads to changes in behavior that results in symptom improvement through various mechanisms of change such as gaining knowledge, changing attitudes and beliefs, motivation, and skill building.

Evidence for Internet-Based Self-Management Programs

Adult Literature

The literature on Internet interventions is rapidly growing with studies on feasibility and utility, as well as evidence of efficacy in improving clinical health outcomes (Cuijpers, van Straten, & Andersson, 2008; Lorig, Ritter, Laurent, & Plant, 2008; Murray, Burns, See Tai, Lai, & Nazareth, 2005; Nguyen et al., 2004; Palmqvist, Carlbring, & Andersson, 2007; Spek et al., 2007; Wantland, Portillo, Holzemer, Slaughter, & McGhee, 2004). Wantland et al. (2004) conducted a systematic review and meta-analysis of 22 randomized controlled trials that compared web-based to non-web-based self-management interventions in adults with chronic health conditions. Use of Internet interventions improved the specified knowledge and behavioral change outcomes compared to non-Internet interventions across a wide variety of chronic conditions. However, they were not able to determine durability of treatment effects (maintenance of gains over time) or cost-effectiveness.

Nguyen et al. (2004) conducted a systematic review and qualitative synthesis of control, comparative and pilot studies (n=17 studies) to evaluate the impact of professionally facilitated Internet-based programs for diverse adult clinical populations on health outcomes, resource utilization and user satisfaction. All of the interventions included a health care professional who either served as a facilitator or therapist for the experimental group through regular telephone and/or email contact. Some outcomes (physical function, emotional and physical symptoms) in certain groups were moderately improved compared to control groups and user satisfaction with interventions was generally positive. However, the level (intense versus brief contact), mode (telephone, email), and type of human support (health professionals, trained personnel, peers) needed to maintain engagement in Internet health interventions is unknown (Nguyen et al., 2004; Barak et al., 2009).

Murray and colleagues (2005) conducted a Cochrane review of Interactive Health Communication Applications (IHCA) (computer-based interventions that encompass health information plus at least one of the following: social, decision-making, and/or behavior change support). 24 randomized controlled trials of IHCAs for adults and children (n=3739 participants) with chronic disease were included. IHCAs had largely positive effects on end-user knowledge and feeling more socially supported, and small to moderate effects on behavioral (adherence) and clinical outcomes (i.e., symptom reduction, improvements in health status/health-related quality of life) and self-efficacy compared to non-users. However, they were unable to determine the effect on emotional and economic outcomes as most studies did not include these as outcomes (Murray et al., 2005). Furthermore, only 1/5 studies targeting children were Internet interventions (others were video-games or CD-ROMs); all had small sample sizes.

Cuijpers et al. (2008) conducted a systematic review of 12 randomized controlled trials of Internet-based CBT for health problems in children and adults (n=1,704 participants). Only 2 studies targeted children and youth. Most interventions used a self-guided format in which the treatment protocol was presented on the Internet and patients worked through it independently. The effects for Internet interventions targeting chronic pain and headaches were comparable to those for face-to-face treatments (moderate to large effects); however, the effects for other target conditions were variable and generally smaller in magnitude. Trial rigor was variable and most studies were under powered to detect small treatment effects.

Pediatric Literature

Despite the evidence of the effectiveness on Internet-based self-management interventions for adults with a wide range of chronic health conditions; there is limited empirical evidence on the availability and effectiveness of Internet interventions to promote self-management in children and youth with chronic health conditions (Cuijpers et al., 2008; Lorig et al., 2008; Palmqvist et al., 2007; Spek et al., 2007; Wantland et al., 2004). A systematic review conducted by Stinson et al. (2009) examined the effectiveness of Internet self-management interventions on health outcomes in youth with sub-acute or chronic health conditions. Only 9 of 29 published articles on Internet interventions met the inclusion criteria (7 randomized controlled trials, 1 quasi-experimental and 1 pilot randomized controlled trial) and were included in analysis. Health conditions included asthma, obesity, traumatic brain injury, recurrent pain and encopresis. All of the interventions were psycho-educational in nature targeting improved health outcomes. However, they varied greatly in content, procedural aspects of interventions (self-guided versus guided self-help with minimal therapist involvement), duration, and number of sessions. Parents were included in 5 studies as active participants of which only 1 study had specific modules for parents. Two studies asked children and parents to complete sessions together. Dropout rates varied from 0 to 28% but tended to be lower than those found in the systematic reviews of adult Internet interventions. While outcomes varied greatly between studies, overall, health outcomes (reduced pain, improved disease control in terms of number of asthma attacks and weight loss) improved in Internet interventions compared to control conditions in 7/9 studies. There was conflicting evidence regarding disease knowledge and health-related quality of life, and evidence was limited regarding decreases in health care utilization. This review concluded that there was some beginning evidence that self-management interventions delivered via the Internet improve selected outcomes in certain chronic childhood illnesses.

DEVELOPMENT OF SELF-MANAGEMENT INTERNET PROGRAMS FOR CHILDREN AND YOUTH

There is currently no consensus or guidelines regarding the best way to develop and evaluate Internet-based treatment programs (Ritterband, Andersson, Christensen, Carlbring, & Cuijpers, 2006). However, a sequential phased approach has been advocated for the development and evaluation of complex behavioural interventions (Craig et al., 2008). This approach should include: (1) an assessment of the unique self-management needs of the target population (end-users); (2) usability testing of the site in terms of user performance (ease of use, errors, efficiency) and acceptability (satisfying to complete); (3) pilot testing the feasibility and acceptability of the program and; (4)

a definitive randomized control trial to determine the effectiveness of the program on child health outcomes in the real world. Below we describe the process and practical tips based on our experience developing and testing an Internet-based self-management program for adolescents with juvenile idiopathic arthritis (JIA) called "Teens Taking Charge: Managing Arthritis Online".

Step 1: Needs Assessment

Traditionally, self-management interventions (regardless of how they are delivered) have been developed by health care professionals with little input from the end-users (top down approach). Few studies have explored the self-management needs of children or adults with chronic illnesses to inform the development of these treatment programs ensuring usable and acceptable end-products. A needs assessment should be conducted to determine the self-management learning needs of the end-users and whether an Internet-based treatment delivery modality would be acceptable. Methods for conducting needs assessments (i.e., surveys, individual and or focus group interviews) and analyzing these data are abundant in the literature and to review them in detail is beyond the scope of this chapter. For this, interested readers are referred to comprehensive texts dedicated to this subject (McGillion et al., 2008). Information gleaned from the needs assessment will inform the development of the program content, need for human support, degree of interactivity needed to keep youth engaged as well as the types of multimedia that should be used in the online treatment program.

We conducted a qualitative study using individual and focus groups interviews to explore the self-management needs of adolescents with arthritis and to determine the acceptability of a web-based program of self-management (Stinson et al., 2008). Adolescents articulated how they developed effective self-management strategies through the process of "letting go" from others who had managed their illness (health care professionals, parents) and "gaining control" over managing their illness on their own. The two strategies that assisted in this process were: (1) gaining knowledge and skills to manage the disease and; (2) experiencing understanding through social support. Five further sub-themes that emerged around skills to manage the disease included: knowledge and awareness about the disease, listening to and challenging care-providers, communicating with the doctor, managing pain, and managing emotions. Adolescents were united in their call for more information, self-management strategies and meaningful social support to better manage their arthritis. They believed that web-based interventions were a promising avenue to improve accessibility and availability of these interventions. Information from this study was used to inform the development of the program content and interactive features of the Internet-based self-management program.

Step 2: Building the Website and Usability Testing

The next step is the development of the website and testing the usability of the site to further refine the prototype. Barak and colleagues (2009) outline four 'essential ingredients' of therapeutic Internet interventions that need to be considered when developing an online self-management program. The first component, program content is considered the "backbone" of the intervention and is intended to educate and/or create a therapeutic cognitive or behavioural change. The program content should be informed by the underlying theories (e.g., social learning, cognitive, behavioural) as well as from an assessment of the self-management needs of the end-users (Step 1). The second component is the use of multimedia such as graphic illustrations, animations, audio and video clips. It is generally felt that including a greater variety of multimedia formats makes for a more engaging and dynamic online intervention.

The third component and likely the most important to consider in developing Internet interventions for children and youth, is the incorporation of interactive online activities. Interactive activities can include things such as weekly goal setting, self-assessments (knowledge quizzes) and self-monitoring tools (diaries) which help to personalize the program. Providing children and youth with an opportunity to participate more interactively in the program is thought to pique their interest and increase their level of engagement as it may facilitate a sense of connectedness to the program through this personalization (Barak et al., 2009). Provision of guidance and supportive feedback is the fourth component of Internet health interventions and often encompasses personalized emails, instant messaging, phone sessions or face-to-face meetings (Ritterband et al., 2009). The amount of external feedback regarding participant progress can range from none to high, whereby specific tailored feedback is provided and is usually generated either via automated programming or by a human. Current research regarding the effectiveness of such external support is conflicting as some studies have found it to improve adherence and health outcomes, and others not (Ritterband et al., 2009). In light of this, the time, effort and cost to incorporate a support component must be considered. Inclusion of a support component also restricts the external reach of the Internet intervention whereas a program without support will allow for a larger external audience to be reached. Thus careful consideration of each of these components must be taken in developing self-management Internet programs for children and youth.

The results from the needs assessment were used to develop the content of the self-management program and inform the interactive features of the "Teens Taking Charge: Managing Arthritis Online" Internet program. The online program is a 12-week multi-component treatment protocol that consists of self-management strategies, disease specific information and social support (discussion board, video clips with peer modeling and stories of hope) that are available in English and French (see Figure 1). It is delivered on a restricted website and through regular telephone contact with a trained coach (non-health care professional). The 12 modules for adolescents include learning about the different types of arthritis, understanding how arthritis is diagnosed, arthritis medications, managing symptoms (pain, stiffness and fatigue), managing stress and negative thoughts, relaxation, distraction, other types of care (exercise, nutrition, splints), self-monitoring and supports, lifestyle issues and looking ahead (education, vocation, transitional care issues). There are 2 modules specifically for parents/care-givers to help them encourage healthy behavior (i.e., the impact of arthritis and helping parents learn to let go). Adolescents and parents are able to view each other's sites and they can work through the modules together (e.g., younger teens) or independently. The aim of this program is to help adolescents identify more active ways of self-managing their arthritis.

The content was developed by a team of experts from across Canada (researchers, multidisciplinary rheumatology and adolescent medicine health care professionals and two consumers), written at a grade 6-7 level and geared to the needs identified by adolescents and their parents in Step 1 (Needs Assessment). The content is multilayered, interactive (animations, video clips, discussion board with 'Ask an Expert' functionality, goal setting, weekly knowledge quizzes, and 'My Journal' to track goals and progress) and allows the adolescent/parent to follow their interest and delve into a topic or deal with the material on a more surface level. (See Figure 2, Figure 3, and Figure 4 for screenshots of a video clip, a click through animation on how we feel pain, and a quiz).

Once the online program has been developed, it should be tested for its usability. Usability measures the quality of a user's experience when interacting with a product or system such as a

Figure 1. Teens taking charge homepage

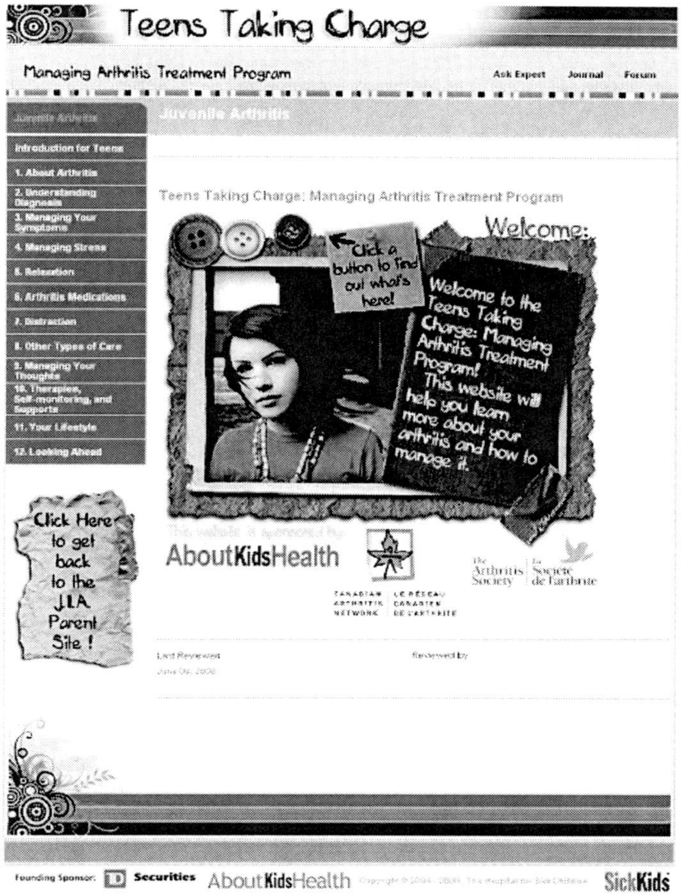
Teens Taking Charge
Managing Arthritis Treatment Program
Ask Expert
Journal
Forum
Juvenile Arthritis
Teens Taking Charge: Managing Arthritis Treatment Program
Welcome
Click a button to find out what's here!
Welcome to the Teens Taking Charge: Managing Arthritis Treatment Program! This website will help you learn more about your arthritis and how to manage it.
Click Here to get back to the JIA Parent Site !
AboutKidsHealth
Securities
SickKids

health website. Usability testing involves soliciting end-user feedback to learn what works, what doesn't, and where gaps in information or functionality exist using iterative cycles to refine the website prototype (Benestad, Vinje, Veierod, & Vandvik, 1996; Palermo, Wilson, Peters, Lewandowski, & Somhegyi, 2009; Ritterband et al., 2003). These factors may impact the frequency of use, understanding, and the likelihood that a user will implement the self-management recommendations. Usability testing can help determine the appropriateness of the website user-interface and content as well as (1) ease of learning; (2) efficiency of use; (3) memorability; (4) error frequency and severity and; (5) user satisfaction with the site. There are many ways to test the usability of a website; readers interested in these methods can refer to more detailed websites (such as http://www.usability.gov/) and publications on this topic (Corry, Frick, & Hansen, 1997; George, 2005; Spool, Schroeder, Scanlon, & Snyder, 1997).

In our case, we used a qualitative approach with semi-structured, audio taped interviews and observation by a trained observer with two iterative cycles to determine user performance and satisfaction with the user-interface of the "Teens Taking Charge: Managing Arthritis Online" Internet intervention to refine the prototype (Stinson et al., 2010b). A purposive sample of English (n=11; mean age = 15.4 ± 1.7) and French (n=8; mean

Figure 2. Video clip from Session 2 "Understanding Diagnosis"

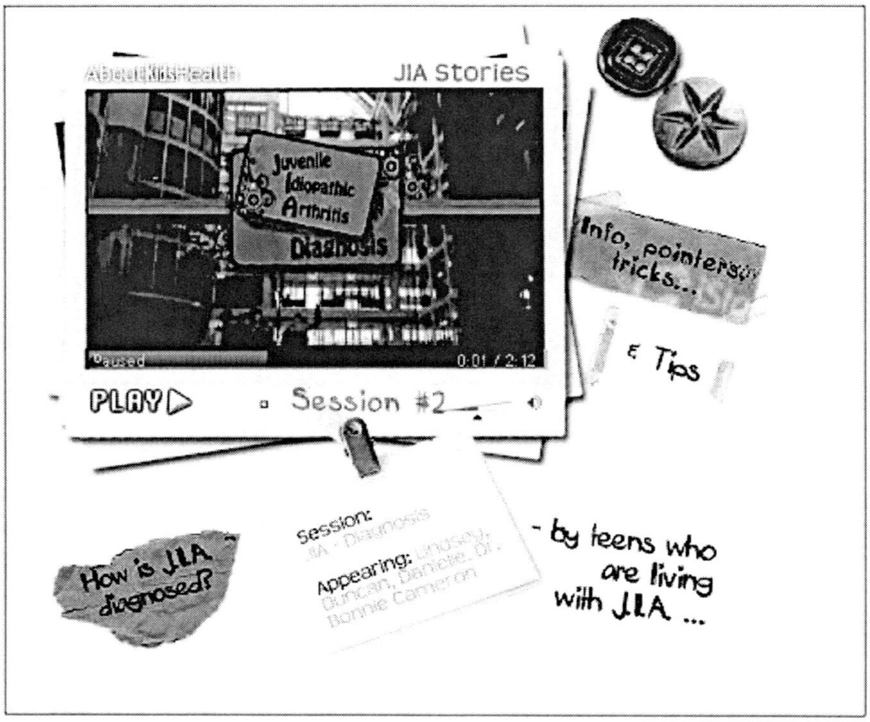

Figure 3. Click through animation on "How we feel pain"

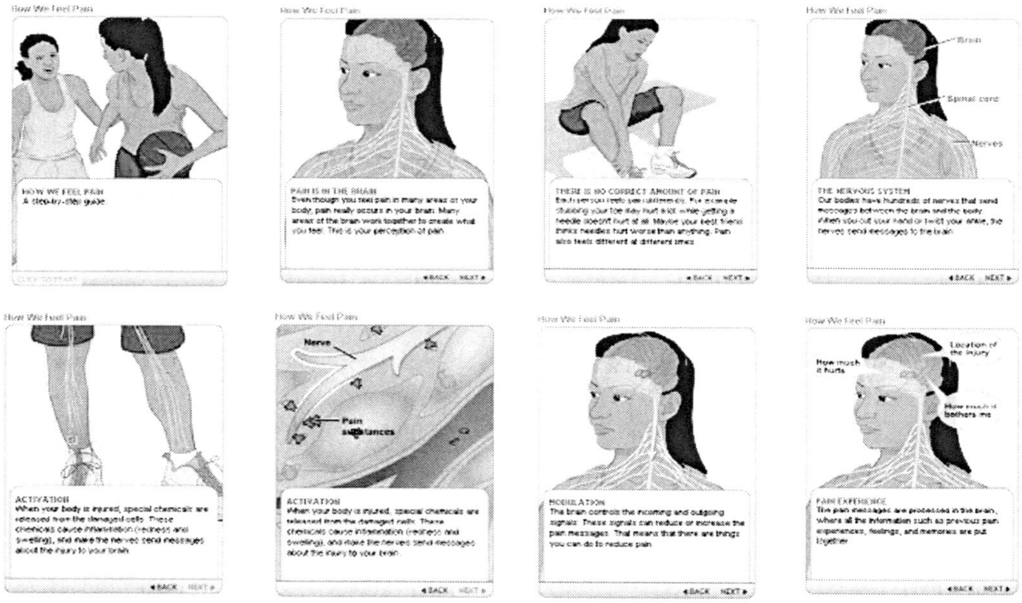

Figure 4. Quiz from Session 1 "About Arthritis"

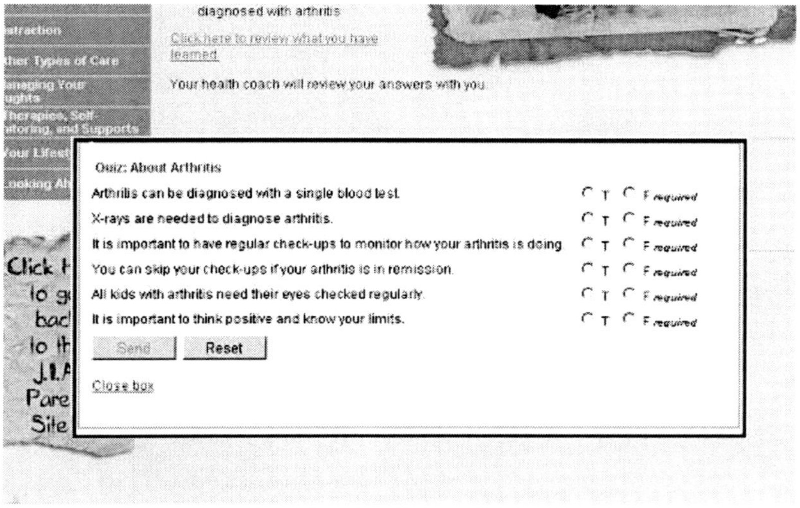

age = 16.0 ± 1.2) speaking adolescents with JIA (73% female) and one of their respective parents/caregivers were recruited from 2 Canadian tertiary care centers (Toronto and Montreal). Thematic analysis using a collaborative and iterative process was used to organize data into categories that reflected the emerging themes. All of the participants had access to a computer/Internet at home; however adolescents were more comfortable using the computer/Internet than their parents. Adolescents and parents provided ideas on how the website user-interface could be improved in terms of its usability (navigation, format and layout). Minor changes to the website user-interface were made and tested in a second cycle of participants. No further problems were identified in Phase 2 testing. Teens and parents responded positively to the content, appearance, and theme of the website (promoting self-management in youth with arthritis) and felt that it was easy to navigate, use and understand. Participants felt content was appropriate and geared to meet the unique needs of both adolescents with JIA and their parents. Most adolescents found the website aesthetically pleasing due to the incorporation of various website layout strategies such as (a) placement of the most important information at the top of the webpage; (b) separation of large amounts of texts into smaller sections and; (c) exemplifying key concepts through the use of animations, illustrations or video clips. The interactive features (discussion board, stories of hope, and video clips of youth with JIA) made them feel supported and 'not alone' in their illness. Most participants felt this program would have been helpful when they were newly diagnosed. Findings from this study highlight the importance of formative usability testing to help ensure the relevance of the content and that the website is user-friendly and acceptable prior to wide scale outcome assessment or implementation.

Step 3: Feasibility Testing

Prior to costly wide scale outcome assessment or implementation, Internet self-management interventions should determine the feasibility of delivering the online intervention. Common feasibility objectives include: rates of recruitment and retention, acceptability, compliance, and determination of sample size estimates to inform future large scale randomized controlled trials.

We conducted a pilot randomized controlled trial to test the feasibility of the Internet intervention across four tertiary level centres in Canada (Stinson et al., 2010a). The feasibility objectives included: (1) piloting the intervention, attention control strategies, and outcome measures; and (2) determining adolescents' compliance with and perceptions regarding the acceptability of and satisfaction with the Internet intervention. The study also provided an opportunity to obtain estimates of treatment effects in primary (health-related quality of life or HRQL), secondary (physical and emotional symptoms), and mediating (JIA specific knowledge, self-efficacy and adherence) outcome measures to inform the calculation of an appropriate sample size for a future randomized controlled trial.

Accrual rates ranged from 26% to 60% of eligible subjects at each site (Mean = 45%). Participants comprised 46 adolescents with JIA ages 12 to 18 years (Mean =14.5 years) and one of their parents who were randomized to the experimental (n=22) or attention control (n=24) groups. Attrition rates were 18.1% and 20.8% respectively from experimental and control groups. Using an intent-to-treat approach, linear mixed models were used to test intervention effects on primary, secondary and other outcomes using an analysis of covariance approach with post-treatment measures compared between groups using baseline scores as covariates. Participants in the experimental group had significantly higher disease knowledge ($p<0.001$, with a large effect size of 1.32) and lower average weekly pain intensity ratings ($p=0.03$, with a moderate effect size of 0.78) compared to those in the attention control group. No differences were found in HRQL, stress, adherence or self-efficacy between groups. The effect size for HRQL was 0.22 which would indicate a small ES for the Internet intervention. Program usage patterns indicated that users completed the program as instructed (high compliance with completing weekly modules; 91%), utilizing communication features, and were actively engaged in the intervention through goal-setting and completing personalized information. Findings supported the feasibility (high acceptability, user satisfaction and compliance) and initial effectiveness of the Internet self-management program in improving knowledge and decreasing pain in youth with JIA (Stinson et al., 2010a).

Step 4: Effectiveness Testing in the Real World Setting

The final step is testing the efficacy (if the intervention is successful when delivered under ideal conditions) or effectiveness (if the intervention is successful in the real world) of the Internet-based self-management program. In clinical medicine, randomized controlled trials (RCTs) are considered the "gold-standard" to assess the effectiveness of a treatment (Eysenbach, 2002). However, if randomization is not appropriate there are other study designs that can be considered for complex behavioral interventions such as self-management programs including individually randomized trials using cluster randomization, stepped wedge designs, preference trials, and N of 1 designs or non-randomized designs (Craig et al, 2008).

If using a traditional RCT design, there are several issues that need to be considered when conducting an RCT of an Internet-based health intervention. First, the trial cannot be conducted in a double-blind fashion as the participant will know what intervention he/she receives. Second, there is considerable risk for contamination which can threaten the ability to detect differences between the groups. For example, control group participants might be disappointed that they did not receive the online intervention and may search the Web for a comparable intervention. To minimize this potential bias, researcher's can ask participants in both groups whether they accessed similar online interventions or monitor their use of other websites directly by using client-side proxy software (Eysenbach, 2002). One can also employ a "sham" control group to minimize the risk of contamination (Ritterband et al., 2003). Basic web conditions (providing static patient education only) are recommended over usual care or wait-list controls as they contain content that individuals could typically find via searching the Web and are routinely provided as part of standard care (Danaher & Seeley, 2009). Furthermore, a recent meta-analysis found that educational Internet interventions had no effect on child or adolescent health behavior or health outcomes; whereas Internet programs that incorporated behavioural methods (self-monitoring, goal setting, immediate feedback, and contingency management) demonstrated large effect sizes for health behaviors (Cushing & Steele, 2010). Credible web-based control conditions also have the advantage of potentially controlling for demand characteristics and participants expectancies better than standard or usual care groups (Danaher & Seeley, 2009).

Another issue is how to assure that the intervention group is actually using the online intervention. For example, individuals may complete the outcome assessment measures and have no to minimal use of the Internet intervention. To address this issue, researchers should ask about the frequency of use or measure it directly using log files (i.e., Google analytics) and or conduct a dose response analysis. Researchers should also consider employing techniques to reduce drop outs (e.g., use of a run-in-period) as well as using an intention-to-treat analysis (Eysenbach, 2002).

We are conducting a RCT to determine the effectiveness of the "Teens Taking Charge: Managing Arthritis Online" Internet program in improving health outcomes (symptoms, adherence, knowledge and health-related quality of life) in a multicentred randomized controlled trial. If the Internet self-management program is effective, it could be the first step in a "stepped care" approach of health care for all youth with JIA. A "stepped care" approach provides adolescents and their family with a simple, accessible intervention for management of their disease and proceeds to more intense (face-to-face) treatments as necessary (Scogin, Hanson, & Welsh, 2003). A self-guided Internet self-management program may help overcome current barriers that prevent adolescents with JIA and their families from receiving these therapies. Moreover, this program is one that could have far-reaching implications for self-management care of other chronic health conditions experienced by youth (Eysenbach, 2002).

FUTURE RESEARCH DIRECTIONS

The full potential of Internet-based self-management programs has not been fully harnessed. Future directions for research in this area need to focus on: (1) teasing out the essential ingredients of Internet-based self-management programs using a theory driven approach; (2) determining the minimum amount of support required to improve outcomes and; (3) the most appropriate person to provide that support (trained non-health care personnel, health care professionals or peers) for children and youth with chronic health conditions. There is also a need to train health care professionals to ensure that patients' self-management abilities are maintained and fostered in clinical settings.

While several models have been developed to help guide the development and evaluation of Internet-based self-management programs; more work is needed to understand how best to develop, operationalize, deliver and evaluate these programs (Ritterband et al., 2009). We also need to conduct dismantling studies to help determine which components result in positive behaviorual changes.

Human support via brief telephone contact has improved motivation and adherence to online health care services which are typically delivered over weeks to months thereby facilitating achievement of desired health and/or behavioral outcomes (Nguyen et al., 2004; Palmqvist, et al., 2007; Spek et al., 2007). However, the level (intense versus brief contact), type of human support (health professionals, trained personnel, and peers) and mode (phone, email, tele-health) needed to maintain engagement in Internet health interventions is unknown (Barak et al., 2009; Nguyen et al. 2004). Future research is needed to determine the minimal amount of human support required with distance treatment programs and the best person to provide that support.

Finally, the broad uptake of efficacious and effective self-management programs is dependent on strong partnerships between researchers and key stakeholders, such as government and consumer groups. Ideally, stakeholder partners from government, health care authorities, and consumer groups should be encouraged to be involved in all phases in the development and testing of Internet-based chronic disease management programs for youth.

CONCLUSION

In summary, Internet-based self-management interventions have a lot to offer to help reduce the burden of chronic diseases in children and youth. As adjuncts to usual care, these interventions are in line with current government emphasis on the need for treatment approaches that focus on helping patients to better manage their day-to-day health in their everyday environment. This chapter has provided an overview of self-management in pediatric chronic health conditions, how the Internet can be harnessed to overcome current barriers to their use, key mechanisms behind successful programs and a framework to develop and evaluate Internet-based treatments using a Canadian-based example. Support for continued research, development and knowledge translation work is critical to the integration of Internet-based self-management interventions into the provision of health care for children and youth living with the burden of a chronic health condition.

REFERENCES

April, K. T., Feldman, D. E., Platt, R. W., & Duffy, C. M. (2006). Comparison between children with juvenile idiopathic arthritis and their parents concerning perceived treatment adherence. *Arthritis and Rheumatism*, *55*(4), 558–563. doi:10.1002/art.22104

Barak, A., Klein, B., & Proudfoot, J. G. (2009). Defining internet-supported therapeutic interventions. *Annals of Behavioral Medicine*, *38*, 4–17. doi:10.1007/s12160-009-9130-7

Barlow, J. H., & Ellard, D. R. (2004). Psycho-educational interventions for children with chronic disease, parents and siblings: an overview of the research evidence base. *Child: Care, Health and Development*, *30*, 637–645. doi:10.1111/j.1365-2214.2004.00474.x

Barlow, J. H., & Ellard, D. R. (2006). The psychosocial well-being of children with chronic disease, their parents and siblings: An overview of the research evidence base. *Child: Care, Health and Development*, *32*(1), 19–31. doi:10.1111/j.1365-2214.2006.00591.x

Barlow, J. H., Shaw, K. L., & Harrison, K. (1999). Consulting the experts: Children's and parents' perceptions of psycho-educational interventions in the context of juvenile chronic arthritis. *Health Education Research*, *14*, 597–610. doi:10.1093/her/14.5.597

Barlow, J. H., Shaw, K. L., & Southwood, T. R. (1998). Do psychosocial interventions have a role to play in paediatric rheumatology? *British Journal of Rheumatology*, *37*, 573–578. doi:10.1093/rheumatology/37.5.573

Barlow, J. H., Wright, C., Sheasby, J., Turner, A., & Hainsworth, J. (2002). Self-management for people with chronic conditions: A review. *Patient Education and Counseling*, *48*, 177–187. doi:10.1016/S0738-3991(02)00032-0

Benestad, B., Vinje, O., Veierod, M. B., & Vandvik, I. H. (1996). Quantitative and qualitative assessments of pain in children with juvenile chronic arthritis based on the Norwegian version of the pediatric pain questionnaire. *Scandinavian Journal of Rheumatology*, *25*(5), 293–299. doi:10.3109/03009749609104061

Bernatsky, S., Duffy, C., Malleson, P., Ehrmann Feldman, D., St. Pierre, Y., & Clarke, A. E. (2007). Economic impact of juvenile idiopathic arthritis. *Arthritis Care and Research*, *57*(1), 44–48. doi:10.1002/art.22463

Corry, M. D., Frick, T. W., & Hansen, L. (1997). User-centered design and usability testing of a website: An illustrative case study. *Educational Technology Research and Development*, *45*(4), 65–76. doi:10.1007/BF02299683

Craig, P., Dieppe, P., Macintyre, S., Michie, S., Nazareth, I., & Petticrew, M. (2008). Developing and evaluating complex interventions: The new medical research council guidance. *British Medical Journal*, *337*, a1655.

Cuijpers, P., van Straten, A., & Andersson, G. (2008). Internet-administered cognitive behavior therapy for health problems: A systematic review. *Journal of Behavioral Medicine*, *31*, 169–177. doi:10.1007/s10865-007-9144-1

Cushing, C. C., & Steele, R. G. (2010). A meta-analytic review of educational and behavioral ehealth interventions for pediatric health behaviors and associated outcomes. *Journal of Pediatric Psychology*, *35*(9), 937–949. doi:10.1093/jpepsy/jsq023

Danaher, B. G., & Seeley, J. R. (2009). Methodological issues in research on Web-based behavioral interventions. *Annals of Behavioral Medicine*, *38*(1), 28–39. doi:10.1007/s12160-009-9129-0

Drotar, G., Greenley, R., Hoff, A., Johnson, C., Lewandowski, A., & Moore, M. (2006). Summary of issues and challenges in the use of new technologies in clinical care and with children and adolescents with chronic illnesses. *Children's Health Care*, *35*(1), 91–102. doi:10.1207/s15326888chc3501_8

Eccleston, C., Morley, S., Williams, A., Yorke, L., & Mastroyannopoulou, K. (2002). Systematic review of randomized controlled trials of psychological therapy for chronic pain in children and adolescents, with a subset meta-analysis of pain relief. *Pain*, *99*, 157–165. doi:10.1016/S0304-3959(02)00072-6

Elgar, F. J., & McGrath, P. J. (2003). Self-administered psychosocial treatments for children and families. *Journal of Clinical Psychology*, *59*, 321–339. doi:10.1002/jclp.10132

Eysenbach, G. (2002). Issues in evaluating health websites in an internet-based randomized controlled trial. *Journal of Medical Internet Research*, *4*(3), e17. doi:10.2196/jmir.4.3.e17

Gall, C., Kingsnorth, S., & Healy, H. (2006). Growing up ready: A shared management approach. *Physical & Occupational Therapy in Pediatrics*, *26*(4), 47–62. doi:10.1080/J006v26n04_04

George, C. A. (2005). Usability testing and design of a library website: An iterative approach. *OCLC Systems & Services*, *21*(3), 167–180. doi:10.1108/10650750510612371

Gray, N. J., Klein, J. D., Noyce, P. R., Sesselberg, T. S., & Cantrill, J. A. (2005). Health information-seeking behaviour in adolescence: The place of the Internet. *Social Science & Medicine*, *60*, 1467–1478. doi:10.1016/j.socscimed.2004.08.010

Griffiths, F., Lindenmeyer, A., Powell, J., Lowe, P., & Thorogood, M. (2006). Why are health care interventions delivered over the internet? A systematic review of the published literature. *Journal of Medical Internet Research*, *8*(2), e10. doi:10.2196/jmir.8.2.e10

Kieckhefer, G. M., & Trahms, C. M. (2000). Supporting development of children with chronic conditions: From compliance toward shared management. *Pediatric Nursing*, *26*(4), 354–363.

Lineker, S. C., Badley, E. M., & Dalby, D. M. (1996). Unmet service needs of children with rheumatic diseases and their parents in a metropolitan area. *The Journal of Rheumatology*, *23*, 104–108.

Lorig, K. R., & Holman, H. (2003). Self-management education: History, definition, outcomes, and mechanisms. *Annals of Behavioral Medicine*, *26*(1), 1–7. doi:10.1207/S15324796ABM2601_01

Lorig, K. R., Ritter, P. L., Laurent, D. D., & Plant, K. (2008). The internet-based arthritis self-management program: A one-year randomized controlled trial for patients with arthritis or fibromyalgia. *Arthritis and Rheumatism*, *7*, 1009–1017. doi:10.1002/art.23817

Marks, R., Allegrante, J. P., & Lorig, K. (2005a). A review and synthesis of research evidence for self-efficacy-enhancing interventions for reducing chronic disability: Implications for health education practice (part I). *Health Promotion Practice*, *6*, 37–43. doi:10.1177/1524839904266790

Marks, R., Allegrante, J. P., & Lorig, K. (2005b). A review and synthesis of research evidence for self-efficacy-enhancing interventions for reducing chronic disability: Implications for health education practice (part II). *Health Promotion Practice*, *6*, 148–156. doi:10.1177/1524839904266792

McGillion, M., LeFort, S., & Stinson, J. (2008). Chronic pain self-management. In Rashiq, S., Schopflocher, D., & Taenzer, P. (Eds.), *Chronic pain: A health policy perspective*. Weinheim, Germany: Wiley-VCH Verlag.

Murray, E., Burns, J., See Tai, S., Lai, R., & Nazareth, I. (2005). Interactive health communication applications for people with chronic disease. *Cochrane Database of Systematic Reviews*, *4*, CD004274.

Newacheck, P. W., Inkelas, M., & Kim, S. E. (2004). Health services use and health care expenditures for children with disabilities. *Pediatrics*, *114*(1), 79–85. doi:10.1542/peds.114.1.79

Nguyen, H. Q., Carrieri-Kohlman, V., Ranki, S. H., Slaughter, R., & Stulbarg, M. S. (2004). Internet-based patient education and support interventions: A review of evaluation studies and directions for future research. *Computers in Biology and Medicine*, *34*, 95–112. doi:10.1016/S0010-4825(03)00046-5

Palermo, T. M., Wilson, A. C., Peters, M., Lewandowski, A., & Somhegyi, H. (2009). Randomized controlled trial of an Internet-delivered family cognitive-behavioral therapy intervention for children and adolescents with chronic pain. *Pain*, *146*, 205–213. doi:10.1016/j.pain.2009.07.034

Palmqvist, B., Carlbring, P., & Andersson, G. (2007). Internet-delivered treatments with or without therapist input: Does the therapist factor have implications for efficacy and cost. *Expert Reviews of Pharmacoeconomics and Outcomes Research*, *7*, 291–297. doi:10.1586/14737167.7.3.291

Phelps, A. (Ed.). (2006). *Chronic health-related disorders in children: Collaborative medical and psychoeducational interventions*. Washington, DC: American Psychological Association. doi:10.1037/11435-000

Rainie, L. (2010). *Internet, broadband, and cell phone statistics*. Retrieved from http://www.pewinternet.org/ Reports/2010/ Internet-broadband-and-cell-phone-statistics.aspx

Rapoff, M. A. (2002). Assessing and enhancing adherence to medical regimens for juvenile rheumatoid arthritis. *Pediatric Annals*, *31*, 373–379.

Ritterband, L. M., Andersson, G., Christensen, H. M., Carlbring, P., & Cuijpers, P. (2006). Directions for the International Society for Research on Internet Interventions (ISRII). *Journal of Medical Internet Research*, *8*(3), e23. doi:10.2196/jmir.8.3.e23

Ritterband, L. M., Gonder-Frederick, L. A., Cox, D. J., Clifton, A. D., West, R. W., & Borowitz, S. M. (2003). Internet interventions: in review, in use, and into the future. *Professional Psychology, Research and Practice*, *34*, 527–534. doi:10.1037/0735-7028.34.5.527

Ritterband, L. M., Thorndike, F. P., Cox, D. J., Kovatchev, B. P., & Gonder-Frederick, L. A. (2009). A behavior change model for internet interventions. *Annals of Behavioral Medicine*, *28*, 18–27. doi:10.1007/s12160-009-9133-4

Sawyer, S. M., & Aroni, R. A. (2005). Self-management in adolescents with chronic illness. What does it mean and how can it be delivered? *The Medical Journal of Australia*, *183*(8), 405–409.

Scogin, F. R., Hanson, A., & Welsh, D. (2003). Self-administered treatment in stepped care models of depression treatment. *Journal of Clinical Psychology*, *59*(3), 341–349. doi:10.1002/jclp.10133

Shaw, K. L., Southwood, T. R., Duffy, C. M., & McDonagh, J. E. (2006). Health related quality of life in adolescents with juvenile idiopathic arthritis. *Arthritis and Rheumatism*, *55*(2), 199–207. doi:10.1002/art.21852

Smith, J. R., Mugford, M., Holland, R., Candy, B., Noble, M. J., & Harrison, B. D. (2005). A systematic review to examine the impact of psycho-educational interventions on health outcomes and costs in adults and children with difficult asthma. *Health Technology Assessment*, *9*(23), 1–167.

Spek, C., Cuijper, P., Nyklicek, I., Riper, H., Keyzer, J., & Pop, V. (2007). Internet-based cognitive behavioral therapy for symptoms of depression and anxiety: A meta-analysis. *Psychological Medicine*, *37*(3), 319–328. doi:10.1017/S0033291706008944

Spool, J. M., Schroeder, W., Scanlon, T., & Snyder, C. (1997). *Website usability: A designer's guide*. North Andover, MA: User Interface Engineering.

Stinson, J., McGrath, P. J., Hodnett, E., Feldman, B. M., Duffy, C., & Huber, A. (2010a). An internet-based self-management program with telephone support for adolescents with Juvenile Idiopathic Arthritis (JIA): A pilot randomized controlled trial. *The Journal of Rheumatology*, *37*(9), 1944–1952. doi:10.3899/jrheum.091327

Stinson, J., McGrath, P. J., Hodnett, E., Feldman, B. M., Duffy, C., & Huber, A. (2010b). Usability testing of an online self-management program for adolescents with juvenile idiopathic arthritis. *Journal of Medical Internet Research*, *12*(3), e30. doi:10.2196/jmir.1349

Stinson, J., Toomey, P., Stevens, B., Kagan, S., Duffy, C., & Huber, A. (2008). Asking the experts: Exploring the self-management needs of adolescents with arthritis. *Arthritis Care and Research*, *59*(1), 65–72. doi:10.1002/art.23244

Stinson, J., Wilson, R., Gill, N., Yamada, J., & Holt, J. (2009). A systematic review of internet-based self-management interventions for youth with health conditions. *Journal of Pediatric Psychology*, *34*(5), 495–510. doi:10.1093/jpepsy/jsn115

Superio-Cabuslay, E., Ward, M. M., & Lorig, K. R. (1996). Patient education interventions in osteoarthritis and rheumatoid arthritis: A meta-analytic comparison with nonsteroidal anti-inflammatory drug treatment. *Arthritis Care and Research*, *9*, 292–301. doi:10.1002/1529-0131(199608)9:4<292::AID-ANR1790090414>3.0.CO;2-4

Turkel, S., & Pao, M. (2007). Late consequences of chronic pediatric illness. *The Psychiatric Clinics of North America*, *30*, 819–835. doi:10.1016/j.psc.2007.07.009

U.S. Department of Health and Human Services. (200). *Usability.gov.* Retrieved from http://www.usability.gov/

van der Lee, J. H., Mokkink, L. B., Grootenhuis, M. A., Heymans, H. S., & Offringa, M. (2007). Definitions and measurement of chronic health conditions in childhood: A systematic review. *Journal of the American Medical Association*, *297*(24), 2741–2751. doi:10.1001/jama.297.24.2741

Walco, G. A., Sterling, C. M., Conte, P. M., & Engel, R. G. (1999). Empirically supported treatments in pediatric psychology: Disease-related pain. *Journal of Pediatric Psychology*, *24*, 155–167. doi:10.1093/jpepsy/24.2.155

Wantland, D. J., Portillo, C., Holzemer, W. L., Slaughter, R., & McGhee, E. M. (2004). The effectiveness of web-based vs. non-web-based interventions: A meta-analysis of behavioural change outcomes. *Journal of Medical Internet Research*, *6*(4), e40. doi:10.2196/jmir.6.4.e40

ADDITIONAL READING

Barak, A., Hen, L., Boniel-Nissim, M., & Shapira, N. (2008). A Comprehensive Review and a Meta-Analysis of the Effectiveness of Internet-Based Psychotherapeutic Interventions. *Journal of Technology in Human Services*, *26*(2), 109–160. doi:10.1080/15228830802094429

Bennett, G. G., & Glasgow, R. E. (2009). The delivery of public health interventions via the Internet: Actualizing their potential. *Annual Review of Public Health*, *30*, 273–292. doi:10.1146/annurev.publhealth.031308.100235

Berman, R. L., Iris, M. A., & Drengenberg, C. (2009). The effectiveness of an online mind-body intervention for older adults with chronic pain. *The Journal of Pain*, *10*(1), 68–79. doi:10.1016/j.jpain.2008.07.006

Bessell, T. L., McDonald, S., Silagy, C. A., Anderson, J. N., Hiller, J. E., & Sansom, L. N. (2002). Do Internet interventions for consumers cause more harm than good? A systematic review. *Health Expectations*, *5*(1), 28–37. doi:10.1046/j.1369-6513.2002.00156.x

Devineni, T., & Blanchard, E. B. (2005). A randomized controlled trial of an internet-based treatment for chronic headache. *Behaviour Research and Therapy*, *43*, 277–292. doi:10.1016/j.brat.2004.01.008

Duarte Macea, D., Gajos, K., Daglia Calil, Y. A., & Fregni, F. (2010). The efficacy of web-based cognitive behavioral interventions for chronic pain: A systematic review and meta-analysis. *The Journal of Pain*, *11*(10), 917–929. doi:10.1016/j.jpain.2010.06.005

Foster, G., Taylor, S. J., Eldridge, S. E., Ramsay, J., & Griffiths, C. J. (2007). Self-management education programmes by lay leaders for people with chronic conditions. *Cochrane Database of Systematic Reviews*, (4): CD005108.

Hicks, C. L., von Baeyer, C. L., & McGrath, P. J. (2006). Online psychological treatment for pediatric recurrent pain: A randomized evaluation. *Journal of Pediatric Psychology*, *31*(7), 724–736. doi:10.1093/jpepsy/jsj065

Kerr, C., Murray, E., Stevenson, F., Gore, C., & Nazareth, I. (2006). Internet interventions for long-term conditions: patient and caregiver quality criteria. *Journal of Medical Internet Research*, *8*(3), e13. doi:10.2196/jmir.8.3.e13

Lewis, D., Eysenbach, G., Kukafka, R., Stavri, Z., & Jamison, H. (Eds.). (2006). *Consumer health informatics: Informing consumers and improving health care*. New York, NY: Springer New York.

Long, A. C., & Palermo, T. M. (2009). Brief report: Web-based management of adolescent chronic pain: Development and usability testing of an online family cognitive behavioral therapy program. *Journal of Pediatric Psychology*, *34*(5), 511–516. doi:10.1093/jpepsy/jsn082

Lorig, K. R., Laurent, D. D., Deyo, R. A., Marnell, M. E., Minor, M. A., & Ritter, P. L. (2002). Can a back pain e-mail discussion group improve health status and lower health care costs? A randomized study. *Archives of Internal Medicine*, *162*, 792–796. doi:10.1001/archinte.162.7.792

Marks, I., & Cavanagh, K. (2009). Computer-aided psychological treatments: Evolving issues. *Annual Review of Clinical Psychology*, *5*, 121–141. doi:10.1146/annurev.clinpsy.032408.153538

Murray, E., Khadjesari, Z., White, I. R., Kalaitzaki, E., Godfrey, C., & McCambridge, J. (2009). Methodological challenges in online trials. *Journal of Medical Internet Research*, *11*(2), e9. doi:10.2196/jmir.1052

Nijland, N., van Gemert-Pijnen, J., Boer, H., Steehouder, M. F., & Seydel, E. R. (2008). Evaluation of internet-based technology for supporting self-care: Problems encountered by patients and caregivers when using self-care applications. *Journal of Medical Internet Research*, *10*(2), e13. doi:10.2196/jmir.957

O'Conner-Von, S. (2009). Coping with cancer: A web-based educational program for early and middle adolescents. *Journal of Pediatric Oncology Nursing*, *26*(4), 230–241. doi:10.1177/1043454209334417

Richardson, G., Gravelle, H., Weatherly, H., & Ritchie, G. (2005). Cost-effectiveness of interventions to support self-care: A systematic review. *International Journal of Technology Assessment in Health Care*, *21*(4), 423–432. doi:10.1017/S0266462305050592

Samoocha, D., Bruinvels, D. J., Elbers, N. A., Anema, J. R., & van der Beek, A. J. (2010). Effectiveness of web-based interventions on patient empowerment: a systematic review and meta-analysis. *Journal of Medical Internet Research*, *12*(2), e23. doi:10.2196/jmir.1286

Strecher, V. (2007). Internet methods for delivering behavioral and health-related interventions (eHealth). *Annual Review of Clinical Psychology*, *3*, 53–76. doi:10.1146/annurev.clinpsy.3.022806.091428

Tate, D. F., Finkelstein, E. A., & Khavjou, O. (2009). Cost effectiveness of internet interventions: Review and recommendations. *Annals of Behavioral Medicine*, *38*, 40–45. doi:10.1007/s12160-009-9131-6

Trautmann, E., & Kroner-Herwig, B. (2010). A randomized controlled trial of Internet-based self-help training for recurrent headache in childhood and adolescence. *Behaviour Research and Therapy*, *48*, 28–37. doi:10.1016/j.brat.2009.09.004

Wagner, E. H., Davis, C., Schaefer, J., Von Korff, M., & Austin, B. (2002). A Survey of Leading Chronic Disease Management Programs: Are They Consistent with the Literature? *Journal of Nursing Care Quality*, *16*(2), 67–80. doi:10.1097/00001786-200201000-00008

Webb, T. L., Joseph, J., Yardley, L., & Michie, S. (2010). Using the Internet to promote health behavior change: A systematic review and meta-analysis of the impact of theoretical basis, use of behavior change techniques, and mode of delivery on efficacy. *Journal of Medical Internet Research*, *12*(1), e4. doi:10.2196/jmir.1376

Wichansky, A. M. (2000). Uability testing in 2000 and beyond. *Ergonomics*, *43*(7), 998–1006. doi:10.1080/001401300409170

Yardley, L., Morrison, L. G., Andreou, P., Joseph, J., & Little, P. (2010). Understanding reactions to an internet-delivered health-care intervention: Accommodating user preferences for information provision. *BMC Medical Informatics and Decision Making*, *10*, 52. doi:10.1186/1472-6947-10-52

KEY TERMS AND DEFINITIONS

Chronic Condition: Prolonged health condition requiring ongoing treatment.

Cognitive Behavioural Therapy (CBT): A type of psychological therapy which aims to change the way in which we think and behave in order to modify the negative impact of underlying health conditions.

E-Health: Health information and services delivered, shared or supported by technology such as the Internet.

Internet Interventions: Interactive websites which combine information with decision support, behavior change support, or peer support.

Internet: Global system of interconnected computer networks.

Self-Management: Ability to independently manage all aspects of one's chronic illness such as associated symptoms, treatments and other physical or psychological consequences.

Youth: School-age children and adolescents.

Chapter 4
An E-Health System for Promoting Wellbeing in the Elderly:
The Butler System

Cristina Botella
Universidad Jaume I, Spain

Rosa M. Baños
Universidad de Valencia, Spain

Ernestina Etchemendy
Universidad de Valencia, Spain

Diana Castilla
Universidad Jaume I, Spain

Azucena García-Palacios
Universidad Jaume I, Spain

Alcañiz Mariano
Universidad Politécnica de Valencia, Spain

ABSTRACT

The disproportionate increase in the world's aged population, especially in developed countries, is one of the biggest challenges for developing health and social development policies. Developed countries are starting to include e-health applications in their health policies; these are effective programs that can reach large numbers of people at a much lower economic cost. The "Butler System" is an e-health application designed specifically for older people and the health professionals who work with this population. The Butler System is a multi-user platform with various levels of action, which includes resources that enhance elderly users' social integration, learning, socio-emotional networks, leisure and training in emotional regulation skills. Furthermore, the platform allows practitioners to continuously monitor older people's emotional states and offers various clinical resources and therapeutic activities. Tools such as the Butler System could become integral to supporting and promoting healthy habits for the elderly and assisting the health professionals who work with this population.

DOI: 10.4018/978-1-60960-866-8.ch004

INTRODUCTION

Two parameters characterize the twenty-first century, particularly in developed countries: the increase in life expectancy and the declining birth rate. As a result of these factors, demographic distributions have changed markedly: many areas are now increasingly comprised of elderly people. This significant demographic shift coincided with the technological revolution that began at the end of the twentieth century, which has redefined the people relate to each other. One result of this rapid change is that the generation gap has increased: older people feel misplaced and unrelated to this "new world" in which photos, music, newspapers, and even communication with their younger family members is increasingly managed in unfamiliar digital formats. Consequently, the elderly have become more vulnerable to adjustment disorders, mood disorders, anxiety problems, etc. Numerous scientific studies have proven the beneficial effects of using Information and Communication Technologies (ICTs) to address these isolation issues in the elderly; they are powerful tools for communication, entertainment, and socialization.

The Butler system, which was designed to bridge the widening gap between current technological realities and the older population, is based on the principles of positive psychology (Seligman, 2002). Our goal was, to facilitate the construction of psychological and social elements that are protective of a healthy quality of life. The project comprises an online multi-user technology platform with assistance lines for elderly users as well as support tools for healthcare professionals.

THE AGING POPULATION AND ITS IMPACT ON HEALTH SYSTEMS

As previously mentioned, global demographics are undergoing clear and rapid transformation, with the aging population emerging as a major worldwide trend. Never before have so many people achieved such advanced ages. The most recent census report conducted by the U.S. National Institute on Aging (Kinsella & Wan, 2009) estimates that between 2008 and 2040 the number of people aged 80 and 85 will have increased by 233% and 165%, respectively; the general population, on the other hand, will only have increased by 33%. By 2040, 1 of every 4 Europeans will be at least 65 years old, and 1 of every 7 will be at least 75. Similar trends are observed in Oceania, Asia, and elsewhere.

The disproportionate increase in the world's aged population, especially in developed countries, is one of the biggest challenges for developing health and social development policies. Reports from institutions such as the WHO (2002) and the American Society of Gerontology (Merck Institute of Aging & Health, 2004) indicate that this demographic transformation will have a strong impact on public health systems, thereby having a economic and social effect on future societies (The Swedish National Institute of Public Health, 2006). According to the U.S. report The State of Aging and Health, elaborated by the Gerentological Society of America (2004), psychological problems in older people will become a significant public health issue, resulting in a dramatic increase in the use and costs of health services.

A report conducted by the Center for Health Workforce Studies (2006), which assesses the implications of population aging on supply and demand in health services, shows that the elderly use a greater amount and variety of health services. Also, it notes that future generations of older people will have higher educational levels, greater access to information and better financial resources in their old age. Given these conditions, the report predicts a change in patterns of health services consumption by this population sector. Future demands on the health system will require a greater number of healthcare workers as well as changes in the way these health services are delivered.

Successful Ageing

Demographic changes are also influencing conceptualization of the elderly and, likewise, in the use of various intervention modes from different scientific fields. The efforts from different field of health aim to increase life expectancy, but also to consider the quality with which solutions will be developed. The field is paying increasing attention to "how" the manner of aging can be influenced, through intervention in the elderly people's living environments and lifestyles (Gutierrez, Serra & Zacarés, 2006).

Technological, scientific and medical advances have allowed humans to live increasingly longer; the challenge now is to determine how these additional years can and will be lived. This change in perspective has led to the concept of "aging healthy": aging is considered as a life-cycle stage in which people can continue to discover and build new social roles in society and in their own life history. This concept goes beyond the goal of preventing disease in the adult population; it aims to optimize the physical, social, recreational and mental health opportunities of older people. In other words, the "elders" will remain an active part of our society and will enjoy an appropriate quality of life, while continually experiencing opportunities for independence and personal development.

A concept closely related to healthy aging is "active aging", proposed by the WHO (1996): "the process of optimizing opportunities for health, participation and security in order to improve quality of life as people age." Active aging highlights the need to enhance the continuity of social, economic, cultural, spiritual and civic life of this population sector.

Social Networks, Health and the Elderly

Studies on well-being and life satisfaction in the elderly population have increased in the past three decades. The literature consistently emphasizes that satisfaction with life in this population is a complex phenomenon, influenced by multiple factors. One of these significant factors is the quantity and quality of social networks comprised of loved ones, such as spouses, grandchildren, neighbors, etc. These sources of social support have a vital impact on the wellbeing and life satisfaction of older people; social networks not only provide them with emotional support (affection, belonging and usefulness), but also instrumental (Florence, 2001, Siu & Phillips, 2000). Hanson's group (Hanson, Sven-Olof, Lars & Sven-Eric, 1989) conducted a study to determine whether there was an association between the causes of mortality and different aspects of social networks, support and social influence networks; they found a high rate of mortality among men who lived alone, who had little social support and low adequacy in social participation.

Upon reaching old age, many people face the possibility of being admitted into a nursing home. However, in many cases this means loss of freedom of movement, loss of family companionship; it can even be defined as a place to wait for death (Tester, Hubbard, Downs, MacDonald & Murphy, 2003). Similarly, remaining in their homes can also result in isolation; elderly living at home can find it difficult to visit friends or maintain social activity (Gilroy, Kellet & Jackson, 2004). However, studies indicate that having social activities, being active and busy and meeting with others are necessary to maintain an interest in life, avoid depression and consequently improve their wellbeing. For example, in 1976 Arling Greg showed that elderly people who had contact with their neighbors experienced less isolation and worry, and had greater feelings of usefulness and self-respect. Davis, Moons and Khan (1981) observed that feelings of integration in the community, within a group of elderly residents, was largely responsible for their perception of independence and the social climate.

Likewise, Holmen and Furukawa (2002) identified a positive relationship between number of friends and high levels of life satisfaction, and a negative relationship between loneliness and low levels of satisfaction. Similarly, Beckett, Goldman, Weinstein, Lin and Chuang (2002) found that poor health, among other factors, was associated with low socio-economic status, a limited network of friends and minimal participation in social activities. Mette (2005) indicated that people who maintained active with friends, acquaintances, etc. suffered significantly less from the negative impacts of reduced social participation.

ICTs and the Elderly

As previously explained, rapid global demographic changes, which coincided with the technological revolution, helped redefined the way people communicate. Technological advances, the advent of the Internet and a wide variety of mobile devices transformed familiar notions of distance and time. ICTs increase the speed of every life while helping satisfy myriad demands, while this very rewarding to those who enjoy the benefits of ICTs, it also segregates and excludes those who cannot understand the rules of this "new world" However, members of the oldest segment of the world's population were born and learned to interact in a radically different reality: letters are no longer written by hand, and hard-copy photos are rarely placed in family albums. People today have unprecedented mobility and communicate with their loved ones in real time via the Internet, from almost anywhere in the world.

This gap between the current social environment and the relatively recent past has had a strong impact on a personal level; the language of our "elders", their methods for communicating and building social networks are becoming increasingly obsolete. This gap produces strong feelings of social exclusion: social interactions are increasingly conducted in electronic formats. This generational gap, compounded by the typical developmental changes of old age (physical changes, loneliness, isolation, social inactivity), exacerbates loneliness, depression, anxiety and adjustment disorders.

To counteract this, several studies investigate how ICTs can have a significant and positive influence on the social lives of elderly people (van de Catering, 2005). Various studies show how ICTs are useful tools for socializing and establishing social networks, and can help alleviate users' social isolation, loneliness and alienation; furthermore, virtual communities can serve as antidotes to the elderly people's decreased community involvement and social capital (Cody, Dunn, Hoppin & Wendt, 1999; Karavas, Lim & Katsikas, 2005). For example, Wellman and Frank (2001) found that older people who participated in virtual communities reduced their levels of isolation; this gain was especially marked in those with reduced mobility. Similarly, Blit-Cohen and Litwin (2004) found older people who used ICTs increased and enriched their social capital. Furthermore, Karavidas et al. (2005) showed that elderly people who were more computer literate were more satisfied with their lives. They concluded that the benefits of understanding computers include increased independence, and better knowledge of issues relating to health and maintaining social networks, among others.

E-Health and the Elderly

The integration of technological advances and health sciences has led to significant progress in health and wellness. ICTs are providing an increasing array tools for improving health and psychological and social welfare. Furthermore, scientific literature indicates that certain factors that characterize an aging society, such as an increase in health care demands and reliance on social security systems and pensions, make the adoption of e-health solutions a priority for some developed countries (Anastasiou, Quarrie & Boulos, 2009). Many works already exist that validate the benefits of technological advances for the needs of the elderly population. For example, the project CAALYX (Anastasiou, et al., 2009), created by six European countries and funded by the European Commission, aims to develop a system for remotely monitoring the vital signs of elderly people. Another effort was the TeleCare project (Camarinha-Matos & Afsarmenesh, 2004), which attempted to design a framework focused on virtual communities to support the elderly in order to help integrate them into society.

Yet another project, Age Invaders (Khoo, Cheok, Nguyen & Pan, 2008), is an interactive game designed to allow elderly people, along with their grandchildren and parents, to play together via the network. These projects show how e-health interventions are effective at meeting the issues related to elderly health and social wellbeing (Proudfoot, 2004; Tse, Choi & Leung, 2008). However, making these ICTs accessible to the elderly is a formidable challenge. The aforementioned digital divide between the elderly and the technological world around them is one difficulty in developing appropriate treatments. In addition, the use of new technologies might actually enhance feelings of isolation, loneliness and disconnection of the elderly from the "new world." For these reasons it is important to create solutions that deliver the benefits of ICTs while considering the specific needs of the elderly population.

THE BUTLER SYSTEM

The Butler system is a multi-user, online e-health platform, which links all of user profiles that exist in the system. Its main objective is to help improve

Figure 1. General structure of the Butler System

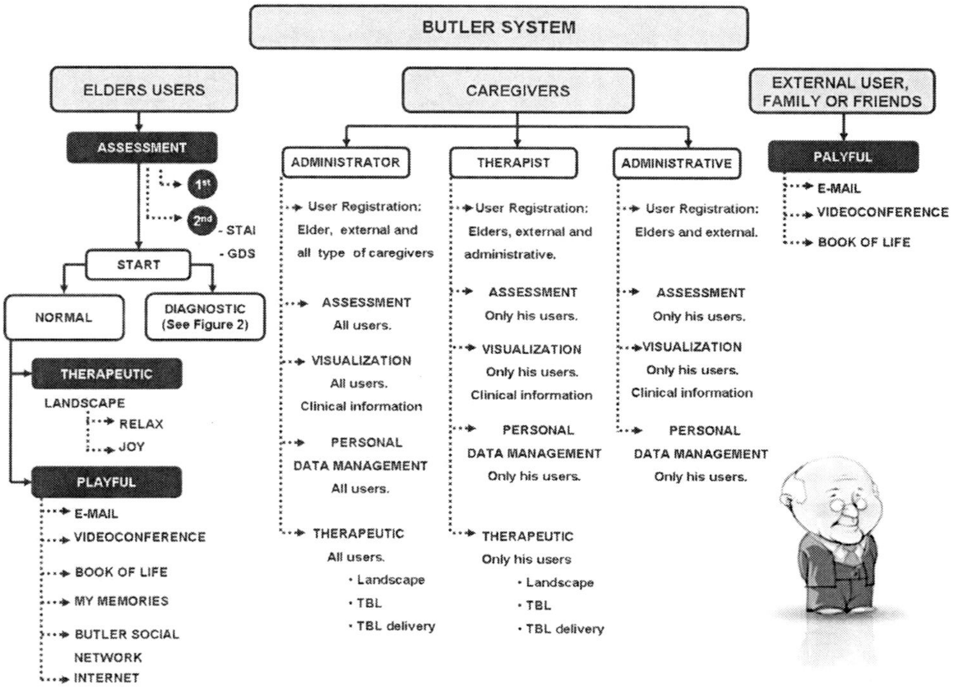

the quality of life of older people, by providing resources that promote their social networks, communication, entertainment, learning, curiosity and their training of positive emotions. Butler includes resources for assisting elderly users as well as support tools for the healthcare professionals who work with this population (see Figure 1). Its structure includes three user profiles: elderly users, health care professionals, and family members or friends of the older users. It comprises three possible levels of action: evaluative, therapeutic and playful. Each user profile can access specific applications within each level of action.

Following is a description of each user profile and the applications that users can access from the various levels of action.

Elderly User

This is the main user profile of the platform, and includes all older people who join the Butler system. Each elderly user has a unique login and password. Members of this profile can access and benefit from all three levels of action.

Assessment Action Level

Every day the older users access the system, the first thing they must do is to answer some questions which help the system gauge their moods (anxiety and depression). The questions are based on the diagnostic criteria for anxiety and depression in the DSM-IV. If the user's answers indicate a clinical situation that is within the normal range, the Butler system will allow the user to access both of the system's other action levels (therapeutic and recreational).

If, however, the system detects any change in the users' mood states (indicating anxiety or depression) it conduct further mood exploration. This second evaluation utilizes scales widely validated and used in psychological assessments, including the Stai-S (Spielberger, Gorsuch & Lushene, 1970) and the GDS-15 (Sheikh & Yesavage, 1986).

After the second evaluation, the Butler system uses a decision algorithm that combines obtained scores, ranges of scores and system resources (therapeutic and recreational action levels); this information enables it to react automatically and in real time to clinical analyses. For example, if the clinical assessment detects levels of anxiety, Butler restricts access to the Book of Life area (defined below), and only allows users to perform exercises on emotional training available through relaxing in "nature"; furthermore, they can access communication and entertainment functions. For more detail on the clinical decision algorithm, see Figure 2.

Therapeutic Action Level

This level includes two therapeutic resources: "virtual worlds" and "therapeutic Book of Life":

Virtual worlds to generate positive emotions: There are two 3D virtual environments (one for joy and one for relaxation), which simulate two natural environments and present the users with a variety of visual and auditory stimuli in order to alter their mood states. The landscapes include a blue sky over an expansive green meadow, various fields, shrubs and flowers, and a central road for the user to travel on. The road includes a stone bridge, where the user can stop to listen the water and observe the reflections in the river. The road leads to the central area of the meadow, a place where the user encounters a crossroads that offers three different paths: to a tree, a creek or a lake; each path leads different emotional training exercises. While the landscape is the same in both environments, each has been adapted to elicit the desired emotion (joy or relaxation), including various aspects of the walk through the meadow, the color of the sky, the grass, the activities to be performed, the audible melody, the voice that guides the tour and the narratives used during the walk. The interaction with the virtual environment is done using semi-directed navigation: users access buttons on the screen, which allow

Figure 2. Algorithm diagnostic

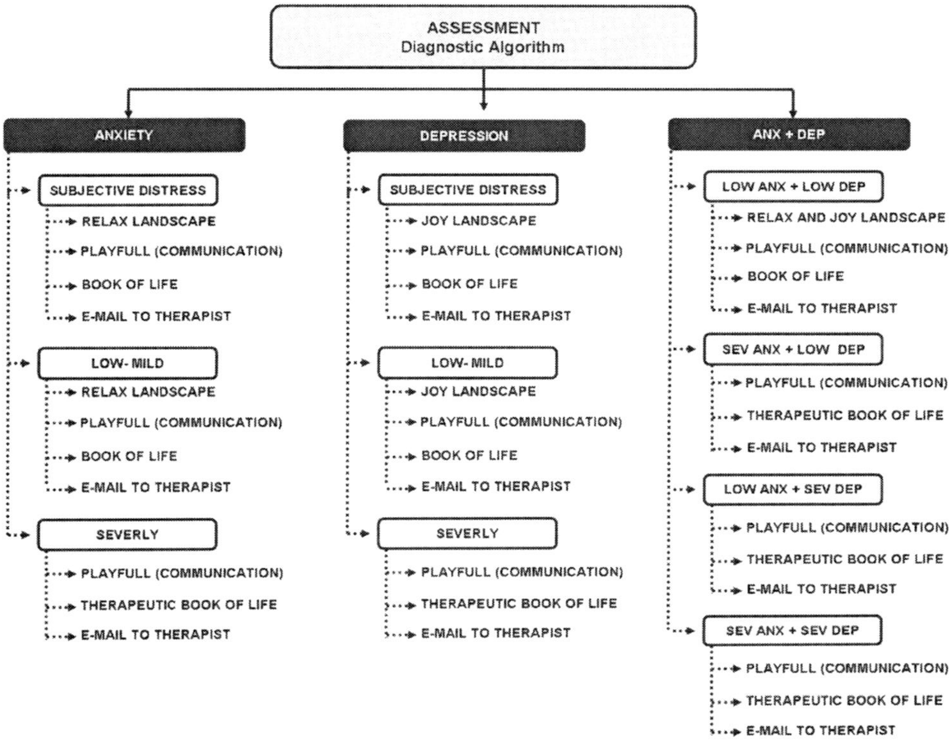

them to stop, walk, look to the left and right and finish the walk.

- **Relaxing Environment:** This begins with a welcome narrative in which the users are is invited to walk through a large, green meadow in which they can enjoy the peace and tranquillity of the surroundings. After a short walk, the users encounter a crossroad where they must choose from three different locations, each of which offers an emotional training exercise in relaxation:
  - **Tree:** This walk leads to a large, ancient, leafy tree, where slow rate breathing is taught and practiced, accompanied by a relaxing melody and birdsong.
  - **Creek:** This is a rock- and grass-lined stream where users can hear water murmuring. There, mindfulness exercises are presented to the elderly users. The instructions tell them to direct all of their attention to the audible sounds for a few minutes, including the water murmuring, music, or anything else they can hear. In addition, they are instructed to recognize and accept any feelings or thoughts that come to them while they are listening, and to simply direct their attention to everything they can hear.
  - Lake: This is a free activity, in which the users observe a scene of a sunrise over a lake; they should let themselves go across the landscape.
- **Joy Environment:** This begins with a narrative that invites users to enjoy a beautiful day, in a meadow full of life and color. As

in the relaxing walk, at the crossroads the users can choose to perform various activities, this time related to training in joy:

- Tree: This element facilitates the recovery of autobiographical memories related to joy. Users are asked to remember funny anecdotes of their life: they should try to imagine all the details of whatever memories come to mind, where the event took place, the temperature, light, who was there, and how everyone was dressed. By describing what happened in detail, they thereby relive their good feelings and experience wellbeing again.
- **Creek:** This is an exercise in mindfulness, in which the users are instructed to focus all of their attention on everything they can see in the environment: the light, the vibrant colours, the green grass, the blue water, the bright sky, and so on. As in the relaxing walk, they are instructed to recognize and accept any thoughts or feelings that come to mind during this period, and to redirect their attention to everything they can see.
- **Lake:** This walk leads to a lake where the people are invited to observe nature while enjoying a beautiful sunrise.

Therapeutic Book of Life (LVT): This tool is a training program for autobiographical memory of specific positive events, developed by Serrano (2002); it is an adaptation of the Life Review program developed by Hight and Webster (1995). This tool is applied by the therapist in the context of psychological therapy, and therefore will be explained in the section on available resources for users.

Playful Action Level

This includes various applications designed to promote integration, communication, learning, socio-emotional networks and entertainment for the elderly. It contains six applications:

- **Mail:** The older people can easily read e-mails in their mailboxes; they can also have their own address book, send e-mails and can also attach their own photographs.
- **Videoconferencing:** Users can talk via videoconference with any of their friends in the Butler network, as well as with family or friends who have the status of "external friend". In this application, the users also have their own address books, which indicate which users are online or offline. To initiate a videoconference, the users need only to click on the name of the contact.
- **My Memories:** This a space where elderly users can assemble, with the help of health professionals, their own multimedia photo albums and music. Whenever they want to view their photos or listen to their favorite music, they can enter this space and easily access their albums, expand their photos and listen to music of their own choosing.
- **Book of Life:** This resembles a personal diary and functions like a blog: the users can write as many pages as they want in the book, and can add photos and music. They enter a title for each chapter they create, add text and attach the multimedia resources they want from the My Memories area. Once they have finished the page, they can choose whether to keep it private, so that only they can read it, or whether to share it with Butler friends as well as with their external contacts (family and/or friends). They can write or read content in their Book of Life, as well as enjoy their friends' own Books of Life. Each book

contains a table of contents that includes the titles of each chapter; the users can choose a link to whichever chapter they would like to read, or can simply read the book pages in order. The tool is designed to improve communication and increase the number of relationships the elderly people have, allowing them to share their vital memories with others.

- **Friends:** Through this resource, users have access to all of the other elderly users who have joined the Butler network. The Friends area is designed to facilitate and promote a virtual community of friends. This space includes photographs of every user and brief descriptions of their profiles. It also has a search engine, through which the users can locate other people by gender, hometown or common hobbies. After the users have selected and read the descriptions of other users, they can send "friendship invitations". The person of interest will receive this request and decide whether to accept or ignore it. If the request is accepted, the person's photo is automatically linked to the address book for exchanging e-mail or videoconferencing. Users who are a part of the network friends are the ones who can enjoy the Books of Life.
- **Internet:** Internet access has been adapted so that older people can easily access the website search engine. From this site they may search for their areas of interest, read the newspaper, enjoy videos, encyclopaedias, etc. The users can surf the Internet wherever they like, but there is always an on-screen option to return to the Butler start menu.

External User

This user profile includes those who comprise the socio-emotional network of the older person, such as family, friends, and others. This user profile requires a unique login and password, but these users only have access to certain applications of the Playful action level; furthermore, they are not part of the virtual community of friends who make up the Butler network. Their participation in the Butler platform benefits the older people by allowing them to strengthen their ties with their closest family members and friends with whom they can send and receive e-mails, video conference or share pages of their Books of Life.

Caregivers

This user profile includes all health professionals who participate in the system and who have clinical responsibilities for the elderly users. There are three possible statuses in this profile: Administrator, Administrative and Therapist, each of which has access to different resources.

Administrator: This is the status of wider application. Other administrators, therapists, elderly users and external users can join the system through this user profile. Administrators can manage the information of elderly users, either by changing personal information, as well as, adding multimedia material to the My Memories application of a user.

- **Evaluation level:** In this level the administrator can see the clinical information of all of the elderly users, can access their health records as a group, or individually, and can view the results of the scales, diagnostics, therapists' annotations, etc.
- **Therapeutic level:** The administrator can see the work between the elderly users and their therapists, in the therapeutic Book of Life. The administrator can also see how often users have accessed the 3D environments for emotional training, which environments were used in each case and how much time was spent on each of the exercises.

Administrative: This profile has the greatest restrictions. The administrative role is to help manage the register of the elderly and external users in the system, and to upload multimedia material to My Memories. They do not have access to users' health records, diagnostic details, or information about the therapeutic Books of Life or what kinds or durations of emotional training has taken place in the 3D environments.

Therapist: This user status includes the therapists or health professionals who are directly responsible for the elderly users. Their access is very similar to administrators, with some restrictions. The therapists can register administrative elderly users and external users and can manage their information; they may also upload multimedia resources to My Memories. What they can not do is generate administrator users or access all of the users' information; they may only access the profiles of those in the system who are their designated patients. For this reason, when new elderly users are registered, the assigned therapist field must be completed. Hence, each therapist only manages the elderly individuals who are their clinical responsibility, while the administrator users can manage the information of all users.

- **Assessment level:** This user status is similar to administrator; however, those on this level can only access the information of elderly users who have assigned them as their therapists. Another important aspect of the program is the alarm system indicating the clinical conditions detected in the elderly users. Specifically, when users enter the system, their mood states are evaluated. If their scores reach a clinical level, the responsible therapist automatically receives an e-mail containing the results and the clinical examination conducted by the Butler system.
- **Therapeutic action level:** This level is similar to administrator, except that the therapists can only access users that are assigned to them. One of the main tools that the therapists manage is the therapeutic Book of Life application (TBL). Following is a brief explanation of how the TBL functions; for a more detailed description see Etchemendy, Baños, Botella & Castilla, 2010. The TBL resembles a personal diary and is used jointly by the therapist and the user. Each page of the TBL includes one of the questions from Serrano's therapeutic program (2002); the questions are designed to evoke specific positive memories of the elderly people's lives. In addition to a question, each TBL page includes a multimedia photograph specifically selected for that question. In each therapy session, the therapists pose the question and then enter the different memories that the elderly people generate into the book. These memories can be general or specific, positive or negative. The therapists' role is to guide the Life Review process so that the users can retrieve specific positive memories for each of their vital cycle stages, using the written questions in the book as a guide. When the therapists determine that the memory evoked by the older person is specific and positive, they progress to the next question. In addition, when the older people generate appropriate memories, the therapists can include specific melodies that the users decide best fit those memories into the book pages. Subsequently, the Butler system enables the therapists to decide which memories evoked in the therapeutic context are suitable to be available later to the elderly users, through the playful application. Hence, when the elderly users access the other resources offered by the system (e-mail, BL, the Internet, videoconferencing, etc.) they will be able to reread the pages and re-evoke the specific positive memories shared with the therapist.

As discussed above, the current challenge is to generate a clinical care structure capable of housing a growing elderly population, beginning with primary intervention levels, which reduce costs and facilitate healthy lifestyles. A previous study in this area showed how different tools derived from ICTs, when used by elderly people, had a positive impact on their communication and social connectedness as well as their affective, physical and emotional world. However such studies have focused on a single technological resource (using videos, music, or the Internet). The Butler system, on the other hand, employs a variety of tools and media in a single program. This may increase its utility and facilitate its implementation, since users can perform various tasks in one system.

Another significant unique quality of the Butler system is that it has been developed in two levels: one for clinical health, and one for the general elderly population. As for the clinical health level, Butler offers a tool for evaluating and diagnosing emotional problems capable of managing interventions for dysfunctional emotions. This keeps practitioners informed of the general status of a large number of patients, with a significant level of detail and speed. Such tools enable more effective and timely therapeutic actions, while reducing health care spending; they also help minimize the workload of health care professionals working with this population.

As for the general population level, Butler has been customized to the needs of the elderly population in general. It aims to promote health, satisfaction and wellbeing through a variety of strategies, including exercising emotional skills, learning new communication skills and ways to make friends, increasing social support networks, strengthening the desire to continue learning new activities, and fostering curiosity and satisfaction by empowering users to try new things.

Various studies have attempted to assess the adequacy of the system for the elderly, using usability protocols that included heuristic evaluation and testing with real users (Botella et al., 2008, Castilla et al., 2008). In addition, studies have evaluated the effectiveness of the system at mood regulation (of positive and negative emotions); they demonstrated that after using the Butler system, users had high levels of satisfaction, low levels of difficulty of use and a significant increase in their mood state and levels of happiness, as well as reduced levels of sadness and anxiety (Botella et al. 2009; Etchemendy et al., 2010).

FUTURE RESEARCH DIRECTIONS

The Butler system is a complex program that offers multiple levels of action. As previously stated, preliminary studies have already been conducted on elderly people who had no clinical signs of anxiety or depression and who only used the recreational resources and VR environments to train positive emotions. The results were very positive and encouraging (Botella et al, 2009; Etchemendy et al., 2010). Nevertheless, they should be considered merely as preliminary findings that must be supported by studies involving larger sample sizes, users with both clinical and non-clinical characteristics; furthermore, the platform must be used for longer periods of time. Currently, the Butler system is being used in various Spanish nursing homes and day centers, and additional data will soon be available. Our next steps are to analyze the impact of the program on this population, and to investigate the available tools that the platform has for health care and the impact of their use on external users. In the future, the Butler system might support a social network designed specifically for elderly people. A significant number of people in this segment of the population might be able to use the Butler system for cultivating friendships, social networking, entertainment, and more, from the safety and convenience of their homes.

CONCLUSION

Addressing demographic transition with a political, social and economical structure for facilitating and promoting active and healthy aging is one of the major worldwide challenges, especially in developed countries. The current demographic distribution and its future trends will have a strong impact on the global economies, cultures, social security systems and health systems, among others. To meet this challenge, several developed countries are realizing the benefits that ICTs bring to the field of the health and wellbeing of the elderly population. ICTs, and telecare applications in particular, are emerging as valuable options for providing assistance to more people with reduced health care costs without sacrificing efficiency. (Barlow, Bayer & Curry, et al. 2005). However, technological and generational gaps pose additional challenges for the elderly population. The application of ICTs to this population can not to hope that this population will suits them, the direction must be inversed. Several scientific studies suggest that ICTs can help improve the wellbeing and quality of life of the elderly.

Furthermore, contrary to the common assumption that the elderly would reject ICTs, scientific studies such as Boni and Perkins (2007) show that the elderly view technology as a significant and positive aspect of our society that can help improve the quality of life of many people.

The Butler system is an e-health application created especially for elderly users and their caregivers. It includes different levels of action designed to improve their wellbeing. The system employs applications useful for promoting health and enabling health professionals to treat different emotional disorders, especially those related to anxiety and depression. The Butler system does not require complex technology, and can be self-administered by elderly people. This is related to a final reflection about the system and its target population: while "elderly" is a term that includes people of different ages and characteristics, our experience is that as long as the users have maintained adequate cognitive and sensory (vision and hearing) abilities, they can use the system without difficulty. In other words, users' cognitive and sensory capacities are more indicative than age of their ability to benefit from using the system. Hence, the Butler system can help to provide solutions to contemporary challenges in the area of the health and wellbeing of the elderly.

ACKNOWLEDGMENT

This study was funded in part by "CIBER of Physiopathology of Obesity and Nutrition, an initiative of ISCIII" and Excellence Research Program PROMETEO (Generalitat Valenciana. Conselleria de Educación, 2008-157).

REFERENCES

American Psychiatric Association. (2000). *Diagnostic and statistical manual of mental disorders* (4th ed.). Washington, DC: American Psychiatric Association.

Anastasiou, A., Quarrie, P., & Boulos, M. K. (2009). Personal location aware care in Europe—The challenge from prototype to product: The CAALYX experience. *E-Health Journal International*, *5*, 18–29.

Barlow, J., Bayer, S., & Curry, R. (2005). Flexible homes, flexible care, inflexible organisations? The role of telecare in supporting independence. *Housing Studies*, *20*(3), 441–456. doi:10.1080/02673030500062467

Beckett, M., Goldman, N., Weinstein, M., Lin, I., & Chuang, Y. L. (2002). Social environment, life challenge, and health among the elderly in Taiwan. *Social Science & Medicine*, *55*(2), 191–209. doi:10.1016/S0277-9536(01)00161-7

Blit-Cohen, E., & Litwin, H. (2004). Elder participation in cyberspace: A qualitative analysis of Israeli retirees. *Journal of Aging Studies*, *18*, 385–398. doi:10.1016/j.jaging.2004.06.007

Boni Li, Y., & Perkins, A. (2007). The impact of technological developments on the daily life of the elderly. *Technology in Society*, *29*, 361–368. doi:10.1016/j.techsoc.2007.04.004

Botella, C., Castilla, D., Lozano, J. A., Alcañiz, M., Breton, J., & Baños, R. … Quero, S. (2008). *The Butler Project: First results of usability validation of a cognitive and emotional teleassistance system for elderly*. (Oral presentation). XXIX International Congress of Psichoterapy. Julio, Berlín (Alemania).

Botella, C., Etchemendy, E., Castilla, D., Baños, R., García-Palacios, A., & Quero, S. (2009). An e-health system for the elderly (Butler Project): A pilot study on acceptance and satisfaction. *Cyberpsychology & Behavior*, *12*(3), 255–262. doi:10.1089/cpb.2008.0325

Camarinha-Matos, L. M., & Afsarmenesh, H. (2004). TeleCARE: Collaborative virtual elderly support communities. *Proccedings of the 1st Workshop on Tele-Care and Collaborative Virtual Communities in Elderly Care*, TELECAR 2004, Porto, Portugal, 13 April 2004.

Castilla, D., Botella, C., Baños, R., Alcañiz, M., Lozano, J. A., García-Palacios, A., … Andreum, S. (2008). *The Butler System: Results about the usability of the system*. 42nd Annual Conventiom Orlando (EEUU) Noviembre.

Center for Health Workforce Studies. (2006). *The impact of the aging population on the health workforce in the United States: Summary of key findings*. Retrieved from http://www.albany.edu/news/pdf_files/ impact_of_aging_excerpt.pdf

Cody, M. J., Dunn, D., Hoppin, S., & Wendt, P. (1999). Silver surfers: Training and evaluating internet use among older adults learners. *Communication Education*, *48*, 269–286. doi:10.1080/03634529909379178

David, T. G., Moons, R. H., & Kahn, J. R. (1981). Community integration among elderly residents of sheltered care settings. *American Journal of Community Psychology*, *9*, 513–526. doi:10.1007/BF00896473

Etchemendy, E., Baños, R., Botella, C., & Castilla, D. (2010). Program of life review support on the new technologies for elderly people: An positive psychology application. *Escritos de Psicología*, *2*, 1–7.

Etchemendy, E., Baños, R., Botella, C., Castilla, D., Alcañiz, M., Rasal, P., & Farfallini, L. (2010). An e-health platform for the elderly population: The Butler system. *Computers & Education*, *56*(1). doi:.doi:10.1016/j.compedu.2010.07.022

Florence, F. M. S. (2001). *An exploratory of informal support and life satisfaction of older persons in Macau*. Unpublished thesis, Lingnan University, Hong Kong.

Gilroy, R., Kellett, P., & Jackson, S. (2004). *Contrasting living arrangements for older people. Conferencia ENHR*. Cambridge, UK: University of Cambridge.

Greg, A. (1976). The elderly widow and her family, neighbors and friends. *Journal of Marriage and the Family*, *38*(4), 757–768. doi:10.2307/350695

Gutiérrez, M., Serra, E., & Zacarés, J. J. (2006). *Envejecimiento optimo*. Valencia, Spain: Editorial Promolibro.

Haight, B. K., & Webster, J. D. (1995). *The art and science of reminiscing: Theory, research method, and applications*. Bristol, PA: Taylor & Francis.

Hanson, B., Sven-Olof, I., Lars, J., & Sven-Eric, L. (1989). Social network and social support influence mortality in elderly men. *American Journal of Epidemiology*, *130*(1), 100–111.

Holmén, K., & Furukawa, H. (2002). Loneliness, health and social network among elderly people a follow-up study. *Archives of Gerontology and Geriatrics*, *35*(3), 261–274. doi:10.1016/S0167-4943(02)00049-3

Karavidas, M., Lim, N. K., & Katsikas, S. L. (2005). The effects of computers on older adults. *Computers in Human Behavior*, *21*, 697–711. doi:10.1016/j.chb.2004.03.012

Khoo, E. T., Cheok, A. D., Nguyen, T. H. D., & Pan, Z. (2008). Age invaders: Social physical inter-generational mixed reality family entertainment. *Virtual Reality (Waltham Cross)*, *12*, 3–16. doi:10.1007/s10055-008-0083-0

Kinsella, K., & Wan, H. (2009). *U.S. Census Bureau, international population reports, P95/09-1, an aging world: 2008*. Washington, DC: U.S. Government Printing Office.

Merck Institute of Aging & Health. (2004). The state of aging and health in America 2004. Retrieved 1 May, 2010, from http://www.aging-society.org/ agingsociety/pdf/ SAHA_2004.pdf

Mette, C. (2005). *Wellbeing and dependency among European elderly: The role of social integration*. FEDEA. Working paper. Retrieved from http://www.fedea.es/ pub/Papers/2005/ dt2005-12.pdf

Proudfoot, J. G. (2004). Computer-based treatment for anxiety and depression: Is it feasible? Is it effective? *Neuroscience and Biobehavioral Reviews*, *28*, 353–363. doi:10.1016/j.neubiorev.2004.03.008

Seligman, M. E. P. (2002). *Authentic happiness: Using the New Positive Psychology to Realize Your Potential for Lasting Fulfillment*. New York, NY: Free Press/Simon and Schuster.

Serrano, J. P. (2002). *Entrenamiento en memoria autobiográfica sobre eventos positivos específicos en ancianos con síntomas depresivos*. [Doctoral Thesis]. Albacete, Spain: Departamento de Psicología. Universidad de Castilla la Mancha.

Sheikh, J. I., & Yesavage, J. A. (1986). Geriatric depression scale (GDS): Recent evidence and development of a shorter version . In Brink, T. L. (Ed.), *Clinical gerontology: A guide to assessment and intervention* (p. 165). New York, NY: Haworth Press.

Siu, O. L., & Phillips, D. R. (2000). A study of family support, friendship, and psychological well-being among older women in Hong Kong. *International Journal of Aging & Human Development*, *55*(4), 299–319. doi:10.2190/2K1W-HWLP-JKD5-LRP6

Spielberger, C. D., Gorsuch, R. L., & Lushene, R. E. (1970). *STAI, manual for the state-trait anxiety inventory*. California: Consulting Psychologist Press.

Tester, S., Hubbard, G., Dowans, M., MacDonald, Ch., & Murphy, J. (2003). *Exploring perceptions of quality of life of frail older people during and after their transition to institutional care*. Retrieved March 6, 2010, from http://www.regard.ac.uk/ research_findings/ L480254023/report.pdf

The Swedish National Institute of Public Health. (2006). *Healthy ageing –A challenge for Europe*. European Healthy Ageing Project. Retrieved from http://www.fhi.se/ PageFiles/4173/ Healthy_ageing.pdf

Tse, M. M., Choi, K. C., & Leung, R. S. (2008). E-health for older people: The use of technology in health promotion. *Cyberpsychology & Behavior: The impact of the Internet. Multimedia and Virtual Reality on Behavior and Society*, *11*(4), 475–479.

van de Watering, M. (2005). *The impact of computer technology on the elderly*. Retrieved March 6, 2009, from http://collab.ist.psu.edu/ future-fall2008/ team-space/life-long-engagement/ life-long-engagment-files/ HCI_Essay_Marek_van_de_Watering.pdf

Wellman, B., & Frank, K. (2001). Network capital multi-level world: Getting support from personal communities. In N. Lin, K. Cook & R. Burn (Eds.), Social capital: Theory and research (233-273). Hawthorne, NY: Aldine de Gruyter.

World Health Organization. (1996). *The world health report: Fighting disease fostering development*. Geneva, Switzerland: WHO.

World Health Organization. (2002). *Active ageing: A policy framework*. Geneva. Retrieved from www.who.int/ hpr/ageing

KEY TERMS AND DEFINITIONS

Active Ageing: This refers to the process of optimizing opportunities for health, social participation and safety in order to enhance quality of life as people age. It allows people to realize their potential for physical, social, and mental wellbeing throughout life and enables them to participate in society, while providing them with adequate protection, security and care as needed (WHO, 2002).

E-Health: This is a recent term referring to healthcare practices which are supported by electronic processes and communication. It is a field at the intersection of medical informatics, public health, and business. E-health refers to health services and information delivered or accessed through the Internet, and related technologies.

Information Communication Technologies: This is a general term that describes any technology that helps to produce, manipulate, communicate, and/or disseminate information.

Internet Based Intervention: This is an intervention that uses the Internet to deliver treatment programs with the objective of improving treatment efficiency.

Positive Psychology: This is a new branch of psychology focusing on the empirical study of positive emotions, and the strengths and virtues that enable individuals and communities to thrive. This field was founded on the belief that people want to lead meaningful and fulfilling lives, to cultivate what is best within themselves, and to enhance their experiences of love, work, and play.

Telecare: This refers to remote care of elderly and vulnerable people, providing the care and reassurance they need to continue living in their own homes. It refers to enabling people to remain independent by providing person-centered reactive technologies to support individuals and their careers.

Virtual Reality: This refers to a computer-generated three-dimensional environment in which users can simultaneously view and manipulate the content of the simulated environment. The virtual environment is presented in such a way that the users have the feeling of being physically present in a virtual world, and can interact with it.

Chapter 5
Do Virtual Communities Have an Effect on the Social Network of Cancer Patients? Empirical Insights from Germany

Jan Marco Leimeister
Universität Kassel, Germany

Karin Janina Schweizer
Microsoft Deutschland GmbH, Germany

Helmut Krcmar
Technische Universität München, Germany

ABSTRACT

This chapter presents the results of a study that investigates the determinants and effects of virtual communities on the development of social relationships within the social network of cancer patients. Influencing factors on the formation of virtual relationships and their effect in the form of social assistance are researched. Following an explorative approach, it is examined whether online communities meet their theoretical potential to provide an environment where social relationships can be established that help cancer patients to cope with their situation. The study shows that virtual relationships for patients are established in VCs and play an important role in meeting patients' social needs. Important determinants for the formation of virtual relationships within virtual communities for patients are general internet usage intensity (active posting vs. lurking) and the perceived disadvantages of CMC. We also found that virtual relationships have a strong effect on virtual support of patients; more than 61% of the variance of perceived social assistance of cancer patients was explained by cancer-related VCs. Emotional support and information exchange delivered through these virtual relationships may help patients to better cope with their illness. Deduced from these results, recommendations for patients using online communities and providers administrating online communities are outlined.

DOI: 10.4018/978-1-60960-866-8.ch005

INTRODUCTION

This research was triggered by the situation of cancer patients in Germany. This situation is negatively influenced by two key components: lacking support from the public healthcare system and problems regarding the societal interaction and acceptance of cancer patients. This proves especially problematic as, to achieve an adequate medical support of cancer patients, it is important to serve both their informational as well as their emotional needs. To meet these needs the social support that patients receive through their social network plays a central role (Eysenbach, Powell, Englesakis, Rizo & Stern, 2004). This support positively affects the process of adjusting to the new situation, the well-being of the patients and their attitude in coping with the disease. But the existing social relationships of a cancer patient are not always able to fulfill the task of providing the necessary support (Holland & Holahan, 2003). In many cases social relationships break apart under the burden of the disease. New relationships have to be established to cover the need for social interaction. Besides real-world self-help groups, cancer-related virtual communities have the potential to offer an environment where these relationships can be established.

This study analyzes the role that cancer-related virtual communities play in supporting the development of social relationships in the social network of cancer patients. Furthermore, the role of social relationships that emerged through the use of online communities is examined.

FORMULATION OF RESEARCH QUESTIONS

Background: Web-Based Services for Cancer Patients

According to a 2002 W3B study, German-language websites related to healthcare are a growing segment (Fittkau & Maaß, 2002). In 2003, 24% of the adult population in Germany consulted the internet to find health-related information (Spadaro, 2003). In addition to pure informational websites, numerous offerings exist that enable their users to interact with each other by means such as mailing lists, newsgroups or chat rooms (Bader, 2000). A study conducted by Daum and Krcmar shows that interaction services are becoming more popular on cancer-related websites: In 2001 they found that most German cancer-related websites are purely informational, whereas in 2002 they discovered that more and more websites support interaction services: 18% of the websites offer a bulletin board or an online forum and chat functionalities are included in 5% of the websites (Daum & Krcmar, 2002). These numbers show the growing importance of health-related online offerings in general and cancer-related online interaction services in the German internet in specific. All the more important becomes the question whether these offerings meet their theoretical potential to support their users in coping with their situation.

Online Communities and Virtual Relationships

Before looking at previous studies investigating the potential of online communities to establish social relationships there, it is important to define the two key concepts used in this research: Online communities and virtual relationships. As there is no common agreement on one specific definition of online communities, for the purpose of this study they are defined using some of the key aspects that are repeatedly mentioned (Doering, 2000; Rheingold, 2000):

- Meeting and interaction of people
- connected by a specific interest
- by means of a technical platform
- where they have the chance to establish social relationships.

Social relationships are characterized by a repeated interaction between two persons whereas the individual interaction is influenced by previous interactions as well as the expectation of future interactions (Doering, 2003). To differentiate between virtual and real-world relationships the place of the first interaction is used (Park & Roberts, 1997): A virtual relationship is a relationship where the first contact took place online; a real-world relationship is a relationship where the first contact took place offline.

Especially during the early research on computer-mediated communication and web-based interaction services numerous scholars questioned whether the characteristics of computer-mediated communication allow social relationships to be established in a virtual environment at all (Parks & Floyd, 1996). However, both the experience of numerous users of online interaction services and the results of several studies in this field of research document that it is possible to establish social relationships in online communities (Rheingold, 2000; Rosson, 1999). For example Park and Floyd come to the conclusion that the emergence of social relationships through online services is common and widespread among its users. But, they also discover that relationships which are initiated by virtual interaction mostly are not kept exclusively within a virtual environment, but are migrated to the real world (Parks & Floyd, 1996). Laying the foundation for the current study two research questions are deduced from these insights transferring them to the specific situation of cancer-related online communities:

RQ1:*Do cancer patients establish social relationships through cancer-related online communities?*

RQ2:*Are social relationships of cancer patients that are initiated virtually transferred to the real world?*

To address these two questions participants in this study were firstly asked to describe up to three persons who are important to them to talk to about their disease and whom they got to know via a cancer-related online community. Secondly, they were asked which means of communication (online and/or offline) they use to cultivate the relationship.

Selected Influencing Factors on the Development of Virtual Relationships

As mentioned above online communities provide a platform for their users to establish social relationships there. However, not all users of such services take advantage of this possibility. Subsequently, the question arises which factors influence whether a person establishes social relationships via online interaction services or not. Parks and Floyd come to the conclusion that socio-demographic characteristics hardly influence the socialising behaviour of users of such online services (Parks & Floyd, 1996). However, it might be possible that this result is due to the type of researched interaction service, as for example Wellman and Gulia mention: "The Net is only one of many ways in which the same people may interact. It is not a separate reality. People bring to their online interactions such baggage as their gender, stage in life, cycle, cultural milieu, socio-economic status, and offline connection with others." (Wellman & Gulia, 2001). Therefore, this study analyses whether socio-demographic factors influence the development of virtual relationships among cancer patients. In addition, the question is addressed whether the type of cancer influences whether cancer patients establish virtual relationships or not, as it can be assumed that persons suffering from uncommon types of cancer might rather turn to the internet to exchange information about their disease than people with widely-spread types of cancer. Hence, the third research question reads as follows:

RQ3:*Do socio-demographical factors and the type of the disease influence the development of virtual relationships of cancer patients?*

According to Parks and Floyd the length of time a certain online offer is used and the frequency of usage are the best indicators on whether users of online services develop virtual relationships or not (Parks & Floyd, 1996). This finding is also confirmed by Wright (Wright, 1999, 2000). Furthermore, Nonnecke, Preece and Andrews observe that active members of online communities who post in boards (poster) develop stronger ties to the community than members who just read postings (lurker) (Nonnecke, Preece & Andrews, 2004). Thereupon research question four can be deduced:

RQ4:*Do characteristics of internet usage influence the development of virtual relationships?*

According to the uses-and-gratification approach in media usage research, people choose to use a certain type of media because they expect some kind of gratification from that usage (Burkart, 1998). Hence, it can be concluded that the motive of the actual internet usage, the gratification they expect, influences the internet usage behaviour. This study focuses on the question whether different motives of internet usage have an influence on the development of virtual relationships of cancer patients (Wright, 2002).

RQ5:*Do motives of internet usage influence the development of virtual relationships of cancer patients?*

Based on a study conducted by Wright, motives of internet usage as defined by Papacharissi and Rubin, are used for the purpose of this study: Interpersonal utility (defined by statements such as "to help other" and "to belong to a group"), pass time (defined by statements such as "when I have nothing better to do" and "to occupy my time") and information seeking (defined by statements such as "to look for information" and "new way to do research") (Papacharissi & Rubin, 2000).

Wright highlights the role of perceived advantages and disadvantages of computer-mediated communication (CMC) on whether users of online self-help groups experience them as fulfilling or not (Wright, 2002). Eventually these advantages and disadvantages do not only influence whether virtual relationships are perceived as fulfilling but, whether a person establishes online relationships at all. Hereon, the question to be addressed in this study is:

RQ6:*Do the perceived advantages and disadvantages of CMC influence the development of virtual relationships of cancer patients?*

Advantages and disadvantages identified by Wright through a survey among participants of online self-help groups are used as a foundation for addressing this question (Wright, 2000). These advantages and disadvantages are complemented by information gained through other studies. The advantages addressed in this study are: Access to a wide-range of different persons and to persons who made similar experiences; chance to interact with persons with whom only loose social ties exist (Turner, Grube, & Meyers, 2001), independency from space- and time; chance to communicate anonymously (Wright, 2000, 2002) and non-existing time-pressure to answer questions (Maloney-Krichmar & Preece 2003; Turner, Grube & Meyers, 2001). Disadvantages addressed in this study are: Absence of human expressions (e.g. gestures), missing possibility for direct contact (e.g. hugging), behaviour of other users that is perceived negatively (e.g. hostile messages) and temporally delayed feedback (Wright, 2002).

Social Support Received through Virtual Relationships

In the last step of this study the potential "result" of virtual relationships defined as social support is researched. Wright revealed that people join online self-help groups for the same reasons and therefore for the same problems for which people join real-world self-help groups (Wright, 1999). According to Turner, the support received through online interaction services is perceived as helpful as support provided by real-world contact persons (Turner, Grube, & Meyers, 2001). Positive effects of online support are also mentioned by Gustafson and Maloney-Krichmar. Both studies report that members of online self-help groups superiorly cope with information about their disease due to the received support; furthermore, their emotional situation improves (Gustafson, Hawkins, Pingree, McTavish, Arora, Mendenhall, Cella, Serlin, Apantaku, Stewart & Salner, 2001; Maloney-Krichmar & Preece, 2003). A study conducted by Loader et al. identifies emotional as well as informational support as types of support provided by virtual relationships (Loader, Muncer, Burrows, Pleace & Nettleton, 2002). This leads to research question seven:

RQ7: *Which types of support are provided through virtual relationships of cancer patients?*

Consolidating all seven research questions the research model presented in Figure 1 emerges.

METHOD

An explorative research approach was chosen to allow the necessary openness for unexpected results (Bortz & Doering, 2002). An online survey was conducted as this research instrument allows reaching a relatively high number of people using cancer-related online communities and therefore allows reaching the goal of this study to explore relationships that were established online.

Important design parameters of the online survey undertaken are summarized in Table 1. For more detailed information please refer to (Schweizer, Leimeister & Krcmar, 2004).

The online survey itself contained six blocks of questions relevant to this study: General internet usage behaviour, usage behaviour of cancer-related online offerings, virtual relationships and their social support, perceived advantaged and disadvantages of computer-mediated communication (CMC), motives of cancer-related internet usage, socio-demographic and cancer-related characteristics. The questions within these different blocks were conducted either from previous research or from a qualitative pre-study within which expert interviews were conducted.

Figure 1. Research model

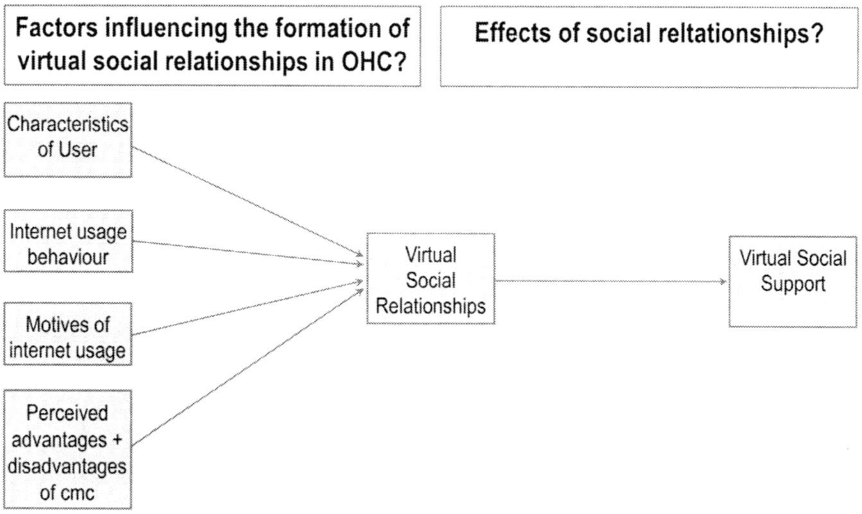

Table 1. Summary of design parameters

Research method	Online-survey
Period	30th March 2004 – 22nd May 2004
Universe	No exact number measurable; in theory all cancer patients that use German-speaking online-offers aligned to cancer-related topics
Sample type	Ad-hoc sample
Approach to contact potential participants	Text with information and link to the survey; posted in 28 German-speaking online-offers aligned to cancer-related topics
Analysable data sets	301

To publish the questionnaire it was written to the managers of all cancer-related online interaction offers found by simulating the behaviour of cancer patients looking for such offers using internet search engines (for the exact process see Daum & Krcmar, 2002). The managers of these interaction offers were asked to publish the link to the online questionnaire. Of 60 offers written to the managers of 28 offers agreed to publish the questionnaire. Altogether 315 people took part in the survey. 301 data sets could be used for the analysis after removing test data sets and data sets filled in by relatives of cancer patients. In these 301 data sets all six blocks of questions were answered as the questionnaire was only saved after being completed.

EMPIRICAL RESULTS

Characteristics of the Survey Participants

Of the 301 cancer patients participating in this survey 204 are female and 97 are male. The age of the respondents varies strongly with the age group of 30-59 years represented the most (n=229). Breast cancer (n=87) was the most common type of cancer the respondents suffered from, followed by haemic neoplasm (n=50). Focusing on the internet usage behaviour of the participants, it is noteworthy that the usage frequency of the internet in general and of internet services with regard to cancer in specific is relatively high. For example, the major part of the respondents uses the internet on a daily base (n=233); in average the participants spend 14 hours a week online.

Results: Virtual Relationships of Cancer Patients (RQ1&2)

The first two research questions that were addressed in this study are whether cancer patients establish social bonds through online communities at all and if they do how these relationships are cultivated. The result shows that virtual relationships established to exchange about cancer are common among cancer patients using online communities: Of the respondents 141 persons (46.8%) describe at least one virtual relationship, 60 participants (19.9%) describe a second virtual relationship and 22 (7.3%) describe a third one. These virtual relationships are described as well-developed and close whereby questions measuring interdependence, depth of relationship and mutual commitment developed by Parks and Floyd were used to measure the quality of relationship (Parks & Floyd, 1996). The information exchange between the cancer patient and his / her virtual relationship takes place on a weekly (47%) or a monthly basis (29%); 72% of the participants exchange non-cancer-related information in addition to information about the disease.

Answering RQ2 Table 2 shows that it is quite common that relationships established via online channels are transferred to the real world and cultivated through both virtual and non-virtual means of communication.

Table 2. Usage of different interaction channels

Means of communication	% of N=232 (all virtual relationships)
Face-to-face meeting	38.6
Via telephone	37.3
Via e-mail	82.1
Via letter	9.9
Online forum	82.1
Via chat	29.6
Other	4.0

Results: Determinants of Virtual Relationships (RQ3-RQ6)

The results to RQ1 show that many, but by far not all cancer patients using online communities develop virtual relationships. Therefore, in the next step influencing factors on whether or not the respondents establish virtual relationships are analyzed.

Socio-Demographical Characteristics and Type of Cancer (RQ3)

To measure the effect of the different socio-demographical characteristics such as gender, age, marital status, education and current occupation on whether the respondents establish virtual relationships or not, chi-square tests were applied. None of the characteristics showed any significant result ($p > .05$). Furthermore, the assumption that persons with uncommon types of cancer rather build up virtual relationships than persons with common types of cancer could not be proven either (chi-square test; $p = .982$).

Internet Usage Behavior (RQ4)

First it was tested whether characteristics of generic internet usage influence the existence of virtual relationships of cancer patients. Chi-square tests showed no significant influence of any of these characteristics ($p > .05$). But, when the influence of the internet usage behaviour with regard to cancer-related topics on the development of virtual relationships was tested, chi-square tests showed significant results: The length of time, since when the internet is used with regard to cancer-related topics, has a positive influence on the existence of virtual relationships. Persons using the internet for cancer-related inquiries for a period of only 0-6 months lack virtual relationships. Cancer patients who have been using the internet for more than two years for cancer-related topics are more likely than average to cultivate virtual relationships ($p = .009$). Also, when cross tabulating frequency and duration of internet usage with regard to cancer-related topics against the existence of virtual relationships the results show that patients who use the internet daily with regard to cancer-related topics and patients who use the internet more than seven hours per week for cancer-related topics are more likely to have virtual relationships than expected values propose. All other groups are less likely than expected values propose. Furthermore, patients actively using online interaction services (posters) are more likely to have virtual relationships than patients only passively using them (lurkers) (chi-square test; $p < .001$).

Motives of Internet Usage (RQ5)

The three motives of internet usage "interpersonal utility" "pass time" and "information seeking" were measured with 12 different questions. Principal-component analysis with varimax rotation was used to measure whether this 12 questions loaded on the expected three motives (eigenvalue = 1.0). Factors were retained on the basis of the "scree" plot and on the requirement that eigenvalue be greater than 1.0. An item was retained if it had loadings exceeding.50 on a factor and no cross loadings exceeding.40. Of the original 12 questions 11 were retained. They loaded as expected on the three motives defined previously by Papacharissi and Rubin. Looking at the three motives of internet usage, Table 3 shows that "information seeking" is the most important motive for using cancer-related internet services, followed by "interpersonal utility". The respondents agreed strongly to both motives whereas the disagreed to use the internet with regard to cancer-related topic to "pass time".

To measure the influence of these three motives on the existence of virtual relationships a correlation analysis was conducted using Spearman's rank correlation coefficient. The correlation analysis indicated a modest positive linear relationship between "interpersonal utility" and the dichotomous variable existence of virtual relationships ($r = .332$, $p < .001$). For the two other motives no significant correlation could be found ($r = .003$ / $r = -.036$; $p = .964$ / $p = .547$). Therefore, it can be concluded that neither "information seeking" nor "pass time" have an influence on the development of virtual relationships whereas, quite logically, "interpersonal utility" has.

Perceived Advantages and Disadvantages of Computer-Mediated Communication, CMC (RQ6)

All measured advantages and disadvantages are perceived as such by the participants of the survey. A correlation analysis using Spearman's rank correlation coefficient was conducted to measure whether perceived advantages and disadvantages influence the existence of virtual relationships. All results of this analysis are shown in Table 4. Significant correlations are marked bold.

Results: Social Support through Virtual Social Relationships (RQ7)

Social support plays a major role in positively influencing the well-being of cancer patients. Social relationships of cancer patients have 'the task' to provide this social support. To measure what kind of social support virtual relationships of a cancer patient provide the respondents were asked 'How does this person support you with regard to your disease? '

Overall, 'to listen' was the most frequently given answer. Moreover multiple participants emphasized how important it is that their conversation partner made similar experiences. One respondent stated: *'The person understands me, because the person was also affected by the disease. Somebody who never suffered from cancer does not understand me this way'* Also, types of emotional support, like 'understanding

Table 3. Motives of internet usage

Motives of internet usage	Mean	Variance	Correlation (r)	Significance (p)
Interpersonal Utility	2.53	0.58	.332	<.001
Information seeking	1.65	0.44	.003	.964
Pass time	4.13	0.78	-.036	.547

Annotation (5-point scale from „Totally agree" = 1 till „Do not agree at all" = 5)

my situation', and 'encouragement' were often mentioned. Furthermore, informational support by their virtual relationships was frequently listed by the respondents.

Although, as the answers to RQ2 show, many of the virtual relationships have been transferred to the real world, practical types of support like visiting or doing errands were only mentioned twice. This shows clearly that, although practical types of support would be possible, informational and emotional types of support clearly dominate virtual relationships.

As a result of the research design the study has to deal with some limitation: Due to the adhoc sampling method the obtained results can not necessarily be regarded as representative. Secondly, the underlying research design only researched those cancer patients using online communities which are per se a lot more likely to establish virtual relationships than oher cancer patients. Furthermore, the study only tested cross effects of variables to a limited extent, whereas the collected data seems to reveal many effects that need to be analysed in more detail. Future research should also focus on potential intermediating variables. Overall, once the social mechanisms taking place in online communities are better understood, the systematic redesign of online communities according to the needs of their users should be in the foreground.

Figure 2 summarizes the findings of this study as to determinants on the development of virtual relationships and the effects of such virtual relationships for cancer patients in Germany.

Recommendations

Virtual communities and virtual relationships can improve the situation of cancer patients by offering them a place to establish social relationships that help them to cope with their situation. But these virtual relationships have boundaries. Like the perceived disadvantages of CMC show (wrong and misleading information), information from the internet generally has to be checked. Also, although virtual relationships offer informational and emotional types of support, they do not seem to offer practical types of support. Therefore,

Figure 2. Results of the research survey

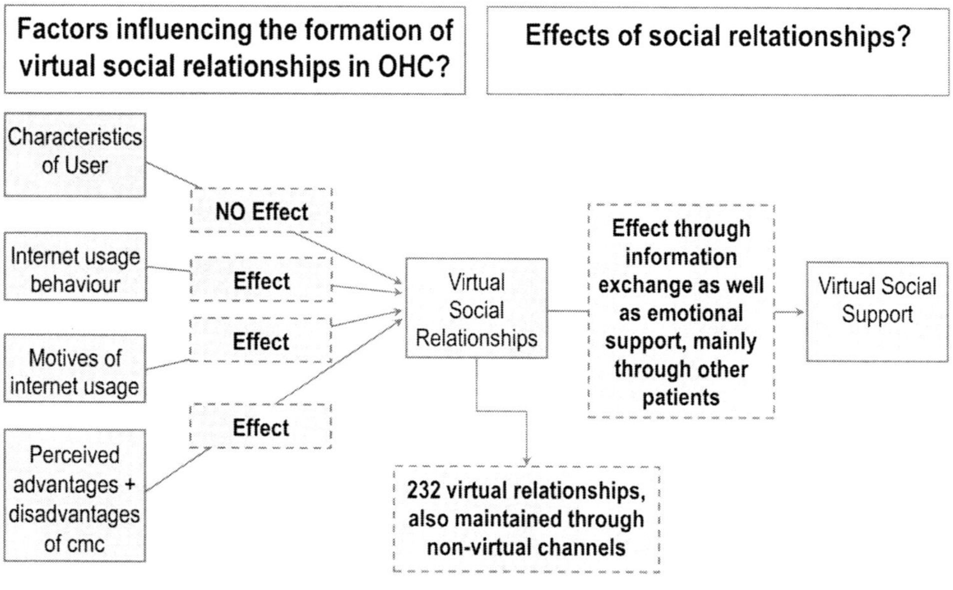

Table 4. Perceived advantages and disadvantages of computer-mediated communication (CMC)

Perceived Advantages and Disadvantages of CMC	Correlation (r)	Significance (p)
Advantages		
The internet allows me to find other people who made similar experiences	.223	.000
I can use the internet independently from time of day	.145	.013
The internet allows me to contact many different persons with a lot of different experiences and information with regard to cancer	.157	.007
I can use internet offerings independently form a specific place	.084	.152
I can remain anonymous	.057	.330
There is no prejudice through others	.001	.990
Answers are more profound than in most face-to-face conversations since people have more time to formulate their answers.	.081	.165
On the Internet it is easier for me to be open	.072	.219
Disadvantages		
It takes longer to get answers than in a face-to-face conversations	-.044	.456
Sometimes people make comments on the internet that are factually wrong.	-.004	.944
Sometimes people make comments on the internet that are misleading.	-.046	.438
My conversation partners are not always accessible since they are not online all the time.	-.046	.435
On the Internet there are no possibilities to touch your conversation partner (e.g. hugging, etc).	.000	.994
Lack of gestures and facial expression can lead to misunderstandings	-.131	.025
There is no possibility to hear your conversation partner's voice.	-.059	.314
The internet makes it difficult to establish personal relationships	-.318	.000
Other people are making remarks that don't have anything to do with the subject	-.062	..296
Other people make hostile remarks	-.019	.746
Perceived Advantages and Disadvantages of CMC	**Correlation (r)**	**Significance (p)**
Advantages		
The internet allows me to find other people who made similar experiences	.223	.000
I can use the internet independently from time of day	.145	.013
The internet allows me to contact many different persons with a lot of different experiences and information with regard to cancer	.157	.007
I can use internet offerings independently form a specific place	.084	.152
I can remain anonymous	.057	.330
There is no prejudice through others	.001	.990
Answers are more profound than in most face-to-face conversations since people have more time to formulate their answers.	.081	.165
On the Internet it is easier for me to be open	.072	.219
Disadvantages		
It takes longer to get answers than in a face-to-face conversations	-.044	.456
Sometimes people make comments on the internet that are factually wrong.	-.004	.944
Sometimes people make comments on the internet that are misleading.	-.046	.438
My conversation partners are not always accessible since they are not online all the time.	-.046	.435
On the Internet there are no possibilities to touch your conversation partner (e.g. hugging, etc).	.000	.994
Lack of gestures and facial expression can lead to misunderstandings	-.131	.025

continued on following page

Table 4. Continued

Perceived Advantages and Disadvantages of CMC	Correlation (r)	Significance (p)
There is no possibility to hear your conversation partner's voice.	-.059	.314
The internet makes it difficult to establish personal relationships	-.318	.000
Other people are making remarks that don't have anything to do with the subject	-.062	..296
Other people make hostile remarks	-.019	.746

Table 5. Overview of deduced recommendations for patients and operators

Recommendations for Cancer Patients
Review information obtained online.
Consult experts to find out which internet sources are trustworthy
Be aware of your own responsibility towards other (e.g. when providing them with information).
Recommendations for Operators
Support quality assurance for health-related content.
Moderate news boards to assure quality of postings.
Require user registration to prevent misleading and hostile remarks.
Provide instructions to community members how they should handle information obtained online.
Implement synchronous interaction services to decrease the perceived disadvantage of delayed feedback.
Introduce personal pages and web-conferences to reduce the problem of missing non-verbal cues.

virtual relationships can play an important role in complementing real-life social relationships, but they can never replace them. Given the diversity of communities in the internet and based on the results of this study, especially how respondents in this study judged advantages and disadvantages of CMC, several recommendations for patients and operators of virtual communities were deduced (see Table 5). For more information see (Schweizer, Leimeister, & Krcmar, 2004).

FUTURE RESEARCH DIRECTIONS

As a result of the research design the study has to deal with some limitation: Due to the adhoc sampling method the obtained results can not necessarily be regarded as representative. Secondly, the underlying research design only researched those cancer patients using online communities which are per se a lot more likely to establish virtual relationships than other cancer patients. Furthermore, the study only tested cross effects of variables to a limited extent, whereas the collected data seems to reveal many effects that need to be analysed in more detail. Future research should also focus on potential intermediating variables. Overall, once the social mechanisms taking place in online communities are better understood, the systematic redesign of online communities according to the needs of their users should be in the foreground.

CONCLUSION

The objective of this study was to examine whether online communities meet their theoretical potential to provide an environment where social relationships can be established that help cancer patients in coping with their situation. Looking at the results of this research, it can be said that, generally, online communities meet these potential and provide a place where cancer patients can interact with other people, exchange information and establish social relationships that supplement their social network. Whether cancer patients using online communities seize this chance depends from different factors. Whereas the process of developing virtual social relationships is not influenced by socio-demographical characteristics of patients, it is influenced by their internet usage behavior, their motives of internet usage and their perception of advantages and disadvantages of online communities.

Concluding, it can be said that virtual relationships among cancer patients who use internet offers are relatively widespread. These relationships play a central role in meeting social needs of patients. Particularly other cancer patients are very important for assuring informational and emotional support, and therefore, in helping cancer patients to cope with their situation.

REFERENCES

Bader, M. (2000). *Selbsthilfenetzwerke und Virtuelle Gemeinschaften - Wirkung und Förderung Neuer Informations- und Kommunikationskulturen in der Gemeinschaftlichen Selbsthilfe*. Dissertation, Universität GH Essen.

Bortz, J., & Döring, N. (2002). *Forschungsmethoden und Evaluation für Human- und Sozialwissenschaftler*. Auflage, Springer Verlag, Berlin u.a.

Burkart, R. (1998). *Kommunikationswissenschaft: Grundlagen und Problemfelder - Umrisse einer interdisziplinären Sozialwissenschaft* (*Vol. 3*). Wien: Böhlau Verlag.

Daum, M., & Krcmar, H. (2002). *Webbasierte Informations- und Interaktionsangebote für Krebspatienten - Ein Überblick*. Working Paper No. 111. Universität Hohenheim, Lehrstuhl für Wirtschaftsinformatik.

Döring, N. (2000). *Virtuelle Gemeinschaft. Lexikon der Psychologie* (Wenninger, G., Ed.). Heidelberg: Spektrum Akademischer Verlag.

Eysenbach, G., Powell, J., Englesakis, M., Rizo, C., & Stern, A. (2004). Health related virtual communities and electronic support groups: Systematic review of the effects of online peer to peer interactions. *BMJ (Clinical Research Ed.)*, *328*(7449), 1166–0. doi:10.1136/bmj.328.7449.1166

Fittkau & Maaß. (2002). *Beauty, Gesundheit & Sport im Internet*. Retrieved April 28, 2004, from http://www.fittkaumaass.de/ stories/storyReader$236

Gustafson, D. H., Hawkins, R., Pingree, S., McTavish, F., Arora, N. K., & Mendenhall, J. (2001). Effect of computer support on younger women with breast cancer. *Journal of General Internal Medicine*, *16*, 435–445. doi:10.1046/j.1525-1497.2001.016007435.x

Holland, K. D., & Holahan, C. K. (2003). The relation of social support and coping to positive adaption to breast cancer. *Psychology & Health*, *18*(1), 15–29. doi:10.1080/0887044031000080656

Loader, B., Muncer, S., Burrows, R., Pleace, N., & Nettleton, S. (2002). Medicine on the line? Computer-mediated social support and advice for people with diabetes. *International Journal of Social Welfare*, *11*, 53–65. doi:10.1111/1468-2397.00196

Maloney-Krichmar, D., & Preece, J. (2003). *An ethnographic study of an online health support community*. Retrieved April 6, 2004, from http://www.education.duq.edu/ institutes/PDF/papers2003/ Maloney-Krichmar.pdf

Nonnecke, B., Preece, J., & Andrews, D. (2004). What lurkers and posters think of each other. *Paper presented at the 37th Hawaii International Conference on System Sciences (HICSS 37)*, 2004, Maui, Hawaii.

Papacharissi, Z., & Rubin, A. M. (2000). Predictors of Internet use. *Journal of Broadcasting & Electronic Media*, *44*(2), 175–196. doi:10.1207/s15506878jobem4402_2

Parks, M. R., & Floyd, K. (1996). Making friends in cyberspace. *Journal of Computer-Mediated Communication*, *1*(4), 16.

Rheingold, H. (2000). *The virtual community - Homesteading on the electronic frontier* (revised edition). Cambridge, MA: MIT Press.

Rosson, M. B. (1999). I get by with a little help from my cyber-friends: Sharing stories of good and bad times on the Web. *Journal of Computer-Mediated Communication*, *4*(4), 1–21.

Schweizer, K., Leimeister, J. M., & Krcmar, H. (2004). *Eine Exploration virtueller sozialer Beziehungen von Krebspatienten*. Working Paper No. 5. Technische Universität München, 2004.

Spadaro, R. (2003). *Eurobarometer 58.0: European Union citizens and sources of information about health. European Opinion Research Group*. EORG.

Turner, J. W., Grube, J. A., & Meyers, J. (2001). Developing an optimal match within online communities: An exploration of CMC support communities and traditional support. *The Journal of Communication*, *51*, 231–251. doi:10.1111/j.1460-2466.2001.tb02879.x

Wellman, B., & Gulia, M. (2001). Virtual communities as communities - Net surfers don't ride alone. In Smith, M. A., & Kollock, P. (Eds.), *Communities in Cyberspace* (*Vol. 3*, pp. 167–194). New York, NY: Routledge.

Wright, K. (1999). Computer-mediated support groups: An examination of relationships among social support, perceived stress, and coping strategies. *Communication Quarterly*, *47*(4), 402–414. doi:10.1080/01463379909385570

Wright, K. (2000). Perceptions of on-line support providers: An examination of perceived homophily, source credibility, communication and social support within on-line support groups. *Communication Quarterly*, *48*(1), 44–59. doi:10.1080/01463370009385579

Wright, K. (2002). Social support within an on-line cancer community: An assessment of emotional support, perceptions of advantages and disadvantages, and motives for using the community from a communication perspective. *Journal of Applied Communication Research*, *30*(3), 195–209. doi:10.1080/00909880216586

Chapter 6
A Content Analysis of an Online Support Group for Survivors of Sexual Violence

Jennifer Yeager
University of East London, UK & Waterford Institute of Technology, Ireland

ABSTRACT

Surviving sexual violence has been described as one of the most traumatic life experiences, and social support is an extremely important coping strategy for survivors. With the rapidly increasing number of available online support communities, understanding exactly what kinds of support survivors need in the context on online social support groups is essential. This chapter presents a study of the types and extent of social support posts exchanged by members of an online social support group for survivors of sexual violence. The Social Support Behavior Code framework was used to code 755 messages that were posted over a 7-day period. Overall, emotional support (42.6%) was the most common support contained in posts, followed by information (21.2%), esteem (20.9%), network (13.1%), and tangible support (2.2%).

INTRODUCTION

The Internet has unquestionably had a profound impact on how people seek support and share experiences related to their health and coping. Specifically, it is the interactivity afforded by Internet communication that has had the most marked impact on virtual communities concentrating on healthcare (Coulson, 2008). Estimates of the number of online support groups range from the hundreds of thousands to millions (Coulson, 2008). Despite this, research specifically examining the role of support groups for survivors of sexual is notably lacking.

DOI: 10.4018/978-1-60960-866-8.ch006

By examining 755 messages that were posted over a 7-day period on Survivors Online[1], an online support group for survivors of sexual violence, this study documented the types and extent of social support posts exchanged by members with Cutrona & Suhr's (1992) Social Support Behavior Code framework. The aims of this study were threefold. Firstly, aim 1 was to document the quantity of social support content in the posts. Aim 2 was to determine how the various types of support manifested in the actual posts. The final aim was to contextualize the findings of this study with previous research using Cutrona & Suhr's (1992) coding framework for use with the online coding of support messages. These aims intended to describe the supports that are of most importance to this population of sexual abuse survivors and to inform mental health professionals and policy makers about how online support can be utilized to promote the welfare of survivors.

BACKGROUND

Sexual Violence and Social Support

Social relationships are important and they can be affected by sexual violence; there is a volume of literature demonstrating that stressful life events generate acute and long-term physical and emotional disorders. The literature on stress and coping also suggests that social support acts as a survival mechanism for individuals under stress and that people's coping methods are strongly associated with all types of social support (Ullman, 1999).

However, few studies have focused specifically on how social support is related to recovery from sexual violence. This is particularly surprising considering that social support has been shown to be a clearly important way of coping with stressful life events in providing emotional support and information that may enhance adjustment. This is further substantiated Herman's (1997) assertion that few human conditions carry more negative weight than surviving rape and that rape survivors are more likely than non-survivors to show subsequent affective and behavioral problems (Rodgers & Gruener, 1997).

While Sanders-Phillips (1997) found that emotional support promoted good adjustment, Popiel & Susskind (1985) established that there were significant differences between the availability of support from different people in their investigation of the role of social support in survivors' subsequent adjustment to sexual assault. In fact, the amount of perceived support varied with how stressful the assault and the amount of overall support did not predict subsequent adjustment. In other words, there were huge individual differences in coping with stress despite a significant relationship between environmental stressors and individual physical and emotional adjustment.

Internet and Social Support

The literature provides compelling evidence that online support groups are beneficial in alleviating the psychosocial sequelae related to sexual victimization; providing emotional support; and facilitating disclosure, all factors which play a key role in successful support and therapy groups on the Internet (Owen, Yarbrough, Vaga & Tucker, 2003; Lieberman & Goldstein, 2005; Braithwaite, Waldron, & Finn, 1999; Finn, 1999; Preece & Ghozati, 2001). The Internet provides survivors of sexual violence with ever-increasing access to online support groups and communities. These communities provide survivors with the ability to engage in asynchronous (bulletin boards) or synchronous (chat rooms) written communication 24 hours a day, 7 days a week (Finn & Lavitt, 1994). Communication is also not restricted by geography; the only requirements to access the online support groups are a computer and Internet connection (Coulson, 2008). Another major attraction to online support for survivors is the potential to access a large and heterogeneous group of survivors, which may not have been possible in the survivors' normal range of social supports (Finn & Lavitt, 1994).

Furthermore, the online social support groups provide survivors with anonymity, which is not possible with face-to-face supports. It has been noted that anonymity is likely to be of particular benefit and attraction to people dealing with stigmatizing conditions (e.g., sexual victimization) as it affords survivors the opportunity to disclose personal experiences while remaining anonymous (Finn & Lavitt, 1994). As a result, online support groups offer an attractive combination of discretion, intimacy, and fun that can sometimes be more empowering that in face-to-face interaction.

In addition, Sherman (2001) and Riva (2002) both report that people do develop strong, interpersonal relationships online. It has been reported that disclosure of personal information is higher online, particularly when participants are anonymous, because they are less concerned about the impression they are making (Sherman, 2001; Riva, 2002); in other words, the lack of cues and reduced evaluation anxiety may lead to more equal participation from low status and shy individuals.

It thus follows that if the Internet experience is a process of negotiation the only way to understand it is to analyze the people involved in it as they go about their daily lives *in situ*. Conducting research on existing social support groups provides important access to undisclosed, marginalized groups of survivors perceive and receive social support. This is particularly important for access to survivors that have not openly disclosed being a survivor of sexual violence. The tendency for members of vulnerable, disadvantaged, and marginalized populations to use the Internet is high, and can be considered a primary source of information and social support for some people (Illingworth, 2001; Mustanski, 2001). It is therefore important to investigate the use of the Internet as a source of support for these survivors.

In the light of these issues presented in the literature, the present study aimed to explore and define the online support experiences of survivors of sexual violence accessing an online support group. Specifically, this research is essential to contribute to the understanding of how survivors access and participate in health and support related online groups.

DATA ANALYSIS

As the site offers a large number of forums and message postings, the significant amount of data downloaded was restricted to messages posted over a 1-week period, totaling 755 posts by 92 members. Data was carefully selected based on the most relevant thread category. This thread was selected based on the large amount of posts, relevant topic matter, and conversational participation by community members. Ethical approval was sought and granted from the Institutional Review Board at the author's affiliated university. Additional permission to access the membership-protected site was granted from the website board moderators, along with consent to perform a content analysis on the data, and to utilize any direct quotes in my research. The moderators posted a message on the site advising participants that data collection would take place over the following week; informing participants about my credentials and research goals; and advising members that they would be contacted directly to provide their consent to use any direct quotes. Due to the anonymous nature of posting online it was not possible to collect data regarding the participants (e.g., in terms of age, gender, etc.). These postings were downloaded and printed for analysis.

The term content analysis has come to describe a "family of analytic approaches" ranging from interpretative to systematic analyses (Hsieh & Shannon, 2005). What is important to recognize is that the appropriate form of content analysis for any given investigation is informed by the theoretical stance of the researcher and issue being studied (Hsieh & Shannon, 2005). The current study employs directed content analysis, which involves the application of existing theoretical categories to a new set of data. Directed content analysis is particularly suitable when the aim of the study is to further contribute to the validation of a theoretical framework (Hsieh & Shannon, 2005). The present study aims to validate and apply Cutrona & Suhr's (1992) theoretical framework of categories of social support to posts on Survivors Online. Coding from an existing framework allows for consistency of terminology and for replicability. The use of constant comparison and verification between the inductive meanings of the posts to the survivors and the theoretical research frame enables an interaction between inductive and deductive approaches. Approaching and analyzing the data in such a way allows for the meanings that the survivors place on their experiences to emerge from the data, while guided by a theory-driven framework of social support.

Coding Framework

Data was initially coded according to a framework designed by Cutrona & Suhr (1992). Cutrona & Suhr's (1992)*Social Support Behavior Code* (Table 1) consists of 5 overall categories of social support, and 22 subcategories.

A coding framework guides coders in which decisions to make when analyzing data, by informing the researcher how to organize data into categories (Hsieh & Shannon, 2005). Hsieh & Shannon maintain that a coding framework provides a "systematic, logical, and scientific" (pp. 1286) method that is essential in establishing trustworthiness in analysis.

The Coding Process

As suggested by Hsieh & Shannon (2005) and Altheide (1987), the posts were initially coded based on the identification of comments that reflect data about support in general. All data that depicted messages of support was highlighted. Step 1 reduced the amount of data to a manageable size, and produced a framework for the next level of analysis.

Table 1. The Social Support Behavior Code (Cutrona & Suhr, 1992, p. 161)

5 overall categories	22 subcategories
Information	Advice Referral Situation appraisal Teaching
Esteem	Compliment Anchorage
Network	Access Presence Companionship Express willingness
Emotional	Relationship Virtual affection Confidentiality Sympathy Empathy Encouragement Prayer Relief of blame
Tangible assistance	Loan Perform direct task Perform indirect task Active participation

The highlighted text was then revisited, and recoded according to the 5 main codes predetermined by the Social Support Behavior Code (Cutrona & Suhr, 1992): information, esteem, network, emotional, and tangible assistance. Where one post included comments relative to multiple categories the data was coded to more than one category. Any text that could not be coded within the predetermined categories was assigned a new code. Step 2 of coding involved returning to the data so that additional concepts or ideas can develop. Again, this step emphasizes the interplay of induction and deduction, where concepts or issues can be derived from either the theory or the data itself.

The text was then revisited for a final time in order to code the data assigned into each of the 5 overall categories into the 22 subcategories. The posts were therefore coded in terms of the existing framework or new codes were formed in the process.

RESULTS

Aim 1: Frequency of Support Behaviors

The first aim of this study was to assess the frequency of the occurrence of the various types of social support in the coded messages on Survivors Online. Table 2 presents the frequency of each category across the 5 overall categories and 22 subcategories of Cutrona & Suhr's (1992) Social Support Behavior Code.

Graphically, Figure 1 illustrates the obvious dominance of emotional posts, followed by information and esteem, network, and tangible support in the obvious minority.

Aim 2: Types of Support Behaviors

The second aim of this study was to determine the types of support behaviors that were present in the coded messages on Survivors Online. In order to accomplish this aim quotes from posts coded into the various categories of support are presented to illustrate how the various types of social support manifested in the context of the actual messages posted on the forum.

Information Support

The overall category of information support included posts that offered suggestions or advice; referrals to other sources of help; situation appraisal; and teaching.

Suggestions/Advice

Posts in the suggestions/advice category generally offered advice for challenges coping with sexual victimization. For instance, one Survivors Online member received this advice about being hurt by her mother's decision to inform family members about her abuse history without her permission:

Have you tried talkin to your mom about it and telling her how it makes you feel?? At least so that kind of thing doesnt get repeated in the future?? Maybe make alist of the reasons why you think its wrong, so it comes across as very logical sounding as opposed to emotional? You have EVERY right to your emotions, and i only mention the letter idea because sometimes people take us more seriously when we have something written down, as opposed to them thinking you are just flying off the handle. Also, she can think about what she has done when she has the letter to read? You can even draft it and put it up on the boards if you want if you re worried about how you ll come across!

Table 2. Frequency of social support within the 755 coded posts

SOCIAL SUPPORT CATEGORIES	FREQUENCY	% OF TOTAL
INFORMATION	512	21.2
Advice	211	8.7
Referral	77	3.2
Situation appraisal	38	1.6
Teaching	186	7.7
TANGIBLE ASSISTANCE	54	2.2
Loan	0	0
Perform direct task	3	0.1
Perform indirect task	0	0
Active participation	4	0.2
Express willingness	47	1.9
ESTEEM SUPPORT	505	20.9
Compliment	164	6.8
Validation	297	12.3
Relief of blame	44	1.8
NETWORK SUPPORT	315	13.1
Access	6	0.2
Presence	24	1.0
Companions	285	11.8
EMOTIONAL SUPPORT	1027	42.6
Relationship	6	0.2
Physical affection	184	7.6
Confidentiality	0	0
Sympathy	231	9.6
Understanding or empathy	376	15.6
Encouragement	226	9.4
Prayer	4	0.2
NUMBER OF MESSAGES	755	
Number of codes across messages	2413	

Figure 1. Graph of support types coded across total posts

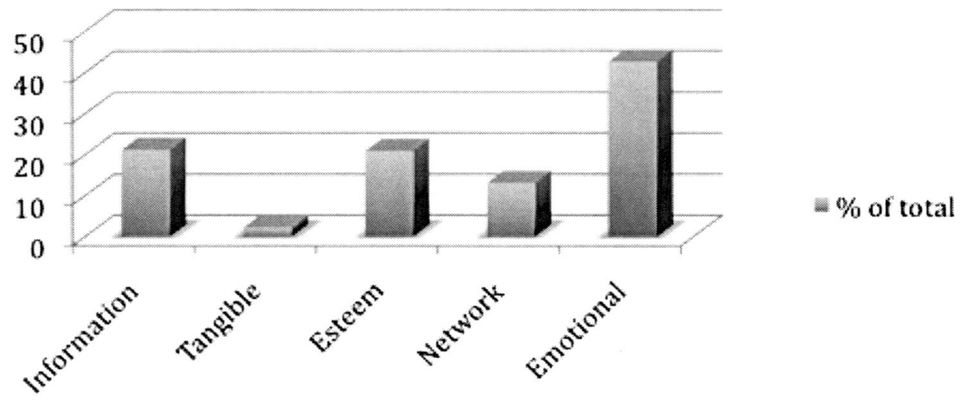

Suggestions and advice also took a very practical focus in providing members with advice of where to go to for help:

is there a crisis center in your area? have you tried looking on rainn.org for a crisis center in your area? maybe they would have some ideas on how to help, or leads on people to talk to. not telling you what to do- just an idea. please be kind to yourself. you are not alone. keep reaching out.

The following two quotes provide examples of suggestions of actions that the members should take to deal with their problems. The first quote suggests the person should take action by setting personal rules, and the second suggests the action of cutting ties to an inappropriate person.

I am sorry you've had to deal with this again and again. How long are you dating for before telling these guys? Maybe you should make a rule for yourself - no telling until date 12, and no opportunity for sex before that either so that they simply can't hurt you? By 12 dates you should have a fair idea of what sort of guy you're seeing. I'm not sure if that helps? You definitely deserve to be safe and whole though, no matter how those bastards might make you feel.

*Please please please please don't ever talk to this man again. He is a complete as*hole, and I am worried for your safety. He called you a whore, blamed you for your rape, put you down, and then took advantage of you when you were drunk. Please don't ever see him or speak to him again.*

Referrals

Posts coded in the referrals category refer the member to some other source of help. For example, in response to a query about not being to afford therapy, one member responded:

Not sure where you are but two ideas came to me...one is to try a training hospital, they might offer low or no charge in exchange for seeing a therapist in training. And the second is to try local churches, there's one near me that offers counseling based on income. The church supplies the room and the psychologist takes whatever fee is agreed upon.

Similarly, another member attempted to refer a survivor to another source of help in concern for the person's coping:

I am sorry this happened to you...

What a difficult time for you at the moment.

Remembering nothing of what happened.

Do you have a therapist or support person.

You need someone right now.

Someone that can support you thought these "blanked out times" and help you reconnected with your entire body.

I suggest you ring a Rape hotline and tell them exactly what you told us here.

In response to another query about locating free therapy options a member posted a list of free Internet-based therapy workbooks.

Im thrilled that you've found someone you can talk to!! The fee is a bummer tho. Have you asked her if she has a sliding scale for fees? Maybe once every week and a half or something? Perhaps budgeting for it?? I do have a collection of therapy workbook links that are free and on the internet!

Here are a few links:

http://www.smartreco...s/toolchest.htm
http://www.ascasupport.org/
http://www.getselfhe...edownloads2.htm
http://ehcounseling.com/materials/

I hope this T gets back to you with good news. Take care

Situation Appraisals

Situational appraisals reassessed or redefined the situation of concern for members. In other words, these posts attempted to reconstruct the situation for the member so they could look at the issue a different way. The following post attempted to reassess a member's concern that she had aborted a child conceived through unprotected sex by taking the morning after pill. The post redefines the situation by providing evidence that the member was unlikely to have been pregnant:

I am so sorry that you feel this way--grieving for the child you never had must be very sad. I don't want you to have to feel like your emotions are in any way invalid.

However, that being said, you're grieving for something that probably wouldn't have happened anyway. The approximate chance of conceiving in a single unprotected sexual encounter is somewhere between 3% and 5%. So it is very unlikely that you would have gotten pregnant even if you hadn't taken the morning after pill.

If you want a child, then maybe this is the time to start exploring your options to have one who's conceived under much happier circumstances (with or without a man)...but don't think of this as a situation where you somehow prevented yourself from conceiving with the morning after pill. There is AT LEAST a 95% chance that you wouldn't have gotten pregnant anyway.

The second quote responds to a member's concern that what she experienced did not constitute rape and did she deserve to be on the site requesting support for her experience. The following post assesses the member's situation:

I'm sorry but that was definitely rape. Even legally, being intoxicated means you cannot consent and means that there was no way he could have legally gotten consent from you, therefore it was rape. Your feelings should prove to you that you were violated and wronged. I'm sorry that this happened to you and hope you can heal from this traumatic event.

The final quote depicting situation appraisal encourages a member to look at her experience in a different light to ensure she is making the right decision. The member encourages the poster to "reconsider" her situation:

If you truly want to walk away from your marriage and your husband that's one thing, but if you're feeling hurt and overwhelmed at the moment and acting out of pain and frustration then please reconsider.

The only mistake here is allowing a very unstable, manipulative MIL to ruin your life. I hope you feel better after some rest and realize that Mr.L chose you for a reason!

Teaching

Teaching posts provide detailed information, facts or skills needed to deal with the situation. The following post provides detailed, factual information in response to earlier query from the woman who was requesting support for the guilt she felt about taking the morning after pill:

If you're having entirely unprotected sex, you are still not fertile for most of the month. The average woman is only capable of conceiving about 3 days per month. Even when sperm and egg are both present during those 3 or so days of ovulation, conception occurs less than half the time, and even if the egg is fertilized and implants, almost half of all pregnancies end in miscarriage during those first few days, before the woman ever even knows she's pregnant at all. Given those statistics, a 3% chance of conceiving from a single unprotected encounter even seems a little too generous. It's probably closer to 2% or so, when you include pregnancies that miscarry unbeknownst to the woman a few days after conception. And miscarriage can be caused to a lot of different things (and sometimes seems to have no cause at all), but stress is a big causative factor of miscarriage. And rape is a big causative factor of stress. Which puts the chances even lower.

I hope this gives you some comfort. It is highly unlikely that taking the morning after pill changed anything at all. You've lost enough because of the rape—you don't have to feel like you've lost a baby too.

Another post provides information on the skills needed to apply makeup and jewelry to a woman who spent years being told by a controlling husband that she was not to wear makeup or jewelry.

I would say when you try out something new - make up, jewellery or clothes - remember, firstly, that this is your choice and you are doing it for yourself and no one else. Keep in mind that you deserve to wear what you like to make you feel strong and confident and feminine because you deserve to feel all those things, not because it will make you more attractive to anyone else, but that you are happy with the face you present to the world. If that means wearing a little make up and a pretty pair of earings then there is nothing wrong, improper or unseemly about that.

Tangible Assistance

The second overall category was tangible assistance. Tangible assistance involved the member offering to take physical action in support of the recipient. The subcategories in this section included offering a loan; performing a direct task; performing an indirect task; active participation; and expressing willingness. No posts offering loans or indirect tasks (e.g. offers to take over a member's responsibilities while under stress) were located in the posts.

Direct Task

Only 1 post offering to perform a direct task was coded. The following message depicts a member offering to locate information for another member:

I am really sorry to hear that. I wish I had some sort of advice for you. The only thing I can think of is maybe try another helpline what country are you from maybe I can look some up for you.

Active Participation

Messages containing active participation offered to join the recipient in action that reduces the stress for the member. The minimal number of posts coded into this category defined offers of "active participation" broadly. While the following two posts offer active participation on behalf of another member, the offer is symbolic in nature, rather that concrete. For example, in the following post a member offers to symbolically accompany another member to a stressful doctor's appointment:

I think that what you are going through is extenuating circumstances. I really can not help here, except to tell you that I am thinking of you. I will be a pocket rider if that helps at all.

Similarly, the member in the following post offers to share her tissues with a fellow survivor:

Go ahead and cry. You deserve a really good one. I will share my Puffs tissue with aloe and a shoulder to cry on with you. Life right now sounds like it is pretty overwhelming for you to do alone right now. Just take a break and cry. We'll be here for you.

Willingness

The posts coded into the willingness category expressed a willingness to help other members, and contained the largest number of posts in the tangible assistance category. The first post expresses willingness to help another member by information the member to PM (private message) her if she needs anything:

I am so very sorry for your loss. Safe hugs if ok. Please know that we are all here and supporting you through this difficult time.

If there is anything I can do to help, even if it's just listen, please dont hesitate to PM me. Again, I am so sorry for your loss, and I am really hoping that you ve got some good support r/l.

Take care.

Similarly, the following two posts express willingness to help another member:

Don't forget we're all here for you anytime that you need us

Please take care of yourself, and keep using this board, we re all hear to support and listen to you

Finally, the last post is a thank you message to member on Survivors Online expressing her gratitude for members' willingness to reach out and help her when she needed it:

I woke up feeling blue today. I started going over the past last night which not only resulted in a terrible nights sleep but also has left a lingering feeling of sadness today. I know there is no point going over the past or dwelling on what might have been, though thats easier said then done, and that is something that all the wonderful people here have taught me. In the same way that they (you) taught me that what happened wasn't my fault and that i deserve to heal.

And feeling like that this morning just made me realize how much I value all the support I have here at Pandys and how incredibly grateful I am. We are all brought here because of such terrible things and yet what has been created is a testiment to our combined and personal strength and compassion.

So I just want to say a huge THANK YOU to everyone here. I really appreciate your support, acceptance and friendship.

I want to send safe hugs to all who want them.

Now, enjoy some smileys...

Esteem Support

Esteem support posts validated the recipient's concept of self and competence through compliments; validation, and relief of blame.

Compliments

Compliments said positive things about members or emphasized the members' abilities. In response to a post from a member describing having to deal with stressful family members while taking care of an elderly mother, this member emphasized and complimented the original poster's abilities in the situation:

All I can really think of to say right now is WOW!!! I am so so proud of you for setting those boundaries and sticking with them. It is great that they listened to you, that must have been really validating I'm sorry that you have so much on your plate right now but it sounds like you are handling it so so well. I think it is amazing that you were able to handle everything going on in a healthy productive way. I hope that you will continue to put yourself first and to take good care of yourself especially during this time.

The following message was posted in response to a member's description of confronting the scene where she was faced with a pedophile that tried to convince her to get into his car:

That 9 year old little you was sooooooooo brave for running off and for not going with them!

And how awesome that you were able to go back and to act out what happened and to see how brave you were, that is a big healing step! Brava to you

The final example of a compliment is from a member emphasizing another poster's abilities to support her through moments of self-doubt:

you are NOT a monster. I've read some of the replies you've written to other people's posts, and they are kind, supportive, gentle and considerate. No monster could have written like that.

Validation

Posts in the validation category expressed agreement with the recipient's perspective on the situation. In a response to a post about a member wanting to tell his mother about the extent of his abuse, this member expresses agreement and understanding about wanting the support of her mother:

It takes a lot of courage to challenge the lies we've been told about who we are and about our responsibility for abuse (you really aren't responsible - you really, truly aren't!) It's definitely not easy or something you can just decide to do and do, I think. But hopefully hearing about my own experiences of that and how I can understand the fear and the pain but also found that what I thought my parents thought or would think wasn't right... well, it was a huge relief for me. So so so scary to ask. But I'm glad I did. I'm lucky to be really close to mum and dad and not everyone has that - I know our relationships are all different. You'll know if you can tell her one day or not. Wanting to, wanting that reassurance and comfort is TOTALLY understandable - we don't lose that with age. It's so normal to want your parents' love and approval - please be kind to yourself about feeling that way, OK? About wanting to share what happened with her and be comforted and cared for. Of just wanting not to have to hold it all inside. That's so normal and understandable!

Another member responds to the same post, beginning her message with "like you, I never told my mom", establishing agreement with the original poster's actions:

Like you, I never told my mom because I was afraid of the pain it would cause her and afraid she would blame herself. I'm sorry. I know it's hard. I know it's cliche, but it's true and we have to be reminded: you did nothing wrong. You are not disgusting or bad. Be good to yourself.

The final post responds to a member's confusion about whether or not she is justified in feeling glad that her mother was sent to a nursing home. The message clearly validates the poster's perspective on what happened.

My dear friend, I've been in a similar situation with my father-in-law, who died last year, so I really do understand what you mean about feeling she'll be safer and cared for more without so much medical intervention. It is very hard to watch someone you love unable to eat or interact properly. Please be really, really gentle with yourself about how you feel, dear mate. Your reactions make sense and are really loving. My husband felt so guilty about wishing his dad peace from the struggles he was going through, because that meant wishing he would die. But it was all from love and respect for his dad. It's natural to wish the end of things that are painful for you all. I know that if you could, and if my husband could have, you'd both wish your mum and his dad alive, well and happy. It's very difficult grieving for someone who's still there with you, but no longer having that quality of life or ability to be present in your life. I don't know if that's the case with your mum - but please be kind to yourself about that whole range of feelings. You're not alone in having mixed feelings and being concerned about her comfort right now as well as her survival - caring about her quality of life as well as the length of it is not being unloving in any way. I'm so sorry that she's so unwell and I hope, if it's possible, she'll recover more. Sending you so many gentle, caring, loving thoughts. I hope you'll all have the best possible quality of life and interaction together for as long as that can happen and a peaceful, painless end when that time is up, whenever that may be. With much love and sympathy and care and glad that your mum's in a better situation now and you'll be spared dealing with your brother as much (I hope?) If OK hugs.

Relief of Blame

Relief of blame described messages that tried to alleviate the member's feelings of guilt about the situation. The four subsequent posts clearly present member's responses to posters situations that present messages confirming the posters' lack of responsibility and blame in their sexual victimization.

I'm so sorry for what you've been through and that you are having such difficulties dealing with all this. I know how easy it is to blame ourselves but please try and remember that what happened was not your fault and leave the blame where it belongs, with him.

You are not evil. You are guilty of nothing. You are doing a sensible, smart, GOOD thing by staying away from him and protecting yourself. I know it's hard when reality seems to be twisted so much by who they seem to be on the outside. YOU know how he is, YOU know WHO he is, when he's alone with you. Don't give him another opportunity to hurt you. You do not deserve to be hurt. Nobody deserves that. Nobody. And you're no different. You deserve to be treated with love and respect, kindness and affection. Do not let anyone convince you otherwise.

Network Support

The third overall category of network support included posts that connected members to others in similar situations through access; presence; and companions.

Access

The access category included posts offering to provide members with access to new companions. Posts included in this coding category did not offer access to new companions outside of Survivors Online, but rather offered access to new friends and support within the Survivors Online community. This was offered mainly to new posters and new members. For instance, one member posted "Oh and I almost forgot! WELCOME!! I'm glad you've found us" in response to a new member's first post. Similarly, the following post supported another new member:

This site it truly a blessing. Everyone here is so kind and supportive. We're here for you. You're in my prayers.

Finally, this post provides a member with access to a new companion by offering herself as a new companion:

I have found that I have been able to get closer to some of the fellow survivors here that will listen when I am struggling. I know it is not RL but to me the emotional support has been wonderful. If you ever need some to listen please feel free to PM me.

Presence

Posts about presence offer to spend time with the person and "to be there". The following four posts show members offering their presence as support to other members.

Please be gentle with yourself as you work through this and continue to reach out to us for support. I know that we've spoken before so please know that you can continue to pm me anytime.

We are here to listen when and if you are ready to explain

Sorry to hear you are feeling so alone. I didn't think you were moaning, just saying how you feel....

I hope you feel better soon.

Hugs

If you want?

sending a butterfly to sit with you.

**sitting with you* Hugs.*

Companions

Posts included in the companions category remind the member of the availability of companions, and others who are similar to themselves. The first two messages emphasize that these members are similar to the poster and are there for them.

I have been (and still am) in your situation. It is hard to hold the ones we care about responsible. We always want to justify their behavior to make it seem less nightmarish than it really was. It is our way of dealing with the abuse.

oh my friend - please dont ever apologize for venting and letting it out. it takes courage to do that and it helps - you arent alone here. i am sorry for what you are having to endure - i can empathize with your pain and not wanting to have to deal with it.

These two posts emphasize primarily the presence of others and availability of support on Survivors Online:

Please keep reaching out and talking about it during the good times and bad. We are all here to support you

In a way, if you had to remember it was good to have it happen at your T's where you are fully supported and safe. Give yourself some time to deal with these new memories and feelings as they come, okay? And know that you aren't alone!

Emotional Support

The fifth and final overall category is emotional support. Posts of emotional support included all messages conveying sympathy or emotion towards members. Specifically messages were coded for content of relationships; physical affection; confidentiality; sympathy; understanding; encouragement; and prayer. No messages of confidentiality were represented in the coded posts.

Relationship

The relationship category included posts stressing the importance of closeness and love in relationship with members. The member in the following quote stresses the importance of how she feels about her children in response to another member's post about a miscarriage.

But I love my children more than anything in the world. I couldn't imagine life without them. I never knew so much love and happiness before they came into my life. So I don't think that anyone is wrong for loving their child, regardless of how it came to be. And I don't believe that no pregnancy takes away your right to grieve. I've had friends who are infertile tell me of similar feelings. Our feelings often don't make sense to us or to others, but they are our feelings. Be well dear

In the next post another member highlights the love she feels for her mother in supporting her:

My mum is an amazing woman. She's dealt with this with so much love, strength and bravery. She's really fronted up, even though it's so very painful and hard. I love her very much and I admire her too.

I just wanted to say that here. Mothers can be AMAZING.

Finally, this last quote shows a member congratulating another member on getting married by emphasizing the importance of love:

I didn't know you'd gotten married! That's a BIG one. I know it can be complicated, but true love is so so GOOD! She's a lucky woman (and it sounds like a very special one too).

Physical Affection

Posts containing physical affection included offers of physical contact (including hugs, kisses, etc.). Many posts on Survivors Online ended with brief statements such as, "safe hugs if ok?" The following three quotes are examples of some of the more detailed offers of physical affection.

((((((((((((XXXXX))))))))))))))))))))))[2]

Sending you lots of hugs hon, I know that life can get very complicated but keep holding onto the fact that it does get better and you can come through to the other side. Keep reaching out whenver you need anything

You can cry on my shoulder

Lots of love and care to you and many gentle thoughts. You're not complaining over nothing at all - it's real, it matters, and so do you. Have a sympathetic virtual shoulder, or just listener.

Sympathy

Sympathy messages expressed sorrow or regret for the recipient's situation or distress. The following three posts all begin with "I'm sorry", conveying sympathy to the members' situations.

I am so sorry that you still find yourself in an unsafe environment. I'm happy to hear that things are going pretty well for you right now and that you will be able to get away for a few days. I know how hard it is to feel trapped in an unsafe situation and I just want to let you know that I am here to listen and that I understand.

I'm really sorry you've experienced this more than once. It is horrible to put yourself out there and feel that vulnerable and someone take advantage. I've never been through this myself and can't imagine what's going on with them, but wanted you to know that I was listening.

im sorry i havnt many words for this but wanted you to know that ive heard you and sending supportive hugs your way, sorry i couldnt help more x i do get you feeling that way and wanting to rant at him, your not alone in anything you have said xx

Understanding/Empathy

Messages in the understanding/empathy category expressed understanding of the situation or disclosed a personal situation that communicated understanding to the member.

The first message emphasizes being "in the same boat" as the poster:

Well, I don't have anything helpful to tell you, except that I'm in the same boat. I've had very similar problems... Every place I go to is so expensive! I can't afford it... But I need it, so I'm not sure what to do from here...So, long story short, I understand your frustration. Can't afford diddly-squat and meanwhile, I'm miserable and only getting worse.

The second post discloses a personal situation of working with other survivors to communicate understanding and empathy to the original message poster:

I understand 100%! I also work with victims everyday for my job, and yet I have told exactly one person in my family a small part of my story. EVERYDAY I talk to victims and for victims, but in my family I have not crossed that hurdle. I would have froze too It is such a big thing to let my family in to see and know the real me, there has been so much pain, and so much not talked about with our family. I also am considered the "put together one", so if I would even think about talking about myself and my issues, it would be quite a shock to my whole family. But that feels so fake and isolating, I am trying to figure out how to be real with my family and if they don't like it well, so be it

Encouragement

Posts of encouragement provide the poster with hope and confidence. The first message provides many instances of providing the poster with confidence, calling the poster "my hero!!!!"

You are doing the absolute BEST you can by bringing this to the authorities and potentially protecting more innocent children. How amazing and brave is that???? You are my hero!!!! If all of us could have had somebody like you in our lives, just think how much better this world could be. You are God's instrument in helping to make our world and our children safer. Focus on the good you are doing. God knows your heart, He knows. One day maybe I can be like you.

This post tells the poster "Don't give up!" and conveys many messages of hope to the recipient:

I've been in the same situation all this last year! Give it time and it will change! Don't give up! I know it's draining...but you can do it! Baby steps! If you are getting so angry that you are finding yourself drained, be careful that it doesn't poison you, because the guy still has control over you...and you don't want him to have any sort of control over you! It will get better! And it's okay to be angry!

Prayer

In the final category, messages of prayer offered to pray with other members. The following three posts present straightforward support in the form of prayer:

My heart aches for you and I wish I could say something to you to make you feel better. You are not alone, and even though I don't know you, I am with you.

I pray you find peace in this horrible situation. It may not be socially acceptable to be vengeful, etc - but honestly, I feel so proud of you!

I'm praying for your family

I'm so sorry for your loss. You're in my thoughts and prayers during this difficult time.

DISCUSSION

The results of this study provide an indication of the types of computer-mediated social support that are exchanged between members of a support group for survivors of sexual violence. In particular, emotional and informational support were the more frequently provided, and appeared to be associated with the unique challenges faced by survivors coping with sexual victimization.

Suitability of the Coding Framework

This study contributes to the existing social support literature, as well as to assessing the suitability of an existing measure of social support (namely, Cutrona & Suhr's 1992 Social Support Behavior Code) and the support present in a computer-mediated support group for sexual violence survivors. Despite being originally created to examine conversations in marital partnerships, the coding framework was nevertheless applied with a reliability figure of.72, very similar to Cutrona & Suhr's (1992) statistics of.76. Only the categories of loan; indirect task; and sympathy were not present in the coded data. While this suggests that a slightly modified version of the coding framework may be more suitable to online data, 19 of the 22 subcategories were relevant to the present dataset. This is also representative of the Social Support Behavior Code being derived from a comprehensive review of the social support literature (Cutrona & Suhr, 1992; Braithwaite *et al*., 1999).

Finally, the application of a coding structure to the data collected here ensured that the analysis was performed within the context of an existing theoretical framework, which provided a well-defined and explicit coding system. This was further supported by the high level of interrater reliability, and the similarity between the findings of this study and others utilizing the framework.

Aim 3: Frequency of Social Support Categories in Other Studies

The final aim of this study was to contextualize the findings of this study with previous research using Cutrona & Suhr's (1992) coding framework for use with the online coding of support messages. The findings of the present study were compared to the results of Braithwaite, Waldron and Finn's (1999) study of people with disabilities; Coulson, Buchanan, and Aubeeluck's (2007) study of participants with Huntingdon's Disease; and Coursaris and Liu's (2009) study of people living with HIV/AIDS. The prevalence of emotional support in this data is somewhat consistent with other studies performing content analyses of online data using Cutrona and Suhr's (1992) framework. Table 3 presents the frequency of the social support categories across the 3 other studies utilizing the framework to code online social support forum messages.

Table 4 presents the data above more simply, in terms of the rank of overall category of support. The chart clearly illustrates how information and emotional supports rank highest across all of the studies, and tangible and network supports are lowest across all studies (except Coulson, Buchanan, & Aubeeluck, 2007, where esteem and tangible support rank lowest).

The dominating presence of emotional and informational support in the present study is consistent with these other studies. Similarly, esteem support ranked third in the present study, as well as in 2 of the other 3 studies, followed by network and tangible assistance. In all of the four studies emotional and informational support ranked either first or second. However, it is important to note that the difference in rank between information and esteem support is small (21.2% and 20.9% respectively), suggesting that these forms of support were almost equal in occurrence on Survivors Online. This is not surprising since the populations across the comparison studies are people with physical conditions. Sexual victimization, on the other hand, is not a physical illness. Validation and relief of blame are two subcategories of esteem support that are particularly important forms of social support for survivors of sexual violence, whereas these supports may not be as essential to the participants across the other studies.

The prevalence of emotional and informational support in this study is also consistent with content analyses of social support forums not specifically using Cutrona & Suhr's (1992) framework to analyze posts on online forums. Again, information and emotional support have been reported as the most prevalent forms of social support across a variety of other studies investigating torn knee ligaments (Preece, 1999), eating disorders (Winzelberg, 1997), irritable bowel syndrome (Coulson, 2005), type I diabetes (Ravert, Hancock, & Ingersoll, 2004), prostate and breast cancer (Gooden & Winefield, 2007), and cancer (Weinberg, Schmale, Uken, and Wessel, 1996; Klemm, Bunnell, Cullen, Soneji, Gibbons, & Holecek, 2003).

The Prevalence of Supports in this Study

The high prevalence of emotional support in this study (accounting for 42.6% of the total codes) highlighted the important function of Survivors Online as a vehicle for providing members particularly with encouragement (9.4%), sympathy (9.6%), and understanding and empathy (15.6%). This is particularly important considering the evidence that poorer adjustment to trauma is related

Table 3. The frequency of Cutrona and Suhr's (1992) social support categories across studies

Social Support Categories	Braithwaite, Waldron, and Finn (1999)	Coulson, Buchanan, and Aubeeluck (2007)	Coursaris and Liu (2009)	Yeager (2010) – Present study
Participants	Disabilities	Huntington's Disease	HIV/AIDS	Sexual Violence
INFORMATION	% OF TOTAL	% OF TOTAL	% OF TOTAL	% OF TOTAL
Advice	31.3	56.2	29.1	21.2
Referral	5.2	41.4	14.2	8.7
Situation appraisal	1.4	21.5	2.8	3.2
Teaching	11.8	7.9	6.0	1.6
	12.8	19.5	9.7	7.7
TANGIBLE ASSISTANCE	2.7	9.8	0.5	2.2
Loan	0	0	0.04	0
Perform direct task	1.7	6.5	0.02	0.1
Perform indirect task	0	0	0.1	0
Active participation	0.001	3.7	0.0	0.2
Express willingness	0.001	14.8	0.4	1.9
ESTEEM SUPPORT	18.6	21.7	5.9	20.9
Compliment	4.6	8.9	2.2	6.8
Validation	13.2	12.9	3.5	12.3
Relief of blame	0.008	2.9	0.4	1.8
NETWORK SUPPORT	7.1	48.4	5.2	13.1
Access	1.2	40.3	0.3	0.2
Presence	1.7	11.8	3.7	1.0
Companions	4.1	4.6	1.5	11.8
EMOTIONAL SUPPORT	40.0	51.9	12.9	42.6
Relationship	4.3	3.9	2.2	0.2
Physical affection	7.1	2.3	0.9	7.6
Confidentiality	0.003	7.1	0	0
Sympathy	2.7	9.0	1.6	9.6
Understanding or empathy	12.8	27.9	3.3	15.6
Encouragement	11.5	30.2	4.5	9.4
Prayer	1.5	14.4	2.8	0.2
NUMBER OF MESSAGES	1472	1299	5000	755

to lower levels of social support (Herman, 1997; Ullman, 1999).

Cutrona & Suhr's (1992) optimal matching model suggested that emotional support is more likely to be offered when the person is distressed about events that are not controllable. In contrast, informational support is most common when the person can control the situation and use the information productively. In the present study, the high level of emotional support (42.6%) supports Cutrona and Suhr's optimal matching model, as most members of Survivors Online are distressed about uncontrollable events related to the experience or sequelae of sexual victimization. This was followed by information support (21.2%) where members provided each other with advice (8.7%) and teaching (7.7%) specifically related to coping with the trauma experienced by victimization.

This data strongly suggests that the online seeking of social support for survivors of sexual violence warrants attention by researchers, mental health practitioners and policymakers as both emotion and information support plays a strong role in affording support on Survivors Online. This suggests that online support sites can become an important method for conveying accurate coping advice and messages to survivors of sexual violence.

Following emotional and information support, esteem support accounted for 20.9% of the

Table 4. Rank of overall category of support across studies using Cutrona & Suhr's (1992) framework[3]

Paper author	**Braithwaite *et al.* (1999)**	**Coulson *et al.* (2007)**	**Coursaris & Liu (2009)**	**Yeager (2010) - Present study**
Rank 1	Emotional	Information	Information	Emotional
2	Information	Emotional	Emotional	Information
3	Esteem	Network	Esteem	Esteem
4	Network	Esteem	Network	Network
5	Tangible	Tangible	Tangible	Tangible
Participants	Disabilities	Huntington's Disease	HIV/AIDS	Sexual Violence

total codes. The primary focus of esteem support posts was to validate a member's feelings and experiences (12.3%), followed by compliments (6.8%). The "fellow survivors" on the board have a personal perspective on the issues posted and can therefore validate other members' experiences by having "been there" themselves. Many posts included messages of validation, along with a compliment to the member to further boost their agreement with the person's perspective (e.g., "I totally agree with what you did, you are so brave!"). Somewhat surprisingly, relief of blame accounted for only 1.8% of posted messages.

Very few posts requesting support contained blaming messages. This is mostly likely due to two issues; firstly, very few new members posted on this forum (and the messages that did contain blaming posts were from new members). Secondly, other forums may be more likely places to have posts relating to the relief of blame. The "My Voice" forum is described on Survivors Online as the place to "share, seek help, discuss survivor related issues: the main forum". Alternatively, the "Moving forward" forum specifically states that "crisis, self-blame, and drama free, the focus of this forum is on the further steps in healing and how to get there". These forums are more likely to contain newer members introducing their story and experiences to other members for the first time, or to attract members struggling with self-blame related to their victimization, possibly accounting for the low occurrences of self-blame posts in the present study.

Network support (13.1%) ranked fourth (out of 5), and often involved members reinforcing the availability of support and help to others, particularly new members. This accounted for 11.8% of the 13.1% of posts. After this initial reinforcement of the availability of support to new members network support decreased dramatically in subsequent postings. Network support was quite rare in the present study, as it was in Cutrona & Suhr's (1992) study. Network support was also quite low in Braithwaite *et al.* (1999) and Coursaris & Liu's (2009) studies. The obvious reason is that participation in an online support group meets network support needs, so members do not make the availability and presence of support a focus of messages posted on the site.

With the least amount of postings (2.2%), the primary focus of tangible assistance posts focused on messages portraying a willingness to help (rather than concrete offers of specific intervention). The occurrence of these types of support were noticeably less than the other categories, most likely due to the nature of online communication, the anonymity and confidentiality afforded through the forum, and the fact that many of the member may be physically located anywhere from a few miles apart to continents apart. Due to the nature of online communication there were no posts offering loans or performing indirect tasks for members (this involves taking over a member's responsibilities while under stress). Only 3 posts offered to perform a direct task, and 4 posts offered to join members in activities to reduce their stress, but these active participation messages were symbolic in nature, rather than actual offers of tangible assistance (e.g., "I will be a pocket rider if that helps at all"). Of the 2.2% of posts related to tangible assistance, 1.9% of the posts (almost all) were expressions of willingness to help other members. These all took the form of offering to "be there" for other members by replying to emails and PMs (private messages).

FUTURE RESEARCH DIRECTIONS

This study was exploratory in nature and analyzed messages posted to one online forum. While this forum is clearly the most active and populated, it is not known if the results of this study are generalizable to other online groups of sexual violence survivors. Future research should compare content analyses of posts from more than one forum to assess the quality and quantity of exchanged social support across forums.

Similarly, this study focused on one message board within the Survivors Online forum. The "My Voice" message board is the busiest on Survivors Online, and was therefore selected for this study. However, it would be of interest to compare the results of this study to similar content analyses of other message boards within Survivors Online to ascertain if the quality and quantity of posted messages remains consistent.

CONCLUSION

This study strongly suggests that online support groups present a solution for survivors of sexual violence, who are often crippled by the need for understanding, empathy and validation as a result of their experiences. A critical understanding of how survivors of sexual violence use support groups to seek social support and coping and health-related information is essential in the evaluation and treatment of the sequelae of sexual victimization. This data can be used to inform mental health professionals and policy makers about how online support can be utilized to promote the welfare of survivors.

REFERENCES

Altheide, D. (1987). Ethnographic content analysis. *Qualitative Sociology*, *10*, 65–77. doi:10.1007/BF00988269

Braithwaite, D., Waldron, V., & Finn, J. (1999). Communication of social support in computer-mediated groups for people with disabilities. *Health Communication*, *1*, 123–151. doi:10.1207/s15327027hc1102_2

Coulson, N. (2005). Receiving social support online: An analysis of a computer-mediated support group for individuals living with irritable bowel syndrome. *Cyberpsychology & Behavior*, *8*(6), 580–584. doi:10.1089/cpb.2005.8.580

Coulson, N. (2008). Health-related virtual communities: An overview. *Health Psychology Update*, *17*(1), 37–41.

Coulson, N., Buchanan, H., & Aubeeluck, A. (2007). Social support in cyberspace: A content analysis of communication within a Huntington's disease online support group. *Patient Education and Counseling*, *68*(2), 173–178. doi:10.1016/j.pec.2007.06.002

Coursaris, C., & Liu, M. (2009). An analysis of social support exchanges in online HIV/AIDS self-help groups. *Computers in Human Behavior*, *25*(4), 911–918. doi:10.1016/j.chb.2009.03.006

Cutrona, C., & Suhr, J. (1992). Controllability of stressful events and satisfaction with spouse support behaviors. *Communication Research*, *19*, 154–176. doi:10.1177/009365092019002002

Finn, J. (1999). An exploration of helping processes in an online self-help group focusing on issues of disability. *Health & Social Work*, *24*, 220–232.

Finn, J., & Lavitt, M. (1994). Computer-based self-help groups for sexual abuse survivors. *Social Work with Groups*, *17*, 21–45. doi:10.1300/J009v17n01_03

Gooden, R., & Winefield, H. (2007). Breast and prostate cancer online discussion boards: A thematic analysis of gender differences and similarities. *Journal of Health Psychology*, *12*(1), 103–114. doi:10.1177/1359105307071744

Herman, J. (1997). *Trauma and recovery*. New York, NY: Basic Books.

Hsieh, H., & Shannon, S. (2005). Three approaches to qualitative content analysis. *Qualitative Health Research*, *15*(9), 1277–1288. doi:10.1177/1049732305276687

Illingworth, N. (2001). The Internet matters: Exploring the use if the Internet as a research tool. *Sociological Research Online, 6*(2). Retrieved June 21, 2008, from http://www.socresonline.org.uk/ 6/2/illingworth.html

Klemm, P., Bunnell, D., Cullen, M., Soneji, R., Gibbons, P., & Holecek, A. (2003). Self-help on-line: An outcome evaluation of breast cancer bulletin boards. *Journal of Health Psychology*, *10*(6), 855–862.

Lieberman, M., & Goldstein, B. (2005). Self help online: An outcome evaluation of breast cancer bulletin boards. *Journal of Health Psychology*, *10*, 855–862. doi:10.1177/1359105305057319

Mustanski, R. (2001). Getting wired: Exploiting the internet for the collection of valid sexuality data. *Journal of Sex Research*, *38*, 292–301. doi:10.1080/00224490109552100

Owen, J., Yarbrough, E., Vaga, A., & Tucker, D. (2003). Investigation of the effects of gender and preparation on quality of communication in Internet support groups. *Computers in Human Behavior*, *19*, 259–275. doi:10.1016/S0747-5632(02)00068-7

Popiel, D., & Susskind, E. (1985). The impact of rape: Social support as a moderator of stress. *American Journal of Community Psychology*, *13*, 645–676. doi:10.1007/BF00929794

Preece, J. (1999). Empathic communities: Balancing emotional and factual communication. *Interacting with Computers*, *12*(1), 63–77. doi:10.1016/S0953-5438(98)00056-3

Preece, J., & Ghozati, K. (1998). Observations and explorations of empathy online. In Rice, R., & Katz, J. (Eds.), *The Internet and health communication: Experience and expectations* (pp. 237–260). Thousand Oaks, CA: Sage.

Ravert, R., Hancock, M., & Ingersoll, G. (2004). Online forum messages posted by adolescents with type I diabetes. *The Diabetes Educator*, *30*(5), 827–834. doi:10.1177/014572170403000518

Riva, G. (2002). The sociocognitive psychology of computer-mediated communication: The present and future of technology-based interactions. *Cyberpsychology & Behavior*, *5*(6), 581–598. doi:10.1089/109493102321018222

Rodgers, C., & Gruener, D. (1997). Sequelae of sexual assault. *Primary Care Update for Ob/Gyns*, *4*(4), 143–146. doi:10.1016/S1068-607X(97)00011-5

Sanders-Phillips, K. (1997). Assaultive violence in the community: Psychological responses of adolescent victims and their parents. *The Journal of Adolescent Health*, *21*, 356–365. doi:10.1016/S1054-139X(97)00165-1

Sherman, R. (2001). The mind's eye in cyberspace: Online perceptions of self and others. In Riva, G., & Galimberti, C. (Eds.), *Towards cyberspsychology: Mind, cognition, and society in the internet age* (pp. 53–73). Washington, DC: IOS Press.

Ullman, S. (1999). Social support and recovery from sexual assault: A review. *Aggression and Violent Behavior: A Review Journal, 4*, 343-358.

Weinberg, N., Schmale, J., Uken, J., & Wessel, K. (1996). Online help: Cancer patients participate in a computer-mediated support group. *Health & Social Work*, *21*(1), 24–29.

Winzelberg, A. (1997). The analysis of an electronic support group for individuals with eating disorders. *Computers in Human Behavior*, *13*, 393–407. doi:10.1016/S0747-5632(97)00016-2

ENDNOTES

1 Pseudonym

2 Parantheses surrounding a person's name [e.g., (((((Jennifer))))] symbolize hugging that person.

3 Cutrona and Suhr's (1992) study focused on offline, marital dyads. The results of their study are therefore not relevant for inclusion here.

Chapter 7
Blogging:
A New Tool for Coping and Accessing Psycho-Social Support for People Living with HIV?

Cecilia Strand
Uppsala University, Sweden

ABSTRACT

Upon learning about an HIV-positive status, the individual is often faced with immense psychological stress. Besides coming to terms with a life-threatening disease, fears of stigma and discrimination are often attributed as stressors. The purpose of this chapter is to explore blogging as a tool to cope with a lifelong and highly stigmatized disease such as HIV/AIDS. A literature review and content analysis of six HIV-positive individuals' blogs indicate that blogging can be regarded as a tool for coping with HIV and potentially a form of self-administered therapy. Due to the ephemeral nature of blogs, the case blogs were revisited after 7 months to determine if they had been maintained. The fact that all six were still being updated regularly indicates that the bloggers found blogging about HIV/AIDS beneficial in one or several ways.

INTRODUCTION

With 33.4 million currently infected with HIV, and with approximately 7000 newly infected individuals every day (UNIADS, 2009), the virus has often been referred to as one of our time's great public health challenges (European Commission, 2010; Lewis, 2005).

HIV is a retro-virus that targets the body's immune system, and in particular its T-cells lymphocytes. As an HIV-infection progresses the number of CD4-positive T-lymphocytes decreases and, unless the infected individual has

DOI: 10.4018/978-1-60960-866-8.ch007

access to anti-retroviral treatment, he/she becomes increasingly vulnerable to a wide range of viral and bacterial infections, often referred to as opportunistic infections (Engel, 2006; Hoffman & Rockstroh, 2010). Without anti-retroviral therapy the individual dies after a variable period of time.

Despite nearly 30 years of research, there is still no vaccine (Hoffman & Rockstroh, 2010). Instead public health efforts have focused on two fronts: prevention of new infections, as well as, treatment and care of those already infected. Despite earlier disputes on disease control priorities, it is increasingly accepted that the earlier prevention vs. treatment dichotomy is not a constructive approach to a comprehensive HIV/AIDS strategy (D'Adesky, 2004; Barnett &Whiteside, 2006). Anti-retroviral treatment is not only life prolonging for the infected individual, but an essential component in motivating individuals to take part in voluntary counseling and to get tested for HIV in the first place. Moreover, prevention of infection will continue to be pivotal in future control strategies as anti-retroviral drugs are still relatively expensive despite recent reductions in prices. Furthermore, HIV with its high mutation rate is particularly well equipped to adapt to both new anti-retroviral treatment regimens and potential future vaccines (Engel, 2006).

Treatment options have improved significantly, in particularly in the developed world where HIV/AIDS is increasingly being regarded as a chronic disease that can be managed rather than a death sentence (Engel, 2006). Anti-retroviral treatment aims at suppressing the HIV-viral load in the body which prevents the virus from weakening the immune system (Hoffmann & Rockstroh, 2010). Anti-retroviral treatment needs to be taken consistently and without interruption to be effective (World Health Organization, 2003). In order to ensure that treatment options continue to save lives in both the developed and developing world, it is crucial to keep adherence rates high. Low adherence to treatment regimens results in HIV builds resistance and the drug eventually becomes useless (Hoffmann & Rockstroh, 2010; World Health Organization, 2003). An important factor for successful anti-retroviral treatment is the individual's acceptance of the situation, as well as access social support (Simoni, Frick, & Huang, 2006; Cornet, 2008; Nachega, Mills, & Mauro, 2010).

Accepting an HIV-infection and reaching out for medical and social support is however often hampered by the high level of stigma and discrimination attached to HIV/AIDS. HIV/AIDS has since it was discovered in the early 1980s' been intimately linked to various stigmatized groups' such as homosexuals, prostitutes and injecting drug users (Stoller, 1998; Engel, 2006). While HIV today also affects much less stigmatized groups, an HIV-positive status is still often associated with socially unacceptable behaviors, such as hypersexuality, promiscuity, prostitution and drug use (Dodds et al. 2004; Engel, 2006). HIV-infection thus continues to be burdened by external and internalized stigma and discrimination (Reeves, 2001; Adam & Sears, 1996).

According to Ray, Lindop and Gibson (1982) "Coping is action directed at the resolution or mitigation of a problematic situation" (p. 385). Lazarus and Folkman (1984) provide an expanded definition on coping as a "person's cognitive and behavioural efforts to manage internal and external demands on the person, which are appraised as taxing or exceeding the person's resources", and outline six different types of coping: rejection, control, resignation, dependency, avoidance and minimization. The act of 'coping' in this chapter refers to a situation where the individual cognitively accepts his/her situation and in particular the HIV infection, as well as behaviorally attempts to access social support in situations which exceed the individual's own resources.

While there are several studies showing the psychological benefits of traditional journal writing in coping with stressful life events, this chapter will review and explore the potential psycho-social benefits with blogging in dealing with a highly stigmatized, lifelong, and in many instances, debilitating disease, such as HIV/AIDS. Based on a literature review and a content analysis of six blogs that are part of an online community for HIV-positive individuals in the US, this chapter end up suggesting that blogging could serve as a tool for coping with HIV, as well as potentially serve as a type of self-administered therapy. Finally, this chapter argues that while there is not yet any research concluding that blogging has psycho-social benefits for individuals living with lifelong and highly stigmatized disease such as HIV/AIDS, there exist enough data outlining both the importance of addressing the non-clinical side of HIV/AIDS and benefits of blogging among other chronically ill individuals, as well as research showing the benefits of traditional journal writing to cope with stress, to motivate further research.

The chapter will begin with exploring the concept of coping and link the concept to HIV, as well as describe why coping is so important in relation to HIV. Blogging as a tool to assist in the process of coping is explored further by analysing six case blogs. The results of the content analysis and the potential implications are presented and discussed in the two final sections.

COPING WITH HIV/AIDS

HIV/AIDS is a taxing disease to live with: socially, due to the stigma and discrimination, physically, due to the deterioration of the immune system and later treatment side-effects, and finally psychologically. Kalichman and Sikkema (1994) conclude in a meta-analysis that HIV-infection and AIDS-related illness are related to a wide range of psychological distress reactions. Notably depression is prevalent in connection with diagnosis of an infection, and frequently reoccurs in connection with HIV-related illness symptoms. The individual's ability to handle these sides of an HIV-infection depends on his/her ability to cope cognitively and behaviourally.

The concept of 'coping' in this chapter refers to a situation where the individual cognitively accepts his/her situation and in particular the HIV-infection, as well as behaviorally attempts to access social support in situations which exceed the individual's own resources. Coping therefore does not always include the act of accessing social support. Furthermore, there is no temporal order between the two components of coping. Cognitive acceptance can be a prerequisite for attempting to access social support, and social support is most likely also an important factor in the process of cognitively coming to terms with an HIV-infection.

The effects of not coping have been investigated in several studies. Starace et al. (2002), conclude that depressive symptoms in people living with HIV are associated with low levels of adherence to anti-retroviral therapy. Leserman's (2008) review of several longitudinal studies from 1997-2007 shows that depression is related to clinical and immunological progression of HIV/AIDS, as well as mortality despite treatment. On that basis Leserman (2008) concludes that HIV treatment often focus on clinical aspects of the disease, and end up pointing out the need for "psychological/psychiatric screening, treatment and referrals to address depression and the psychological squeals of past trauma as part of standard HIV care" (p. 544).

Given that HIV is stressful from a social, psychological, and physiological perspective, HIV-positive individuals need to access not only appropriate clinical care, but social support. Kalichman et al. (1996, in Reeves, 2000) present three distinct types of social support utilized and needed by HIV-positive individuals: emotional, informational, and instrumental. Emotional support consists of "affection, comforting, and encouragement that results in a sense of belonging and personal worth"; and informational support entails increasing one's knowledge base; and finally, instrumental support provides "practical assistance with daily living" (Kalichman et al., 1996, p. 590, in Reeves, 2000). These three types of support help alleviate the psychological stress that accompanies a stigmatized and chronic illness such as HIV/AIDS.

Other research focusing on HIV-positive individuals' Internet use and their coping ability found that acquiring information online, helping and supporting others, as well as the social support available through virtual networks increased the users' ability to cope (Reeves, 2000). Virtual network was particular important as unlike people, it was always there. Moreover, in a subsequent study, Reeves (2001) found two other reasons to use the Internet: advocating and escaping. The informants in Reeves' (2001) study all relied heavily on online resources to stay updated on the latest treatment developments, as well as to locate and communicate with individuals in a similar position with whom the informants could identify. Participants in the study reported that these were important tools in coping with life as HIV-positive.

In a survey of HIV-positive individuals in the U.S, Kalichman et al. (2003) also found that health-related internet use was associated with active coping in the form of information seeking and accessing social support. They note, however, that health information is not equally accessible to poorly educated, economically disadvantaged, and socially marginalized individuals. In two separate studies (Kalichman, Benotsch, Weinhardt, Austin, & Luke 2002; Kalichman et al. 2006) it was found that people living with HIV/AIDS who use the Internet, frequently consulted online sources for additional health information such as finding news and clinical trials outcomes. These individuals displayed an active health information seeking behaviour. Active health information seeking behaviour and problem-focused coping style is, according to research by Devins and Binik (1996), associated with health benefits for some people with chronic medical conditions. Moreover, Kalichman et al (2005) found that, "Individuals who used the internet for health information were less likely to miss taking their HIV medications and this difference was not accounted for by other demographic characteristics" (p. 446). Kalichman et al. (2006) conclude that the "Internet is therefore broadening the available active coping resources for some people living with chronic diseases, including HIV infection" (p.209).

BLOGGING: A TOOL FOR COPING AND SOCIAL SUPPORT

A blog is defined as a web page with a series of dated entries presented in reversed chronological order, often run and frequently modified by a single individual (Blood, 2002; Baker, Psych, & Moore, 2008). While many blogs are like online unlocked diaries, there is a growing number of professional blogs with several contributors providing information and commentary on various topics.

Nardi (2004) identifies five main motivations for why individuals blog: (a) documenting one's life, (b) providing commentary on issues of importance to the blogger, (c) expressing and handling thoughts and emotions, (d) articulating and developing ideas through writing, and (e) forming and maintaining virtual communities. Trammell, Tarkowski, and Sapp (2006), guided by a user and gratification perspective on blogging, found that among bloggers in Poland the main motivation for blogging was self-expression rather than social interaction, entertainment, passing time and satisfying information needs. Other studies have, however, found that blogging is often motivated by a wish for social interaction (Baker, 2008; Nardi, Schiano, Gumbrecht, & Swartz, 2004).

Depending on the content, and features of the blog, blogging offers opportunities for dialogue, yet the blogger is able to escape the sometimes intensive feedback associated with, for example, face to face communication. Gumbrecht (2004) finds that such a lack of co-temporality provides a type of protection from immediate and sometimes unwanted social reaction. The blog allows the blogger to anonymously vent with few restrictions in content. In short, blogging offers a protected space to communicate subject matters that might otherwise be difficult to express in regular social interaction (Gumbrecht, 2004).

Journal writing as a therapeutic device has been well documented and shown to lead to "significant improvements in the author's physical health, psychological well-being, psychological functioning and overall functioning" (Baker, Psych, & Moore, 2008 p. 81). Baker et al. (2008) also found that blogging seemed to not only relieve isolation and alienation, but improve sense of community. Accordingly, they suggest that blogging has beneficial effects on well-being, specifically in terms of perceived social support.

A few studies have focused on the potential benefits of blogging and participation in online communities for individuals with a chronic illness, most notably cancer patients (Leimeister, Schweizer, Leimeister, & Krcmar, 2008; Kim & Chung, 2007; Chung & Kim, 2008). Gonzalez and Lengacher (2007) conclude in a study on individuals with breast cancer that "Non-disclosure of emotions has been shown to inhibit individuals' adjustment to illness and formulation of adequate coping mechanisms". Chung and Kim (2007, 2008) conclude that blogging and the sharing of personal experiences helped cancer patients and their friends and families to better cope with their cancer-related health conditions. Moreover, blogging facilitates individuals linking up to the social support that is found when connecting to others afflicted by the same condition and thus relieves feelings of isolation.

Nguyen, Carrieri-Kohlman, Rankin, Slaughter and Stulb (2003) concluded that access to virtual support can be very important to those whose disability impairs their mobility. "The online community eliminates geographic constraints, allows for anonymity, 24-h access to search for information that may help in feeling more in control of a situation, and possibly minimize feelings of isolation" (Nguyen, et al., p. 96). Jacobs and Goodman (1989) identified that the most important therapeutic features of self-help groups were the way these provided access to individuals who experience a common problem (i.e. 'homogeneity of concern') and access to a normative community where the individual is transformed from being abnormal in their surrounding society to normal within the group. According to Jacobs and Goodman (1989), these two functions of self-help groups can empower individuals in a way that cannot be re-created by professional counselors. Leimeister et al. (2008), however note that the intensity of Internet usage (active posting vs. lurking) was a significant factor in determining the rewards of online community participation.

In conclusion, based in the reviewed research there is good reason to believe that blogging—when it leads to regularly disclosing emotions and expressing thoughts, commenting on issues of importance to the blogger, sharing information and finally, finding and maintaining virtual networks of support—has the potential to improve an HIV-positive blogger's general psycho-social well-being, and support him/her coping with the disease.

EXPLORING COPING AND SOCIAL SUPPORT IN 6 CASE BLOGS

In order to further explore blogging as a tool to coping with HIV, the coping concept was operationalized using the research findings from the literature review. By merging the three types of social support: emotional, informational, and instrumental identified by Kalichman et al. (1996), with the findings of Gonzalez and Lengacher (2007), and Chung and Kim (2007, 2008) on disclosure of emotions in order to adjust to illness and formulate adequate coping mechanisms, as well as the findings by Reeves (2000, 2001) on advocacy and social networking; four new categories was constructed that was believed to capture the multi-dimensionality of coping with a chronic

Figure 1. Screen shot of the POZ portal

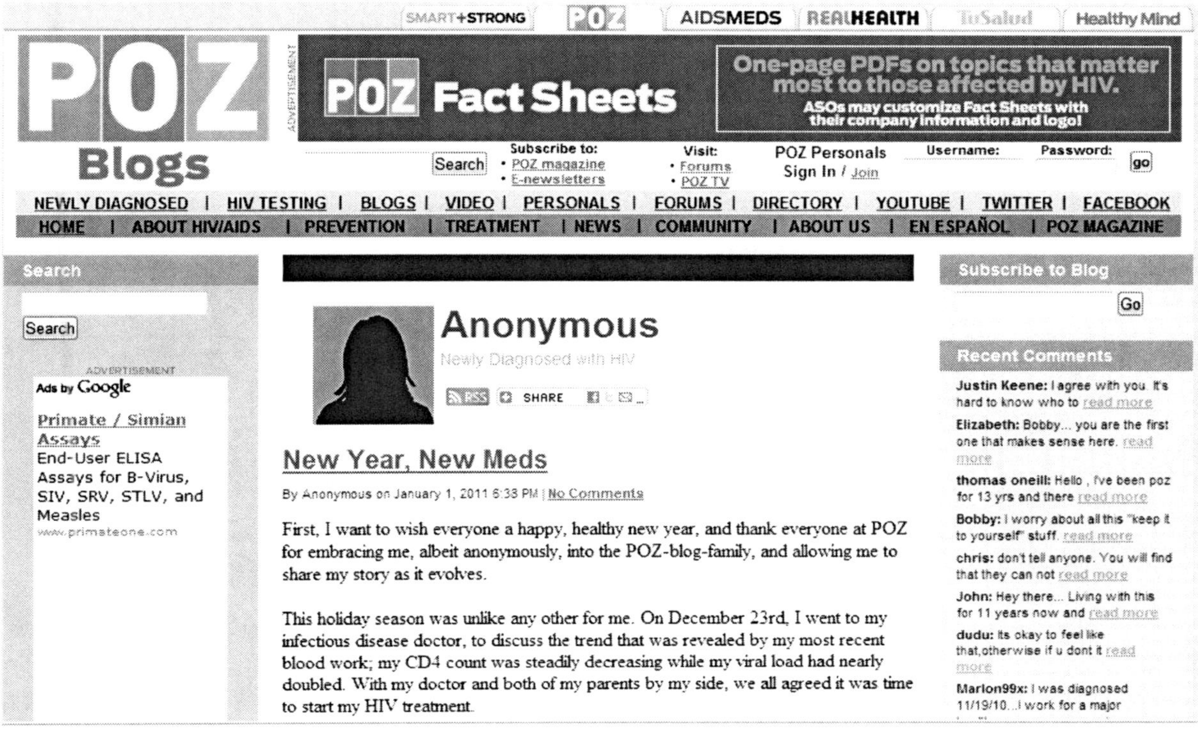
SMART+STRONG
POZ
AIDSMEDS
REALHEALTH
Healthy Mind
POZ
Blogs
ADVERTISEMENT
POZ Fact Sheets
One-page PDFs on topics that matter most to those affected by HIV.
ASOs may customize Fact Sheets with their company information and logo!
Search
Subscribe to:
• POZ magazine
• E-newsletters
Visit:
• Forums
• POZ TV
POZ Personals
Sign In / Join
Username:
Password:
go
NEWLY DIAGNOSED | HIV TESTING | BLOGS | VIDEO | PERSONALS | FORUMS | DIRECTORY | YOUTUBE | TWITTER | FACEBOOK
HOME | ABOUT HIV/AIDS | PREVENTION | TREATMENT | NEWS | COMMUNITY | ABOUT US | EN ESPAÑOL | POZ MAGAZINE
Search
Search
ADVERTISEMENT
Ads by Google
Primate / Simian Assays
End-User ELISA Assays for B-Virus, SIV, SRV, STLV, and Measles
www.primateone.com
Anonymous
Newly Diagnosed with HIV
RSS
SHARE
New Year, New Meds
By Anonymous on January 1, 2011 6:38 PM | No Comments
First, I want to wish everyone a happy, healthy new year, and thank everyone at POZ for embracing me, albeit anonymously, into the POZ-blog-family, and allowing me to share my story as it evolves.
This holiday season was unlike any other for me. On December 23rd, I went to my infectious disease doctor, to discuss the trend that was revealed by my most recent blood work; my CD4 count was steadily decreasing while my viral load had nearly doubled. With my doctor and both of my parents by my side, we all agreed it was time to start my HIV treatment.
Subscribe to Blog
Go
Recent Comments
Justin Keene: I agree with you. It's hard to know who to read more
Elizabeth: Bobby... you are the first one that makes sense here. read more
thomas oneill: Hello , I've been poz for 13 yrs and there read more
Bobby: I worry about all this "keep it to yourself" stuff. read more
chris: don't tell anyone. You will find that they can not read more
John: Hey there... Living with this for 11 years now and read more
dudu: Its okay to feel like that,otherwise if u dont it read more
Marlon99x: I was diagnosed 11/19/10...I work for a major

disease. The hypothesis is that the existence of the four new categories:

1. social interaction,
2. information sharing,
3. self-expression and,
4. social commentary

in blogs written by individuals living with HIV, would at least in theory make blogging beneficial to the blogger from a psycho-social perspective, and subsequently support his/her coping with HIV. Six blogs by HIV-positive individuals were used to explore the concept empirically.

As this study is explorative, it relies on a purposive sample procedure. Purposive sampling entails "selecting information rich cases for in-depth analysis related to the central issues being studied" (COL undated: 47). The case blogs were selected through an active online community: the POZ.com and their bloggers. The POZ portal offers daily news, treatment updates, blogs and an online social network that includes personal ads; a moderated community forum; and a private, peer-to-peer mentoring program (see Figure 1). The objective of POZ is to address the wide spectrum of needs of people living with and affected by HIV/AIDS.

The POZ blogs section describes the blogs in the following way: "These are the autobiographical stories, rants, raves, mental machinations and poetic waxings of people living with or affected by HIV/AIDS. The POZ bloggers hail from all corners of the HIV community" (blogs.poz 2010, unnumbered webpage). In November 2010 the portal had grown to host 30 bloggers, four women, 25 men, and one anonymous individual.

Analysing blog content carries several benefits. Blogs provide publicly available information that are not tampered with as there are few restrictions imposed on what material a blogger or blog followers can post. Hookway (2008) argues

Table 1. Coding sheet used for each blog

Blogger ID:			
Number of entries: 1/3-1/6 2009			
Content Categories	**Description of category**		
Social interaction	**Facilitation of social interaction Y/N:** **If yes: Number of Social interaction accomplished (e.g. Received comments):** **Attempts to engage with readers by posing (non-rhetorical) questions in blog entries?** **If yes: number of blog entries containing questions to the readers**		
Information sharing	Blogging to share HIV/AIDS information and/or HIV/AIDS related news. News /information shared, but mainly un-commented by the blogger.	n:	Illustrative ex:
Self –expression	Blogging to share personal information on life as HIV positive. Blogging to communicate and handle personal feelings and thoughts on events. Blogger provide an inside view on how an event was perceived by the blogger.	n:	Illustrative ex:
Social Commentary	Blogging to provide commentary on social issues or news of importance to the blogger. The phenomena is commented and evaluated according to the bloggers stand point.	n:	Illustrative ex:

that the anonymity of the online context enables bloggers to write more honestly and candidly. The anonymity allows the blogger to ignore the social conventions directing face-to-face interaction, and thus remain relatively unselfconscious about what they write. Moreover, because the interactions are logged in their entirety, the information are in one sense complete and unmediated by, for example, an interviewer and un-directed by interview or survey questions. When analysing blogs a researcher can "assume the role of lurkers who unobtrusively observes community engagement, which preserves the purity of the data" (Kvasny & Igwe, 2008 p. 8). In short, blogs offer a wealth of uninfluenced data.

Selection Criteria

The following selection criteria were applied to select case blogs: a) the blog had to be active March 1st to June 1st, 2009, b) the blog had to contain more than five entries during that timeframe, and c) the blog had to have been updated during May 2009, thus ensuring that it was still active. In total six blogs fulfilled the selection criteria.

Coding Sheet and Coding Procedure

A coding sheet was developed to capture the basic quantitative features of the blog such as gender of blogger, number of entries, as well as, the four categories.

Social interaction was assessed by measuring (a) the provision of tools for personal interaction such as provision of a comment function, private email, Facebook, Twitter id etc., (b) whether or not the blog author probed for interaction by posing non-rhetorical questions to his/her readers, and (c) rate of accomplished interaction, e.g. number of comments (See Table 1 for coding sheet).

The second category *information sharing* captures the existence of HIV and health related information in the blog. The third category, *self-expression,* attempts to capture disclosure of thoughts and feelings in relation to HIV; finally, *social commentary* attempts to capture elements of advocacy and commentary on issues or news of importance to the blogger.

Each blog's basic features were recoded onto the coding sheet, and each entry was read and coded to include up to two content categories. That is, the entries which contained several content categories were recorded to contain the two most prominent categories. Moreover, only the blog's text, and not pictures, U-tube clips, links to music, hyperlinks, etc. was included in the interest of time.

The Blogs Revisited 2010

If a blog is continued over time and is not the result of paid employment or a commercial enterprise, it is assumed that the blogging process is rewarding and fulfills one or several of the blogger's needs. Therefore, the case blogs were revisited seven months after the initial study was completed. The return to the blogs in January 2010 sought to establish; a) if the blogs were still being maintained, and b) if anything set the surviving blogs apart from the blogs that had not been maintained.

Limitations

The small sample size and the fact that they all belong to the same established on-line community is a considerable limitation. Moreover, being purposively selected, the sample is clearly biased. Levy (1988 in King 2004) elaborates on the methodological dilemma in researching the therapeutic role of self-help groups. Active members are, for the most part, made up of people for whom the group has at least a minimum therapeutic value and as a result; "Outcome results are thus always positively biased in favour of the group being helpful" (Levy, 1988 in King, 2004 p. 10). It is highly likely that the same effect would prevail in blogs that are updated regularly and maintained over extended time periods. In addition, the purposive sample in this study resulted in a limited sample variation in terms of age and gender.

Another limitation is that the study does not include interviews or any other interaction with the bloggers. Interviews exploring the bloggers' own perceptions would have provided important insights into blogging as a tool to cope with HIV/AIDS and access social support.

RESULTS

While the POZ.com community includes some female bloggers, none of them were active according to the selection criteria. Subsequently, the sample of six case blogs turned out to be entirely dominated by males, and in most cases openly gay. This result of overrepresentation of homosexual men is most likely not only a result of the POZ portal being hosted in the US, but has historical roots. American male gays were the first group to be hard hit by HIV/AIDS in the 1980's (Engel, 2006). Due to prevailing discrimination against homosexuals at that time, they were forced early on to organize themselves around HIV/AIDS in order to demand their rights to treatment, care and respect. Their overrepresentation in this sample can thus be an effect of the fact that the male gay movement has an established cultural pattern of Internet use for organizational purposes.

This section will present the results on the four main categories: *social interaction, information sharing, self–expression*, and *social commentary,* as well as provide some illustrative extracts from the blogs.

Social Interaction

All bloggers provided their readers with the opportunity for interaction either through posting of a comment, or more private communication channels such as, Face Book page, personal email or Instant Messenger id. All bloggers also received comments to various degrees (Table 2). One blog did however receive far more comments than any other blog. A key feature of this popular blog was its clear focus on self-expression. It candidly shared intimate information on life as HIV-positive, and the blog's personal style in addressing its readers could be the reason behind its popularity. As for prompting interaction by posing non-rhetorical questions to the readers, few bloggers used this tool to probe further interaction. Moreover, there seems to be no clear connection between blog

Table 2. Level of social interaction by blogger

Social interaction						
Blogger by initial and number of entries.	**DW (7)**	**RF (12)**	**PS (6)**	**DC (8)**	**OG (30)**	**PD (23)**
Facilitation of Social interaction: Comments solicited through feedback forms, twitter, FB page, email and provision of Instant Messenger id, etc.	yes	yes	yes	yes	yes	yes
Prompt interaction by posing questions to the readers. Number of entries containing questions.	2	4	2	3	1	3
Social interaction accomplished: Number of online comments	15	99	45	28	26	28

entry frequency and level of feedback from the readers. Instead of diligent updates, it appears that the blog's style is a much more important predictor for interaction between blog author and reader.

Information Sharing, Self–Expression, and Social Commentary

While five out of six blogs included information sharing, self-expression, and social commentary content to various degrees, each blog emphasized different content features (See Figure 2 for blog profiles).

Self-Expression

Self-expression is a feature in all blogs. For some bloggers, the blog is clearly an outlet to express emotions and thoughts and on being HIV positive. Some blog entries appear to be pure venting exercises, where the author in a candid and raw manner vents his distress, sense of isolation and lack of social support. The following is a transcript from one of the case blogs.

There's not going to be any positive spin on this blog, no patina of optimism, or light on the end of the tunnel. AIDS sucks. Can I be miserable for a month or so? Actually I really haven't been happy for years. I was certainly a great liar in my writing telling stories about spinal taps and diapers with a smile. Yes, I'm having an Official Pity Party for One. The combination of losing my internship at POZ, a major screw up on my Social Security Disability and Medicare (which thankfully has been resolved,) new and different medication side effects… Facebook friends are alway there, but you can't cyber-cry on someone shoulder. My face ain't looking so great either. I was told to return for another treatment, but because of lack of funds and the swine flu outbreak everything it on hold. Forget about dating or having sex, you don't even want to know the last time I was intimate with someone, or you probably wouldn't believe it anyway. I'm actually glad my testosterone is so low it helped me steer clear of a lot of rejection, and stopped me from thinking with my dick. And what is my goal, my purpose in life, besides paying too much for rent to live in Manhattan? Feeling alone, immobile and frustrated, thanks for letting me regurgitate on your blogosphere. (D.C, May 1, 2009)

The entry below was commented 17 times.

Can someone explain to me why I feel like shit? Here is the deal. I am 53 years old, work out 6 days a week and it shows, my "numbers" are excellent, I do not drink, smoke, or drug at all. I eat well, pray, meditate, go to church every Sunday, and try not to fuck up other people's lives as general rule. I am nearly 99.9% adherent to

Figure 2. Content distribution between bloggers and number of entries within parenthesis

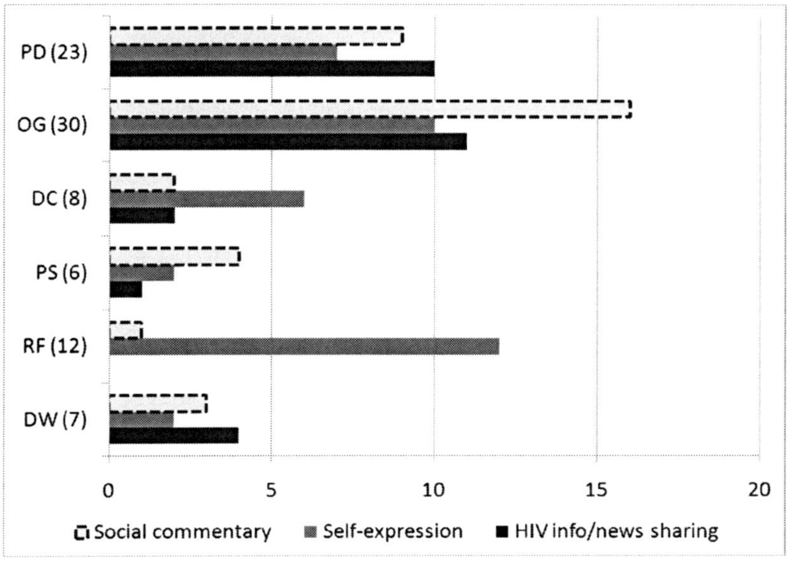

my HIV medications, and my only other medical problem is an enlarged prostate; yet I feel like shit some days. I have been talking and writing about this for years. I call these days of total and unexplained pain, exhaustion, fatigue, and other bullshit "AIDS days". So I am tired of talking about them now and I want someone to give me an answer. Better yet... how about a solution? (R.F April 20, 2009)

Below is a selection of comments R.F received:

I wanted to respond to you regarding your blog. I also do have "AIDS Days" all the time. For me, it is just a day to review all the bad that I have done. The hows and whys that I contracted this disease. I have been positive for 3 years, and I am still having issues with it. So I wish there was something that could be said, but the best thing for anyone to do is to just work thru it. (Joe, 29 April 2009)

WHAT I CAN ADVISE YOU IS, ACCEPT JESUS CHRIST IN YOUR LIFE IN TRUTH AND IN SPIRIT (SAMBO 29 April 2010)

probably the meds. I felt the same way on every regimen for the past 20 years. I was out of options several times, as I am sure you have been and often thought it wasnt worth living feeling so sick and wretched. the came a miralce for me, prezista. yeah, its still a fucking poisonous protease inhibitor but it does not make me sick. It still causes hideous fat deposits, lypodystrophy, and I cant eat any carbs but I have never felt better in my life. (Jack, 4 may 2009)

Information Sharing

Five out of six blogs regularly shared HIV-related news and information. A majority of the information in this content category was oriented towards sharing news on new treatment options and new drugs. Given the life-long medication needs, the complexity of the disease and its ability to mutate, and the constant evolution in medical research, keeping abreast with the developments of new treatments is an important component in coping with HIV. Ensuring oneself and the readers that there is constantly newer and better medicines being developed is most likely not only a way to cope with adverse side effects of current treatment, but also a way to ensure that even individuals with long treatment histories is not running out of treatment options.

The drug KP-1461 has long fascinated me (1, 2). It's novel mechanism- called Viral Decay Acceleration attempts to treat HIV infection by coaxing the virus into mutating itself to death. Years ago, I met with Koronis, the company developing the drug, as the were ramping up their development program. Fascinated by the sheer audacity of this mechanism, I have followed this drug a bit more closely than other drugs at similar stages of development ...Last week Koronis issued a press release- copied below- claiming that their scientific advisory board had reviewed all of the clinical trials and laboratory data on KP-1461 and confirmed that it has measurable anti-viral activity and development of this compound will move forward. As is typical, the press release is short on details. It states that 'recently completed passaging experiment' confirmed results from earlier, similar work. It was those passaging studies that were in question- the first set showed activity, a second set did not, and now apparently this third set confirms the first set of results. I am not satisfied. I am awaiting a formal presentation of these results. (P.D on May 23, 2009)

People living with HIV could soon monitor their own condition at home using a hand-held device, similar to ones used by diabetics. Scientists at three of London's largest research centres have been granted £2m to develop a hi-tech, finger prick blood-testing gadget. The device's tiny mechanical sensors - microcantilever arrays - measure HIV levels to warn of impending flare ups. A display then alerts the user if there is any need for them to visit a doctor. (D. W, May 6, 2009)

Social Commentary

Social commentary, that is, commenting on the surrounding society response to the HIV epidemic, or lack thereof, appeared with a surprising high frequency. This might be the result of the gay community's history of mobilization and collective action, where criticism of existing policies and demand for better health care services formed an important part of the movement's overall campaign strategy, and success.

In the wake of this week's defeat in the special election California's Governor Schwartzeneger, or as many like him the Governator, has proposed cutting all general fund money for AIDS- meaning massive cut back in prevention, early intervention programs, and ADAP. It would also likely threaten some Federal money- Ryan White- which is tied to certain state funding requirements. The state of California has long been a leader in the response against HIV/AIDS- but that is now threatened. Have no doubt, this will be fought tooth and nail. (P.D May 22, 2009)

Finally, all blogs were revisited in January 2010 to see if some or all were being maintained. All blogs were up and running and had had various degrees of activity. While there is an inherent bias in the sample due to the selection criteria, it is interesting that all of the case blogs were being maintained. This result contradicts blogs' usual ephemeral nature and indicates that this type of blogging is rewarding in one or several way.

DISCUSSION

As discussed earlier HIV is "special" in terms of the psychological challenges it places on infected individuals. Nevertheless, the individual's level of psycho-social well-being and ability to cope, is closely linked to adherence to anti-retroviral treatment, and disease progression, and thus of great importance. This chapter have explored blogging as a tool to cope with HIV and to access psycho-social support.

The research by Leimeister et al. (2008) on the importance of active participation (as opposed to lurking) to reap the rewards of online community participation, and the findings by Gonzalez and Lengacher (2007) that non-disclosure of emotions inhibits the individuals' adjustment to illness and formulation of adequate coping mechanisms, and research carried out by Chung and Kim (2007, 2008) highlighting the importance of sharing personal experiences via blogs among cancer patients to better cope;, and finally, research by Kalichman et al. (1996) and Reeves (2000, 2001) on the importance of access to social support indicates that blogging could be a tool and prime candidate to provide positive psycho-social benefits to the blogger.

But is blogging merely a tool? Returning to the definition of coping as an "action directed at the resolution or mitigation of a problematic situation", would rather indicate that blogging is also simultaneously a quiet active act of coping. The case blogs contain rich narratives dealing with acceptance of HIV/AIDS, disclosure of intimate feelings and self-expression, venting to relieve psychological stress, receive and share HIV -related health information, attempt to influence social policy, as well as, attempts to reach out to virtual social support. The case blogs' would thus indicate that the very act of blogging about life as HIV-positive includes acts of mitigation and attempt at resolving issues of importance.

Blogging is not a magic bullet suitable for everyone, and should not be seen as a quick fix for acute or chronic depression and deep social isolation. Rather blogging could perhaps function as a form of self-administered therapy and complement to other forms of support for those who are isolated from traditional means of social support, such as family, friends and community-based support organizations due to geographical constraints, fear of discrimination or medical circumstances. More research is needed to determine if blogging should be recommended as part of a package of interventions seeking to support the psychological well-being among people living with HIV. The fact that HIV is a highly stigmatized disease does, however, indicate that blogging is particularly suitable for this group and their non-clinical needs.

FUTURE RESEARCH DIRECTIONS

Even if this study's convenience sample is small and not representative in any way for people living with HIV, this chapter argues that there is an unexplored and untapped potential for blogging as *one* tool to assist coping with HIV/AIDS. Moreover, taking into account the costs connected with psychological health care, many health care systems prioritize medical interventions, leaving psycho-social aspects of illness to other actors or to the individual. Accordingly, there are several reasons why the therapeutic role of blogging warrants further research, and preferably through a standard randomized control group research design, with a treatment of e.g. blogging group and a non-blogging control group.

While the reviewed cases do not include any youth bloggers, there are compelling reasons why HIV-positive youth should be prioritised in further research of the psycho-social benefits of blogging. First of all, youths are often in the early stages of their HIV infection and in many instances have not yet begun anti-retroviral treatment. Accordingly, they have less regular contact with the formal health sector services (Flicker et al. 2004). Nevertheless, their needs for health information and psycho-social support are no less pressing than those of adults. Secondly, they are going to live and be sexually active with the virus for a long time. In short, it is important to promote physical and psychological self-care, as well as prevention messages aiming to avoid re-infection and infection of others. Promoting blogging and/

or the reading of other individuals living with HIV and their blogs could potentially improve young HIV-positive individuals' ability to cope with a life as HIV positive, and alleviate their sense of isolation by connecting them to virtual normative communities battling similar issues.

CONCLUSION

HIV/AIDS-related stigma and society's discrimination of people living with HIV makes it more difficult for people to come to terms with an HIV-positive diagnosis, and subsequently manage their illness by both accessing appropriate HIV treatment and make full use of care (Sayles et el. 2009). Coming to terms with a stigmatized, lifelong and possibly fatal disease such HIV/AIDS, entails not only accepting the physical consequences of an HIV-infection, but also finding ways to accept and cope with the social and psychological aspects. Living a full life despite of HIV is dependent on the individual's ability to cope, which entails not only cognitively accepting the condition, but reaching out and accessing social support in situations where the need exceeds the individual's own resources. The results of the literature review and case study presented in this chapter show that blogging embodies several of the coping concept's components and accordingly has a potential to deliver a range of psycho-social benefits for the blogging individual.

REFERENCES

Baker, J., Psych, M., & Moore, S. M. (2008). Distress, coping, and blogging: Comparing new Myspace users by their intention to blog. *Cyberpsychology & Behavior*, *11*(3), 81–85. doi:10.1089/cpb.2007.9930

Barnett, T., & Whiteside, A. (2006). *AIDS in the twenty-first century: Disease and globalization*. New York, NY: Palgrave Macmillan.

Blood, R. (2002). *The weblog handbook: Practical advice on creating and maintaining your blog*. Cambridge, MA: Perseus Publishing.

Brashers, D., Haas, S., Neidig, J., & Rintamaki, L. (2002). Social activism, self-advocacy, and coping with HIV illness. *Journal of Social and Personal Relationships*, *19*(1), 113–133. doi:10.1177/0265407502191006

Chung, D., & Kim, S. (2008). Blogging activity among cancer patients and their companions: Uses, gratifications and predictors of outcomes. *Journal of the American Society for Information Science and Technology*, *59*(2), 297–306. doi:10.1002/asi.20751

Commonwealth of Learning Center Asia (COL). (n.d.). *Manual for educational media researchers-know your audience*. COL. Retrieved October 1, 2010, from http://www.cemca.org/ books/

Cornet, M. (2008). *Overcoming barriers in ART-adherence: Experiences from Uganda*. IS Academy. January 2008. Retrieved December 1, 2010, from http://www.minbuza.nl/ dsresource?objectid=buzabeheer:50355&versionid=&subobjectname=

D'Adesky, A. (2004). *Moving mountains: The race to treat global AIDS*. London, UK: Verso.

Dodds, C., Keogh, P., Chime, O., Haruperi, T., Nabulya, B., Ssanyu, S., & Weatherburn, P. (2004). *Outsider status: Stigma and discrimination experienced by gay men and African people with HIV*. Sigma Research. Retrieved October 1, 2010, from www.sigmaresearch.org.uk/ downloads/report04f.pdf

Engel, J. (2006). *The epidemic: A global history of AIDS*. New York, NY: Smithsonian Books/Collins.

European Commission. (2010). *EU research fighting the three major deadly diseases: HIV/AIDS, malaria and tuberculosis*. Research EU, 1st edition EU projects 2007-2010. Retrieved December 13, 2010, from http://ec.europa.eu/ research/ health/ infectious-diseases/ poverty-diseases/ doc/ prd-catalogue-fp7_en.pdf

Flicker, S., Goldberg, E., Read, S., Veinot, T., McClelland, A., Saulnier, P., & Skinner, H. (2004). HIV-positive youth's perspectives on the internet and e-health. *Journal of Medical Internet Research*, *6*(3), e32. doi:10.2196/jmir.6.3.e32

Gonzalez, L., & Lengacher, C. (2007). Coping with breast cancer: A qualitative analysis of reflective journals. *Mental Health Nursing*, *28*(5), 489–510. doi:10.1080/01612840701344472

Gumbrecht, M. (2004, May). *Blogs as protected space*. Paper presented at the 13th International Conference on World Wide Web, New York, NY. Retrieved June 3, 2010, from www.blogpulse.com/ papers/ www2004gumbrecht.pdf

Hoffmann, C., & Rockstroh, J. (2010). *HIV 2010*. Hamburg, Germany: Medizin Fokus Verlag.

Hookway, N. (2008). Entering the blogosphere: Some strategies for using blogs in social research. *Qualitative Research*, *8*(1), 91–113. doi:10.1177/1468794107085298

Jacobs, K., & Goodman, G. (1989). Psychology and self help groups: Predictions on a partnership. *The American Psychologist*, *443*, 536–545. doi:10.1037/0003-066X.44.3.536

Kalichman, S., Benotsch, E., Weinhardt, L., Austin, J., & Luke, W. (2002). Internet use among people living with HIV/AIDS: Association of health information, health behaviors, and health status. *AIDS Education and Prevention*, *14*(1), 51–61. doi:10.1521/aeap.14.1.51.24335

Kalichman, S., Benotsch, E. G., Weinhardt, L., Austin, J., Luke, W., & Cherry, C. (2003). Health-related Internet use, coping, social support, and health indicators in people living with HIV/AIDS: Preliminary results from a community survey. *Health Psychology*, *22*(1), 111–116. doi:10.1037/0278-6133.22.1.111

Kalichman, S., Cain, D., Cherry, C., Pope, H., Eaton, L., & Kalichman, M. O. (2005). Internet use among people living with HIV/AIDS: Coping and health-related correlates. *AIDS Patient Care and STDs*, *19*(7), 439–448. doi:10.1089/apc.2005.19.439

Kalichman, S., Cherry, C., Cain, D., Weinhardt, L., Benotsch, E., Pope, H., & Kalichman, M. (2006). Health information on the internet and people living with HIV/AIDS: Information evaluation and coping styles. *Health Psychology*, *25*(2), 205–210. doi:10.1037/0278-6133.25.2.205

Kalichman, S. C., & Sikkema, K. J. (1994). Psychological sequelae of HIV infection and AIDS: Review of empirical findings. *Clinical Psychology Review*, *14*(7), 611–632. doi:10.1016/0272-7358(94)90001-9

Kim, S., & Chung, D. S. (2007). Characteristics of cancer blog user. *Journal of the Medical Library Association*, *95*(4), 445–450. doi:10.3163/1536-5050.95.4.445

Kvasny, L., & Igwe, F. (2008). An African American weblog community's reading of AIDS in Black America. *Journal of Computer-Mediated Communication*, *13*(3), 569–592. doi:10.1111/j.1083-6101.2008.00411.x

Lazarus, R. S., & Folkman, S. (1984). *Stress, appraisal and coping*. New York, NY: Springer.

Leimeister, J. M., Schweizer, K., Leimeister, S., & Krcmar, H. (2008). Do virtual communities matter for the social support of patients? Antecedents and effects of virtual relationships in online communities. *Information Technology & People*, *21*(4), 350–374. doi:10.1108/09593840810919671

Leserman, J. (2008). Role of depression, stress, and trauma in HIV disease progression. *Psychosomatic Medicine*, *70*, 539–545. doi:10.1097/PSY.0b013e3181777a5f

Lewis, S. (2005). *Race against time*. Toronto, Canada: House of Anansi Press.

Nachega, J., Mills, E., & Schechter, M. (2010). Antiretroviral therapy adherence and retention in care in middle-income and low-income countries: Current status of knowledge and research priorities. *Current Opinion in HIV & AIDS*, *5*(1), 70–77. doi:10.1097/COH.0b013e328333ad61

Nardi, B. (2004). Why we blog. *Communications of the ACM*, *47*(12). Retrieved from http://darrouzet-nardi.net/bonnie/pdf/Nardi_why_we_blog.pdf. doi:10.1145/1035134.1035163

Nardi, B., Schiano, D. J., & Gumbrecht, M. (2004). Blogging as social activity, or, would you let 900 million people read your diary? *Chi Letter*, *6*(3).

Nguyen, H., Carrieri-Kohlman, V., Rankin, S., Slaughter, R., & Stulb, M. (2003). Internet-based patient education and support interventions: A review of evaluation studies and directions for future research. *Computers in Biology and Medicine*, *34*(2), 95–112. doi:10.1016/S0010-4825(03)00046-5

Ray, C., Lindop, J., & Gibson, S. (1982). The concept of coping. *Psychological Medicine*, *12*(2), 385–395. doi:10.1017/S0033291700046729

Reeves, P. (2000). Coping in cyberspace: The impact of internet use on the ability of HIV- positive individuals to deal with their illness. *Journal of Health Communication*, *5*(Supplement), 47–59. doi:10.1080/10810730050019555

Reeves, P. (2001). How individuals coping with HIV/AIDS use the Internet. *Health Education Research: Theory and Practice*, *16*(6), 709–719.

Sayles, J., Wong, M., Kinsler, J., Martins, D., & Cunningham, W. (2009). The association of stigma with self-reported access to medical care and antiretroviral therapy adherence in persons living with HIV/AIDS. *Journal of General Internal Medicine*, *24*(10), 1101–1108. doi:10.1007/s11606-009-1068-8

Simoni, J., Frick, P., & Huang, B. (2006). A longitudinal evaluation of a social support model of medication adherence among HIV-positive men and women on antiretroviral therapy. *Health Psychology*, *25*(1), 74–81. doi:10.1037/0278-6133.25.1.74

Starace, F., Ammassari, A., Trotta, M. P., Murri, R., De Longis, P., & Izzo, C. (2002). Depression is a risk factor for suboptimal adherence to highly active anti-retroviral therapy. *JAIDS Journal of Acquired Immune Deficiency Syndromes*, *15*(31), S136–S139. doi:10.1097/00126334-200212153-00010

Stoller, N. (1998). *Lessons from the damned: Queers, whores, and junkies respond to AIDS*. New York, NY & London, UK: Routledge.

Trammell, K., Tarkowski, A., Hofmokl, J., & Sapp, A. M. (2006). Rzeczpospolita blogów [Republic of Blog]: Examining Polish bloggers through content analysis. *Journal of Computer-Mediated Communication, 11*(3), Article 2.

UNIADS. (2009). *Global epidemic update*. Geneva, Switzerland: UNAIDS.

World Health Organization. (2003). *Adherence to long term therapies: Evidence for action*. Geneva, Switzerland: World Health Organization. Retrieved June 13, 2010, from http://www.who.int/chp/ knowledge/publications/ adherence_report/en/

Chapter 8
Can Stored Data Answer All Questions:
A Study of Questions on Eating Disorders

Jacob Palme
Stockholm University, Sweden

ABSTRACT

One often hears statements such as eighty percent of the questions can be answered by twenty percent of the answers, or other similar statements, indicating that a small set of answers are enough to answer most of the questions in a particular topical area. To investigate this statement, a set of 630 questions, which were sent to an on-line service, were analyzed. All the questions were about eating disorders and obesity. The conclusion is that the statement, which was investigated, was not true. There was a large variation of different questions, and even though some questions did appear more than once, it was much less than eighty percent of all questions. The chapter offers insight into different types of questions posted on-line in the area of eating disorders. From the study follows that to provide satisfactory answers to a large part of the questions, it is necessary to have humans answering the questions.

INTRODUCTION

A common statement is that 80% of the questions can be answered by a small set of perhaps 20% of all answers. The primary object of this chapter is to investigate the truth of this statement, by studying if 630 actual questions in the eating disorders area can be answered by a small set of answers to common questions.

Suppose you are writing a book about eating disorders, or planning a web site about eating disorders, or want to review such a book or web site. Your goal may be to give good answers to all kinds of questions, which your readers will have

DOI: 10.4018/978-1-60960-866-8.ch008

about eating disorders. It will then be important to know which kinds of questions people want answers to in regards to eating disorders. A secondary object of this chapter is to provide input for such planning work.

SOURCE DATA

To get an overview of which are the most common questions, which people ask about eating disorders, this study is based on an analysis of 630 questions, which were sent to an on-line question area, where people with different psychological problems could send their questions and get free answers by an expert psychologist. 630 questions will of course not cover every question anyone may ask about eating disorders, but it will probably give a good basis for a main organisation of such a book or web site.

Eating disorders are a common set of psychiatric disorders, where a person eats too little (anorexia nervosa), too much (binge eating disorder) or too much combined with compensatory activities like purging and fasting (bulimia nervosa). In the worst cases, these disorders can lead to death, but more commonly causes unhappiness and unhealthy eating. There are no reliable statistics on the incidence of eating disorders, because most people suffer in secrecy and do not come into contact with health care providers. Some studies indicate that between 10 and 35% of young women suffer from bulimia nervosa, severe anorexia nervosa was in another study found for about 1% of teenage girls. 70% of people suffering from eating disorders are women (Beat, 2007). Web4Health is a web site originally developed with support from the European Community (Web4Health, 2011). It contains about one thousand informational texts about different psychological problems. The site is meant to answer questions about psychology, psychiatry and psychological questions. Most of the texts are available in German, English and French, some of them also in Greek, Italian, Finnish and Polish. The Web site was first opened in 2004. It has about 600 000 visitors a month.

On the web site is an area where people can send in questions and get personally tailored answers by a human expert. This service is presently available in German and Swedish, but was until April 2008 also available in English. This study is based on a collection of 12622 such questions in Swedish and English. German questions were not used for this study. Of these 12622 questions, 630 or 5% were found to relate to the area of eating disorders and therefore selected. This selection of 630 questions is the basis for this chapter.

These 630 questions were first roughly categorized into four categories: Anorexia nervosa, bulimia nervosa, binge eating/overweight and other/unspecified eating disorder. However, many questions did not fit very well in these four category groups, and they were then assigned to the group which was closest to their problem. According to this rough classification, the questions had the distribution shown in Table 1.

Table 1. Gross distribution of eating disorders and problems

Numbers				Percentages		
English	Swedish	Total	Category	English	Swedish	Total
41	93	135	Anorexia nervosa	14,7%	26,6%	21,4%
67	52	119	Bulimia nervosa	24,0%	14,9%	18,9%
132	141	273	Binge eating, overweight or obese	47,3%	40,3%	43,3%
39	64	103	Other or unspecified	14,0%	18,3%	16,3%
279	350	630	Total	100,0%	100,0%	100,0%

This rough classification was done in two stages. In the first stage, questions containing any of a number of words or word beginnings which are typical of eating disorders were detected. In the second stage, a manual classification was done of each entry found in the first stage. The list of typical eating disorders word contained 32 words like words containing the strings diet, bulimia, thin (but think as excluded), feed, gain, drink, pounds, etc. This automatic detection was only done for the English questions, for the Swedish questions every single question was analyzed manually. It may mean that a few English eating-disorder questions were missed in this selection process.

The division into the two categories anorexia nervosa and bulimia nervosa was made as specified in DSM-IV (American Psychiatric Association, 1994), which means that people with a bulimic behaviour but with a low BMI were put into the anorexia nervosa category. Binge eating was defined as bulimic eating but no compensatory behaviour like purging or fasting. Often, the information in the question was not enough to make a perfect split of the questions into the four main categories used, and in very unclear cases, the category Other or unspecified was used.

The people asking questions in English were distributed all around the earth where people speak English or know English, but a majority of them came from North America. The differences between the Swedish and English people in Table 1 are thus probably mainly a difference between Sweden and North America. It is well known that obesity is very common in North America, so it is natural that English-language question askers more often ask questions about binge eating, overweight and obesity problems. But it is not obvious why English-speaking people more often asked questions about bulimia nervosa and less often about anorexia nervosa. One can note that there is some relation between anorexia nervosa and bulimia nervosa. Some anorectic people live a bulimic life of switching between eating, purging and fasting. Such people are often classified as anorectic and not bulimic just because their weight was subnormal, and since DSM-IV says to classify such people into the anorexia nervosa class (American Psychiatric Association, 1994). It is also not uncommon that the same person first becomes anorectic and then later in life switches to bulimia nervosa, according to eating disorders expert Gunborg Palme who answers questions online at the Web4Health site (Web4Health, 2011).

But there is more to be gained from the set of questions in this study. A more detailed investigation of the questions give a fuller view of what people most often ask questions about in relations to eating disorders. Each question was first roughly put into one category, as described above, and then the questions in each category were overviewed. Each question was usually 2-15 lines long. An exception from this were questions where the writers gave long detailed description of their life or situation and then asked questions like What is wrong with me or What shall I do or something similar. Except for these life-story questions, the remaining questions could rather easily be abbreviated to one single sentence as shown in the next section of this chapter. Or, of course, into several single sentences if the question actually contained several separate questions. The next chapter shows this abbreviation of all the questions into one single sentence comprising the major issue of each question.

ABBREVIATED LIST OF QUESTIONS ASKED

This section presents analyses of on-line questions related to the four categories of eating disorders: anorexia nervosa, bulimia nervosa, binge eating/overweight and other/unspecified eating disorder.

Detailed Analysis of Questions in the Main Category of Anorexia Nervosa

Of the 630 questions, 133 were classified into the main category for anorexia nervosa. Within this group, questions were further split into subcategories. Note that the total below adds up to more than 100%, since questions often contained multiple related or unrelated subquestions. All the percentages in this section are percent of these 133 people.

Causes of Anorexia: 14% of All Anorexia-Related Questions

Most common were questions about body-image-related causes like "I feel too thick, get anxiety when I eat. Single questions about how anorexia might be caused by family relations, harassment and child abuse, loss of boyfriend, whether anorexia is contagious, why women have anorexia more than men.

Diagnosis of Anorexia: 29% of All Anorexia-Related Questions

20% of the questions were people who wanted help to diagnose themselves. 5% wanted help to diagnose a particular person other than themselves.

Several questions were about diagnostic criteria, and 7% asked questions about why other people say I have anorexia, when I do not agree. Single questions were about relation of anorexia to BMI, alcoholism, happiness and depression. Example of diagnosis questions: how can I get people to understand that I do not have anorexia? (from a person with a BMI of 15.8!). I am slightly underweight, but happy, am I anorectic? How can you see if someone has anorexia? I have not been eating for three days now, do I have anorexia?

Effects and Symptoms of Anorexia: 18% of All Anorexia-Related Questions

Most common were questions of effects on the body, and risks for damage, like for example hair loss, loss of menstruation (3%), loss of ability to get pregnant (3%), incontinence, damage to muscles and skeleton, eyesight, lameness. 2% asked whether anorexia is related to compulsive disorders. Example: When does menstruations reappear after gaining weight and after ended an anorexia eating disorder.

Professional Treatment of Patients with Anorexia: 22% of All Anorexia-Related Questions

Most common (8%) were questions giving a long detailed life history and then asking How can I get well? 2% wanted advice on choice of treatment, 2% asked how successful treatment was expected to be, 2% asked whether enforced treatment is effective. Examples of questions: Should she be committed to a clinic? Help me reduce my weight even more (asked by an already anorectic woman), How to help a person who does not want to get well, Are there medicines for depression caused by anorexia?

Non-Professional Handling of People with Anorexia: 34% of All Anorexia-Related Questions

13% asked for advice on handling anorectic friends, example: She claims she has no problems, but..., She says she wants to lose 10 pounds, How to get anorectic girl-friend to stop vomiting? 10% asked for advice on handling anorectic children, for example Child who refuses to eat, She gets angry and cries when I say that she should eat more. 3% asked about how to treat themselves, for example How can I achieve a sound relation to eating, food and physical exercise? 6% asked questions about diets, most common were questions about diets to gain weight in a healthy manner for an anorectic.

Detailed Analysis of Questions in the Main Category of Bulimia Nervosa

Of the 630 questions, 119 were classified into the main category for bulimia nervosa. Within this group, questions were further split into subcategories. Note that the total below adds up to more than 100%, since questions often contained multiple related or unrelated subquestions. All the percentages in this section are percent of these 119 questions (as asked by 119 probably different people).

Questions about Purging Behaviours (Laxation, Vomiting, etc.): 6% of All Bulimia-Related Questions

2% were how-to questions, such as Where do you buy laxatives? Why can some people retch? Other questions were about how dangerous this is, Do you recommend vomiting do reduce weight? How to stop retching?

Causes of Bulimia Nervosa: 3%

Questions about body image causes, Is it hereditary? Why have I developed bulimia?

Diagnosis of Bulimia Nervosa: 15%

All these questions were asking for help for self-diagnosis. Examples: Why do I eat nothing on some days and binge on other days? How do you know if you have an eating disorder? What kind of eating disorder do I have? I force myself to throw-up after every meal.

Effects of Bulimia Nervosa: 8%

Examples: My throat is swollen and hurts, have I damaged my body permanently? Can this cause death, Can a marriage with a bulimic wife succeed?

Secrecy: 3%

Examples: Should I tell other people, Should I tell my doctor, Will people believe me if I tell them, I told my husband, now he tells other people.

Symptoms: 12%

Examples: Why does cutting make me feel good? Period not coming, when will it come back? Why do people switch between different addictive disorders? Why do I not want food in me? Have my teeth been harmed? One pro bulimia question: I am happy being a bulimic, what is wrong with me? One question was about statistics on the prevalence of bulimia nervosa.

Self-Treatment When You Have Bulimia Nervosa: 31%

A common type of question (19% of all these questions) was a detailed description of a person's behaviour and sometimes even life history, followed by a question such as What shall I do? or What is wrong with me or something similar. 3% of these questions were related to self-control: Should I make daily limits, How can I stop vomiting, How can I stop eating all the time? 9% about dieting: Rapid weight reduction diet. Why does no diet have any effect on me? Do you recommend a low-calorie diet? What diet do you recommend? Other treatment questions: How should I think to get well? Two questions were about physical exercise: Why is training and eating so important for me? Is one hour physical exercise enough or excessive?

Treating Other People with Bulimia Nervosa: 27%

For example treating friends, relatives, children, She misses school, but does not want help!, How to approach a person who does not want help, She steals food and vomits everywhere, what shall I do? I got her to go to a doctor but he just said it was nerves!. 4% were about people unwilling to get treatment, example My husband becomes abusive when I try to get him to get help for his bulimia.

Professional Treatment of Bulimia Nervosa: 22%

6% were about psychotherapy, such as Should I see a therapist? Is group therapy better than individual therapy? What kind of therapy is best? 7% asked about the prognosis of treatment, such as How long time does it take to get well? Can I ever get well? Will I ever be able to live a normal life? After treatment, can you have a healthy baby? Some believe this international web site has directories of specialists everywhere: Where can I get treatment for free in San Diego? (Question asked to our specialist in Sweden, Europe). 6% were questions about drugs, such as laxatives, SSRI medicines, ADHD stimulant medicines for eating disorders, 2% were questions about the drug ephedrine. (SSRI is short for Selective Serotonin Reuptake Inhibitor which are a group of medicines originally for the treatment of depression, but which have been found to be useful for many other psychiatric diagnoses than depression.)

Detailed Analysis of Questions in the Main Category of Binge Eating Disorder and/or Obesity

Of the 630 questions, 273 were roughly classified into the category Binge Eating and/or Obesity. Many of the questions below also included What to do about it? or Do you agree? or What are your opinions of this? in different variants, these additions are not repeated below.

Professional Treatment

Many questions described different kinds of abnormal eating habits, leading to a normal weight, and asked if this is accepted as an eating disorder and can I get professional treatment, even though their weight was normal. Such descriptions of abnormal eating behaviour are described below, for example in the paragraph beginning with Diagnosis: or Where to go for help? or Can I get help for binge eating from my local medical center? The people asking these questions obviously did not have a feeling for how wide and international the internet is, they expect us to know about local medical organisation in the country and state where they live.

Gastric Bypass Surgery

Two asked What is the weight limit for getting surgery for obesity? further two asked Can I get pregnant and have a child after gastric bypass surgery? and single questioners asked: What is the lower age limit for getting surgery for obesity? Where to go to get surgery for obesity? Should I support my girl friend who wants lap band surgery? and How long time before I can get gastric bypass?

Medicines

Two persons asked: My doctor wants me to take a medicine called XXX, is it dangerous? for different medicines XXX, single questions such as: What medicines will help me lose weight? Which medicines are allowed while breast-feeding? I weigh 350 pounds and my doctor prescribed Lorazepam, is this right treatment for me? and A friend is overusing ADHD medicines, what will happen if he reduces dose to normal?

Self-Treatment

Many questions contained How to lose weight? in combination with other information or questions, sometimes specified, for example four asked How to lose weight rapidly? three asked about diet during pregnancy, three asked How to get started? three asked How can I reduce my weight in untraditional method? two asked I need to lose a specified weight before a specified date, two asked How to stop binging? two asked Why does a lot of exercise not cause me to lose weight? and single questions were:

- I eat only healthy food and still cannot obtain a desired weight
- How can I lose weight in untraditional method?
- What calory intake to obtain a certain desired weight?
- Where to start?
- How to lose weight without exercising?
- What diet is right for me to lose weight?
- Suggest a diet to lose weight but still allowing physical exercise?
- How to handle uncomfortable feelings in other ways than eating?
- What kind of training is best to lose weight?
- How to make myself vomit?
- I am lazy and eat bad food
- How to handle stress-related eating?
- I play soccer 5-6 times a week, how to lose weight?
- Is physical exercise good for weight loss?
- My weight is 90 kg, should I lose weight?
- I have lost 38.5 lbs by use and abuse of laxatives, so why do people say this is not good?
- Do you get abstinence symptoms if you lose weight?
- How to get motivation to lose weight, how to get started.
- What are the pros and cons of slimming?
- What are the best ways to lose a few pounds?
- How to find the will power to start reducing my weight?

Treatment of Relatives/Friends

In this category three people asked: What can a pre-school teacher do with a child who binges? Further three asked I have problems watching fat people eat. And single questions were:

- My five year old brother is 10 kg overweight!
- Diet for overweight five-ear old daughter.
- How to help wheel-chair dependent overweight person?
- My husband has gained weight and has excuses for not exercising or eating less, what can I do for him?
- My gf wants me not to have snacks, candy etc. in my house, is this right? (gf = girl friend)
- My bf refuses to lose weight, should I accept that he weighs 35 kg too much? (bf = boy friend)

Causes of Binge Eating and/or Obesity

Three asked Is obesity caused by food, medicines or because of not exercising? two asked Why increased weight after pregnancy? two complained I eat the same as before, but now I am gaining weight. Single questions were:

- I have stopped exercising and now I am gaining weight.
- Can being the victim of childhood sexual assault cause binge eating?
- Can obesity be a way of preventing unwanted advances?
- I have been taking Lexapro, could this be cause of my weight gain?
- Is obesity caused by using eating as a drug?

- What is the relation of life style and obesity?
- I eat when i am lonely!
- I do not eat because I am hungry, but because I feel that I must eat.
- When I have eaten a normal meal, I just want more.
- I have ADHD and know that eating helps to keep me cool, when I stop eating the text I read gets confused.
- What are the relations of life style and obesity?
- What are the main cause of overweight - cookies, food, lack of exercise, or side effects of medicines?

Effects of Treatment

Single questions were:

- I have lost 60 kg, and now I am depressed.
- I was overweight as a child and this has given med lack of social confidence.
- What are the pros and cons of weight loss?
- What are the risks of obesity?
- Is obesity caused by inherited genes?

Diagnosis: (Self or for Other People, Such as Relatives)

- I have a normal weight, but does not want to eat, force myself to eat because my body needs it, is this an eating disorder?
- In periods I eat too much, then eat nothing for a period, is this an eating disorder?
- I eat when bored.
- My mother increases in weight, sleeps all day, does not pay bills, what is wrong with her?
- Am I overweight, my weight is <specified amount> and I am <specified height> cm tall?
- Sudden gain of <specified amount of> pounds in <specified number of> months, why?
- I wake up in the middle of the night and eat, Do I have NES (Night Eating Syndrome)?
- Family says I live in my own world, do I have ADHD?

Hunger

Many questions contained Why am I always hungry? combined with various other information, for example three asked I think about food and eating all the times, and single questions were: I am not hungry, but eat a lot and often, and I feel very bad, am depressed, hungry and overweight.

Harassment

Two questions were about harassment, examples are People harass me because my mother is fat, and Get knocked back by someone saying I am fat.

Not in Any of the Categories about was a Single Question

Is sexual intercourse dangerous when overweight?

Detailed Analysis of Questions in the Main Category of Other or Unspecified Eating Disorder

In this category is included questions which do not clearly belong to any of the categories anorexia nervosa, bulimia nervosa, binge eating disorders or obesity. Most of them had one of these disorders, but did not give enough information in the question to clearly indicate to which group they belonged.

A few had genuinely specified non-standard eating disorders, like several who had problems with eating together with other people, but not when eating alone. Many of the questions below also contained How can I get well? or Do I have an eating disorder? or How can I get rid of my eating disorder? or How to lose weight? or What is wrong with me? Many people said that they used different medicines, usually SSRI-s, diazepams or sleeping pills.

Eating Disorders in General

One question in this category: What are the negative effects of eating disorders?

Questions about Causes of Obesity or Eating Disorders

Two questions can be abbreviated as What are the causes of eating disorders? two as Will gastric banding mean I will be raped again, as I was before I got fat? and single questions were:

- Might fasting in a fund-raising campaign against hunger cause an eating disorder?
- I have eating disorder since my parents divorced, when I was 14 years old.
- I have an all meal plan, where I can eat as much as I want without higher cost.
- My weight mushroomed every time I got pregnant.
- Can sexual abuse cause binge eating?
- How will hormone imbalance at menopause cause rapid weight gain?
- Can overweight cause anorexia?

Questions about Professional Treatment

Three asked variants of After one year taking medicine YY, I gained XX kg, could this be caused by YY? Single questions in addition in this category were:

- Why is it so difficult to find someone to talk to at a reasonable cost?
- Can a psychologist give a certificate of previous eating disorder?
- Is it dangerous to take Reductil when having a normal weight?
- Weight limit to get gastric banding.
- Can my house doctor arrange for treatment of binge eating?
- Age limit to get gastric banding surgery.
- I am 24 weight 350 pounds, is the Lorazepan which my doctor prescribed really right for me?
- Where to go to get gastric banding, can I get it privately?
- Should I start with psychotherapy?
- I need someone to talk to about what is wrong with me when I feel like I am fat and people do not understand me.
- How can I discontinue using Zoloft without terrible abstinence/cessation symptoms - have tried step-wise discontinuation and it only made the pain last for a longer time.

Questions Related to Self-Treatment

There was a large variety of questions related to self-treatment, a total of 72 questions. All from the general exclaim of how life is against you in the not-so-easy answered question: I have an eating disorder, no treatment helps for me, why?

Two people asked how to achieve a thinner body shape after having achieved a desired weight.

Only a single question directly about body image: Should I lose weight or change my belief that I am fat, if so, how?

Five questions were about how to treat an eating disorder: How to get rid of eating disorders? How to treat my eating disorder? I have a normal weight but do not eat well, how can I treat this? I have an eating disorder, how can I get well? and What is the worse part of overcoming an eating disorder?

Six questions were about eating regular meals: Two just asked: How important is it to eat regular meals at regular times? one person asked: How important is it to eat regular meals, should I eat even if I do not feel hungry? another asked: How to eat to reduce weight, tried eating only once a day but got dizzy? another asked: I have started to skip meals to reduce my overweight and one person said: I know this is wrong, but I feel such a power when I skip a meal.

Eight questions were about food, diets and calories:

- I am not overweight, but it requires a lot of effort to keep a normal weight, a friend of mine has no problems at all. How many calories per day should I eat to lose weight?
- Is a diet based on calories or on grams of carbohydrates best?
- What diets are right when wanting to lose weight while training a lot?
- What ideal foods get digested the fastest?
- What is a healthy diet?
- What is the ideal food in order to release fat fastest?
- What should my calorie intake be when I weight XX, am ZZ years old and YY tall?
- I am an extreme dieter, controls all I eat, has normal weight, need help with food plan.

Two questions about fasting: (1) How many pounds a week can you lose by not eating anything at all? and (2) If I fast, will my body switch to no-food expectation?

In seven questions, life problems and feelings were the main issue in the question:

- 14 year old boy don't want to eat anything because I am sad.
- I have nausea every day, can't go to school, please help me, but no psychologist, please.
- 21 year old, slightly overweight, have never had any serious bf, how to get one?
- How to overcome food addiction which is related to my involvement with another person?
- I'm repulsive, not in control, please help me.
- My husband has a lover, but I still love him, now I have anxiety and an eating disorder.
- Unhappy, depressed, people say I am fat, what to do?

Ten questions were about food addiction and binging, each with its own twist of this issue:

- How to overcome my food addiction?
- How to stop thinking of food all the time?
- Do I have to stop eating cookies completely to get rid of my eating disorder?
- Eat well during day, but cannot relax at night without chewing something.
- How common is sugar addiction?
- How do you get rid of sugar addiction (twice).
- How to avoid the enticement of unhealthy food around me, especially at Christmas time?
- Sometimes I eat and eat and eat, no stopping it, other times I don't want to eat at all.
- What to do instead of binging?
- How can I stop eating junk food?

Two questions were about bad living habits: I love to sit in front of the TV and eat, have no friends outside school, want to reduce my weight 22 kg, what to do? and I spent the summer eating and watching TV, now I cannot get into my previous clothes any more, please help!

One question was about ideal weight: I weigh 50 kg, is 12 year old, is 160 cm tall, have an 83 cm waist circumference, should I lose weight?

Five questions were about maintaining an ideal weight: Three people asked different variants of: After having achieved my ideal weight, how do I maintain it? Two questions asked the same issue with some added twist to it: How can middle age and menopause people avoid the weight gain which is normal at those ages? and I have problems keeping a normal weight and avoiding weight loss, how can I stabilize my weight?

There were five questions about medicines: Weight loss pills to use while nursing a baby? Which diuretics will allow me rapid weight loss? Which tablets will help me to lose weight? I take Reductil and have normal weight, is this dangerous? and Will I gain weight if I start taking Fontex?

Three questions related to pregnancy: Diet while wanting to get pregnant? Normal weight gain during pregnancy? and Want to get pregnant, dare not exercise, then I gain weight, what to do?

One question was about the important issue of satisfaction: How to learn to feel satisfaction when I have eaten enough?

There were seven questions about training and exercise: Three people asked: How to eat to lose weight while training, Two asked: Is walking or jogging best for weight loss? and one each asked: Am I exercising too much, followed by long list of daily exercises and diet, and Is training enough to become more thin and look better in a bathing suit?

Vomiting as weight control method was the issue of seven questions. Four asked variants of How to make myself vomit? and one asked each of the following questions: How can I get rid of anxiety after eating, when I have tried to throw up after eating, but not succeeded. Why does my body sometimes not let me throw up? and I eat almost nothing and then make myself throw up.

Two people apparently were tired of advice recommending more physical exercise, they explicitly asked for help on how to lose weight without training, one said that she could not exercise for medical reasons, one did not have time for training. Four gave a few facts about themselves, such as 13 years old, obese or Weight watchers helped me lose 60 kg, but now I cannot lose any more weight or I am fattest in class, students make fun of me and then should I lose weight? or how to lose weight. A total of eight people asked different variants of this kind of question.

One asked for a prognosis of effect of dieting, and said After how long time with a 1200-1400 kcal/day diet will my waist begin to get more narrow?

Question about Other People's Eating Disorders

Many people asked questions regarding eating disorders or weight problems of friends or relatives such as husband, wife, boyfriend, girlfriend, daughter, son, boss etc. a total of 28 questions.

Three people asked different variants about how to behave when meeting with a person who has an eating disorder, a friend, an employee, meeting with in general.

Two questions were claiming that people they know have a body image problem, I have a friend who says he is fat, even though he is not. and Why does my dad feel overweight when he is not? Note that such body image problems were much more common in other people than when people talk about themselves - is this something other people can see in you, but you cannot recognize in yourself?

Two questions were about child care, one about how to handle overweight children, another how to handle a child who, according to the questioner, eats too much.

Five questions were about people who are controlling and perfectionists in four very different ways, one boy friend who also has an eating disorders and has a controlling mother, one about a daughter who also has a shopping addiction, another about a daughter who also throws up, showers for 20 minutes and cuts things into tiny piece, one about a boyfriend who wants to be perfect in everything.

Two questions were about people who cannot eat except when they are alone, one a daughter, the other a girl friend.

Two questions were about people who eat nothing except a few simple specified foods.

Two questions were posted by wives who are concerned about their husbands overweight and lack of interest in eating right.

Single questions were about a friend who eats nothing over the weekend, will she become an anorectic? one about risks of fasting in a fundraising campaign, one with a fat mother who is harassed, one about a daughter who has had an eating disorders for four years (age 26 to 30), one about an obese person sitting in a wheel-chair, one about a mother who has changed and put on weight, one about a friend who sets an alarm clock at night to make herself vomit again, one asking of men with an eating disorder and who are homosexuals if they have problems with their sexuality.

Questions Related to Self-Diagnosis

There were 45 questions about self-diagnosis in different variants. One just exclaimed Am I a hopeless case?

Two just quoted weight and height and asked if they were overweight, others said they feel fat or feel thin while the mirror says otherwise, what is the diagnosis of this? Many asked Am I fat or normal with for example a BMI of 23.5 or even believing they were fat with a BMI of 20.0. Better were those who at least knew they were thin when feeling fat.

Most questions described various feelings or behaviour where the obvious first answer is You are not unique, many people feel or react like you.

Some quoted different eating behaviour, like no solid food, cannot swallow solids, eating nothing except a few apples

Several people quoted problems (like the shakes or nausea) when having to eat together with other people.

Several reported various bad feelings after eating, like blaming themselves, or feeling terrible ad having to exercise vigorously, or feeling they should eat more healthy food.

Several reported skipping some meals.

People sometimes think they are unique when in reality many people are similar, for example thinking like an anorectic while having normal weight.

Some described how catastrophes in life (like parents abandoning children, quit my boyfriend, panic attacks) causing eating disorders, and wanted a diagnosis of such sad life stories.

I just want to be happy, some exclaimed who obviously were not happy.

Six people reported vomiting and problems related with vomiting and asked if this was an eating disorder.

Other questions related to self-diagnosis:

- I am very slim but I am always hungry!
- My weight is normal, but I want to lose at least 12 lbs. and now all food feels repugnant.
- 'I have been gaining weight rapidly and now I have lost all hunger, is this an hormone imbalance, I am 47 years old.
- People tease me for being overweight, I am afraid to talk because people might say I am dumb.
- I do not eat because I do not feel like eating, and this is not because I am afraid of getting fat, and my BMI is 17.4, do I have an eating disorder?
- I sometimes am not hungry and cannot eat, other times am hungry, is this an eating disorders?
- I know that I am not normal, but want to be normal in my eating behaviour.
- I cannot stop pulling my hair and have problems keeping my weight normal.
- I get dizziness and hair loss and everything related to food is distasteful to me - is this a short term problem which will go away?
- I have normal weight but feel strongly that I should lose weight.
- Recently retired, 57 years old, been sober for 22 years, starving after eating.
- Why do I wake up at night and eat sweats?
- I eat, get satisfied, but still eat more, why?
- Medical causes of fast weight gain?

- I know that I am fat (quoting length & height indicating 20,4 BMI) so why do I want to get treatment for anorexia?
- Got depo shot, gained weight, why always wanting to eat?

Four questions about ortorexi: People wanted to know what it is, how common it is, etc.

General Diagnosis Questions

- Does there exist an eating disorder where a person wants to gain weight?
- How long after a person has started on an eating disorder will it be visible on the person?
- Is a weight of 65 kg normal for a 16 year old girl?
- Can you be anorexic even if you are not underweight?
- Can an anorectic binge eat?
- What is the difference between bulimia and anorexia and which is most dangerous?
- Does it exist an eating disorder where people get fat because they want to?
- How long does it take before eating disorder is obvious?
- Can you be anorectic without being underweight?
- Have you heard about sadorexia (sadomasochism+anorexia)?
- What is the difference between Bulimia and Nervosa?
- How common is sugar addiction, and who are afflicted.
- Can eating healthily cause an eating disorder?
- Is this diet right (describes an extremely low-calorie diet)?

Diagnosis of Friends and Relatives:

- Why does my dad believe he is overweight when he is not?
- My girl friend told me she has an eating disorder, we were very much in love, but now she has broken off, says she needs to be herself.
- My daughter has started cut food into pieces, then shower for 20 minutes after eating.
- She eats a lot on fridays but nothing on weekends, and she is shrinking, does this mean that she has anorexia?

More Diagnosis, Eating-Related Problems

- I have a problem watching overweight people eat.
- I sweat and my hands shake and I have nausea when I eat together with other people (2 questions).
- My girl friend refuses to eat together with me.
- Can eating disorders (refusing to eat) cause an increased sex drive?
- I have problem keeping my weight up, the weight tends to go down.
- I don't care about life and want to stop eating completely. When I have started eating, I cannot stop.
- Why do I wake up and eat at night?
- I cannot sleep well unless I eat too much before going to bed.
- How is life for a person with an eating disorder?
- I have suddenly gained almost 50 pounds in 3-4 months, why, when I eat the same as before (2 questions)?
- After how many days of fasting will the body switch to starvation mode?

- I have a friend who is able to eat whatever she wants and still stay slim, she makes me feel worse.
- Can I get a certificate so that I do not have to pay study scholarship back, not having produced study results because of eating disorders.
- Can an obese person develop anorexia?
- It started with eating disorders, ended with drinking one bottle of wine a day for several months - will I get difficult abstinence if I quit?
- Getting more and more stress-sensitive, could not stand smell of raw onions and hot oil in restaurant.
- Statistics about eating disorders among young men, how is this influenced by media?
- I ate a lot when feeling down, bad feelings, loneliness, sadness.
- Identify emotions: (Often combined with What is wrong with me or How can I get well?)
- Previously I had an eating disorders, now when I should be angry or sad, instead I feel restless and anxious.
- I feel that people dislike me unless I lose weight.
- I never feel satisfied, regardless of how much I eat.
- I get dizzy and feel unwell when eating.
- I can only feel restlessness and worry, never sorrow or anger.
- I turn everything into negative feelings.

Effects of Eating Disorders

- How will an hormone imbalance at menopause influence eating (2 questions)?)
- What are the negative effects of eating disorders (2 questions)?
- Did she break off our relationship because she felt I was controlling her?
- Can a rapid weight loss cause a person to become emotionally instable?

FUTURE RESEARCH DIRECTIONS

One possible future research area would be to look at some existing web sites which claim to give a lot of information about eating disorders, and check how many of the questions could find an answer within such web sites, and which conclusions the result of such an investigation could result in.

CONCLUSION

The main conclusion of this study is that the common statement 80% of the questions is answered by 20% of the answers, indicating that one can satisfy a large part of the needs with a small number of answers, is wrong. There are a few questions which occur more than one time, but they are definitely much less than 80% of the questions.

And the belief that one can construct a computer service, which will answer most of the questions, which people have in a psychology/psychiatry area, is probably wrong. To provide satisfactory answers to a large part of the questions, it is necessary to have humans answering the questions.

This study only looks at 630 questions, and it would of course be possible that if the number of questions analyzed was increased, then one would suddenly find that the rest of the questions, the questions not analyzed in this chapter, would suddenly only repeat the questions studies in this chapter. But this seems unprobable. With all probability, a larger set of questions would just contain a larger difference of different variants of questions. The amount of variability in what people think about and ask about in a psychology-related area is immense. And constructing a machine to provide good answers to all of these questions is probably impossible.

However, it might be possible to design a mixed human-machine answering service. Such a service would analyze the questions and return a draft answer. Such a draft answer could contain links to web pages which might help the person asking the question. A human could then review the draft answers and rewrite it into a good answer. This might be possible. But the human at the end is necessary to provide good answers.

One way of looking at this issue is to note that there are mainly two kinds of activities on the internet. One activity is collections of pages containing information, both short answers and long papers, on an immense amount of facts. This area also contains a lot of entertainment services, like e-books, games, videos, etc. The other is tools for human-human communication, all from e-mail to advanced groupware systems like facebook. The human-human use of the internet is sometimes called internet 2, even though it has been available on the internet even from the beginning.

And systems for advanced answering of questions belong to the second area, the internet 2 area. It is a human-human communication task, not a human-machine communication tasks.

REFERENCES

American Psychiatric Association. (1994). *Diagnostic and statistical manual of mental disorders (DSM-IV)*. Washington, DC: American Psychiatric Press.

B-eat. (2007). *Some statistics*. B-eat: Beating eating disorders. Retrieved February 2011 from http://www.b-eat.co.uk/ PressMediaInformation/ Somestatistics

Web4Health. (2011). Psychology free online medical advice website. Retrieved February 2011, from http://www.web4health.info/

Chapter 9
Dynamic Stress Management:
Self-Help through Holistic System Design

Åsa Smedberg
Stockholm University, Sweden

Hélène Sandmark
Mälardalen University, Sweden

ABSTRACT

Different kinds of applications for self-help are available on the Internet today. Some aim to intervene with users' life patterns such as negative stress exposure. It is not always an easy task to manage stressful life situations and to develop and maintain healthy living. It involves learning how to balance perceived demands from working and personal life, and to question underlying thoughts and beliefs. E-health communities can assist in this process through continuous interactions between community members. However, previous studies have shown that combining knowledge of health experts and the experiences of peers can create a good synergy. The question is how these findings can be applied to the area of stress management. In this chapter, the authors present a web-based self-help system for stress management based on a holistic view of actors and their different types of support. The system offers the user information in the form of research and real life stories, practical exercises (both text- and video-based), and the opportunity to interact with health experts and peers, all in an integrated way.

INTRODUCTION

Today, many people are on sick leaves due to high levels of stress (Henderson, Glozier & Holland, 2005; Dekkers-Sánchez, Hoving, Sluiter & Frings-Dresen, 2008). In Sweden, the stress-related diseases have even become the second leading cause of sickness absence (Holmgren, Dahlin-Ivanoff, Björkelund & Hensing, 2009; Sandmark, 2007; The Swedish Social Insurance Agency, 2010). There are different factors that affect stress-related health problems. In previous studies it has been found that high or unclear demands, low control and low social support at work increase the risk

DOI: 10.4018/978-1-60960-866-8.ch009

of "job stress". If this state is prolonged, the risk of poorer health is overwhelming. Role conflict in the balance between work and family can occur when demands from one sphere do not conform to the demands of the other, or when the individual's efforts to fulfill his or her role at work is disrupted by the demands of the family. In working life, it is shown that a disturbed balance between work and family can be a precursor to mental illness and impairment of wellbeing (Sandmark, 2007; 2009). Besides control and demands, social support is an important factor to counteract negative stress symptoms. Social support at work or in private life has a mediating effect of perceived stress and can to some extent prevent negative stress.

When dealing with stress-related health problems, Internet with its facilities for both information sharing and continuous interactions can play an important role. Open web-based systems allow people with high levels of stress to get in contact with health professionals and peers for support and guidance on a continuous basis. Self-help groups on the Internet have emerged in different health areas, and issues related to stress is one of them. There are also different types of web-based intervention systems that use different types of models for dealing with people's stress. However, existing systems tend to focus on either information or communication and do not look for holistic ways to combine these two. Most intervention systems also tend to have a separate chat for the users that is held apart from the rest of the system and not analyzed for patterns of communication or used for improvements in the overall intervention system. This is where this chapter begins. The chapter introduces a web-based stress management system that applies a holistic and communicative approach to intervention. This system is based on group interaction, information sharing and integration of different actors' knowledge.

BACKGROUND

It is becoming increasingly common for people to connect to and communicate with others through the many open communities on the Internet. Especially in the health field, the online communities as well as the visitors of these have rapidly increased in number during the latest years. Whatever health goals people have, they can find like-minded people to collaborate with. Through the online communities people can give and receive support, ask questions, vent problems, share experiences and exchange information and advice.

The use of the Internet has shown to enhance patients' and citizens' knowledge and also their confidence in relation to health care (Fox, Ward & O'Rourke 2005; Mehra, Merkel & Bishop, 2004). It is now easier to find information and advice from several sources (Preece, 2000; Ellis & Bruckman, 2001; Maloney-Krichmar & Preece, 2005). The public's use of various medical sources on the Internet has made people find alternative medical advice or information on issues that their doctors cannot handle so well (Kling, 2000). While surgeons can be very good at operating, it is not certain that they are equally good at explaining how the aftercare and rehabilitation work. Such a gap can be filled by skilled and experienced people who share information and experiences on the Internet, for example in online health communities. A general characteristic of online communities is that they allow groups and individuals with common interests to meet virtually to collaborate, share resources and support each other (Preece, 2000). The online communication can help people widen their social circles (Sproull & Kiesler, 1991). Patients included in the self-help groups on the Internet have also expressed that they feel in touch with other patients as an important aid to cope with their diseases (Josefsson, 2007; Walther, Pingree, Hawkins & Buller, 2005).

There are online communities for self-help groups with various mental and physical illnesses, and also for people suffering from issues related to life patterns and how to cope with daily situations. One example is health communities for people who experience stress in their lives: their working lives, their private lives, or both. In order for us to understand these online communities and to what extent they enable participants to learn how to change their lives in some ways, we need to study the various postings and ways to communicate. Through patterns of speech acts, we can better understand how people work together for a common interest (Austin, 1962; Winograd & Flores, 1987). The way the users of online health communities use speech acts to ask questions and respond to each other (if they agree, offer advice or give counter-ideas, etc.) is of importance in order to understand these communities (Smedberg, 2008a-b). Also, for the purpose of learning together, questions and conversations on practical situations, experienced and foreseen difficulties as well as motivational issues need to be addressed (Smedberg, 2008a-b).

New topics and new ideas can easily be introduced in online communities if different health experts are invited to the online conversations. Also people who have managed to recover from difficult and stressful life situations can contribute with their insights. Thereby the platform can include both strong and weak tie relations (Haythornthwaite, 2007). While the strong tie relations tend to emphasize support of existing ideas and understanding, weak tie relations can more easily offer outside perspectives and even opposing ideas. At the same time, one important characteristic of well-functioning online communities is their ability to foster social and empathical communication (Preece, 1999; 2000), something that is more related to strong tie relations. In a stress management system, the two – social and learning activities – need therefore to be used in combination.

In the health care area there is another type of public system for online interaction and that is the so-called Ask-the-expert system. In this type of system, information can be sought out by the user through the stored user questions and expert answers. These questions and answers (Q&As) are stored and published in a way that makes them possible to browse. Users can also submit their own questions directly to the system, and the questions are then answered by an expert (Budzik & Hammond, 1999). The health experts in such a system are physicians, psychologists, physiotherapists and dietitians, for example. Who will be appointed to answer the question depends on the subject at hand. According to studies, online expert services in health care can be of great value to the ones seeking health information and who need guidance and knowledge (Marine, Embi, McCuistion, Haag & Guard, 2005). Users can get recommendations and advice from a medical expert, and the system offers also a new kind of ongoing relationship between patients and medical experts (Marco, Barba, Losa, de la Serna, Sainz, Lantigua & de la Serna, 2006). This type of relationship is of importance in lifestyle interventions.

Comparative studies of the use of online health communities and Ask-the-expert system have given insights into how users would benefit from the combination of information, advice and support from both types of systems. Raised issues in an online community on overweight and corresponding questions in an Ask-the-expert system in the same area were analyzed (Smedberg, 2008b). The systems were also compared in terms of information and advice given in the answers. Questions and answers were analyzed to determine similarities and differences between the two types of systems. Both quantitative and qualitative analyses were done. The results showed that common questions about diets, exercises and weight loss medication in the Ask-the-expert system were met with similar issues and also similar responses in the online peer conversations. In general, the studies showed that the community members had good basic insight into various health issues and problems.

The studies showed examples of online community conversations concerning group challenges that aimed at encouraging and motivating the community members. Suggestions regarding how to strive for common fitness and weight goals were presented, for example. Among the postings were also greetings and other issues aimed at increasing social bonding. These were examples of conversational topics among peers that had no equivalent among the Q&As. There were also other differences between the systems. When comparing postings on the same subject, it appeared that the way they were presented differed between the systems. While the postings contained similar types of information and advice, the level of detail was different. The Ask-the-expert system offered information and descriptions about the food's content, physical effects on the body in a more detailed manner and also medical terms. The community conversations, on the other hand, contained reports on the members' own experiences with treatments, food and exercises. The results showed that the two types of systems had different and complementary characteristics. The consistency between the Ask-the-expert system and the online communities was more extensive than was the case with the reverse relations, i.e., between the community conversations and the Q&As. One reason for this was the large volume of conversations, which increased the chances of finding a match. The second factor had to do with properties of the community conversations. There were a lot of community conversations that focused on empathy and sympathy, and there were also examples of issues related to motivational contests and requests for face-to-face meetings. Some of the Q&As with no counterpart in the community conversations were related to specific medical conditions.

When one is heading for a new way of life, both comprehensive expert information and experiences and practical advice from others in the same situation are beneficiary. This indicates that it can be a relevant recommendation from medical experts to advise the users to join the online conversations for peers as well. The conclusion from the studies of Ask-the-expert and e-health community systems was that their various features and additional strengths could be exploited more by the users, if the systems were more clearly linked together (Smedberg, 2008b).

The usage of the e-health communities for peers and e-health systems for communication with health experts has changed the conditions for health promotion. Typical characteristics of health promotion are that it supports personal and social development through providing information and education for health, and to enhance life skills. Thus it aims to increase the options available to people to exercise more control over their own health and environment, and to make choices conducive to health. It is a process which aims to enable people to increase control over their lives and improve their health (WHO, 1986). Enabling people by empowerment is a central part of the health promotion process (Gottwald, 2006), and changes of patterns of life, work and leisure could be significant for positive health development. Empowerment helps people to increase control and manage their lives according to their needs and preferences, and thereby increase their own power in order to get a better health. The key question is how to build on and reinforce authentic participation ensuring autonomy, feelings of value and sense of mastery in decision-making. Learning and problem solving abilities are important assets, and the educational approach to health promotion is much concerned to enable people to make informed choices and get more knowledge on health promotive actions. The preventive approach is also trying to achieve behavior changes: Internal locus of control is a key factor in efforts to create empowered environments and empowered individuals (Tones & Green, 2003; Rootman, Goodstadt, Potvin & Springett, 2001).

In the following chapter sections we will firstly present an overview of the area stress management and online stress interventions, secondly we move on to a presentation of the holistic and communication-based system for stress intervention on the web, and finally we introduce a model for how to evaluate this system.

STRESS MANAGEMENT AND WEB-BASED APPLICATIONS

Stress and Stress Management

People's reactions to stress are closely linked to flexibility and the ability to manage worklife as well as life balance, and also the balance between these spheres. Among individuals, there is a great variety of how to perceive and respond to circumstances and demands of the environment, both at work and in private and family life. Factors that are perceived as negative to the health by some people can be perceived as stimulating and positive challenges that promote health and wellbeing by others (Cooper, Dewe & O'Driscoll, 2001). It has been shown in studies that physical, mental, social and organizational conditions can contribute to an individual's experience of "job stress". Different models and theories of how individuals respond to exposure to stressors have been presented.

A sociological model (Karasek & Theorell, 1990), the demand-control model, has since the early 1990s been the dominating model for explaining and analyzing the psychosocial work conditions and its relationship to health. The model explains the relationship between perceived demands and perceived control in the work situation as critical to whether work cause a negative or a positive reaction in the individual. A combination of high demands and high control often leads to a positive state which can facilitate development and learning. The greater control an individual experiences the higher requirements from the environment can be accomplished without adverse effects, while low decision latitude (opportunity) and high demands have been shown to be associated with adverse stress reactions that can lead to impaired health. Requirements are defined as psychological stressors in the work situation, such as time pressure, high workload or demands from superiors. Control is defined as the degree of self-control and self-determination. The model has subsequently been supplemented by a third factor, namely social support. Social support at work or in private life has been shown to have a mediating effect of perceived stress, and it can therefore act as a buffer against negative stress. The social perspective also gives that people with similar living conditions are not necessarily affected in the same way. It shows that stress reactions are also dependent, at least in part, by a person's mind or way of thinking.

The ability to manage stressors (= coping) and the individual's way of dealing with stressful experiences and stress reactions are the result of interactions between internal factors within the individual and external factors and situations. Lazarus and Folkman (1984) developed a stress model in which psychological stress is described as a relationship between the individual and the outside world. The individual continuously makes assessments of the outside world, and finds it manageable or stressful and something that exceeds his or her resources. Coping ability makes it easier to manage stressors, and means that you have cognitive and behavioral strategies to control and reduce factors that might impair your health. Individuals make a primary assessment of the situation which is based on the individual's experience, knowledge, beliefs, goals and expectations. A stress reaction occurs when the individual is experiencing a difficult situation as a threat and not being able to cope with it (Lazarus & Folkman, 1984).

In another stress model presented by Siegrist, mechanisms behind the negative stress reactions are described (Siegrist, 1996). Siegrist has shown that if there is a recurring imbalance between work effort and reward, such as a low appreciation of work, or low payment (effort-reward imbalance), there is an increased risk of adverse reactions that ultimately can affect the mental and physical health.

Stress Management Techniques

Individual intervention or prevention of dysfunction due to negative stress exposure progressive muscle relaxation was originally designed by Jacobson to guide people through successive tensing and relaxation of the body muscle groups from toe to head to achieve overall body relaxation (Jacobson, 1938). This process is easy to learn and teach, safe, non-threatening and noncompetitive. Since then it has been concluded that the effectiveness of the interventions varied according to the health-outcome measure used (Murphy, 1996). Cognitive-behavioural skills were more effective for psychological outcomes, whereas muscle relaxation techniques were more effective for physiological outcomes. Using a combination of techniques; muscle relaxation and cognitive-behavioural skills seemed to be more effective across outcome measures than using a single technique (Murphy, 1996; Jones & Johnston, 2000).

Deep, diaphragmatic breathing is known to counteract the fight or flight response symptoms that are often associated with anxiety and negative reactions on stress exposure (Seaward, 2002; Mayo Clinic Special Report, 2005). Also meditation can be used to counteract stressful situations, as it is a technique to develop concentration and awareness to produce a calming effect. Here diaphragmatic breathing is central to any meditation practice (Seaward, 2002; Mayo Clinic Special Report, 2005; Benson, 2001). It has been found that there could be a lowering of blood pressure during deep breathing (von Schéele, von Schéele, Hansson, Winman & Theorell, 2005), which is interesting to consider in stress management. Work coaching and counselling is a relatively new, but increasingly sought after method for helping people to improve, develop, learn new skills, find personal resources, achieve aims and manage life change and personal challenges such as work-related stress and achieving work life balance. Occupational coaching might be effective for situations, whether in personal life, career, corporate or business life (Beecham, Dammers, van Zwanenberg, 2004; Hannah, 2004). It is well established among business and management executives, but has not been used much on an individual level among gainfully working men and women in the general population (Vaartjes, 2005). These programmes have not been scientifically evaluated regarding primary or secondary prevention for stress related disorders or as a health promotion measure for gainfully working people.

Self-Help Stress Management Online

When effects of a program for web-based stress management were measured, the results showed that the program had better effects on the participants than was the case for the control group (Hasson, Anderberg, Theorell & Arnetz, 2005). The target group consisted of 303 employees from four IT companies and two companies in the media sector. The participants were randomly selected into two groups: an intervention group and a reference group. The difference between the groups was that the intervention group was able to use the web chat and interactive self-help exercises. Examples of self-help exercises were training techniques for relaxation, time management and cognitive training. The exercises were presented as text files, PDFs and flash animations. Activities and tools given to both groups were popular scientific information on stress and health, and a diary that all participants used aimed to improve their self-knowledge and how their health and wellbeing were affected by various events. Indications used to measure changes in stress levels were both physiological markers and psychological assessments of health, recovery and general wellbeing. A follow up study was done after six months to measure the short-term effects. Levels of cortisol were found to be lower in the intervention group than in the reference group. Also self-reported eating habits, memory capacity, physical activity level, self-esteem and job satisfaction were improved. The evaluation continued after 12 months (Hasson, Arnetz, Theorell & Anderberg, 2006). The results of this long-term intervention showed that both intervention and reference group improved their scores of self-related health (SRH). However, no statistically significant difference could be seen between the two groups. No function for online counseling was implemented in the web-based intervention system. Furthermore, no measurements of the online conversations via chat, or other quantitative or qualitative study of communication patterns, were included in the studies. The role of communication as a means to support stress management was not considered whatsoever. This is a challenge for further research and shows the demands of interdisciplinary, or at least transdisciplinary, research within this area.

Other studies of online intervention programs have solely focused on designing and evaluating web-based counseling functions. For example, one study compared the effect of an IT-based stress-management program with the effect of an identical intervention program via traditional face to face format (Pollak Eisen, Allen, Bollash & Pescatello, 2008). The results showed that both groups responded well to the relaxation exercises. The results gave, however, that the group who used the IT-based program experienced a lower impact on their stress level than the group who used the traditional intervention program.

Internet-based cognitive behavioral therapy (CBT) has shown to be just as effective for panic disorder - repeated panic attacks - as traditional CBT treatment in group. In mild to moderate depressions Internet-based CBT can work well (Bergström, 2010). In a randomized clinical trial of 104 patients who suffered from panic disorders, efficiency of Internet-based CBT was compared to traditional CBT treatment in group. The treatment continued for 12 weeks. Both types of treatments turned out to work very well. There was no significant difference between CBT in groups and internet-based CBT, neither immediately after treatment nor at the six-month follow-up study. The treatment was supported by textual material and exercises that the participants could do on their own at home. Once a week the participants had follow-up contact with an experienced therapist via the Internet.

A HOLISTIC AND LIVING STRESS MANAGEMENT SYSTEM

This chapter section will introduce our web-based stress management system based on holistic ideas. Systems theory differentiates systems by their holistic properties. The holistic properties originate from all system parts working together as to form a whole (Churchman, 1968; Schoderbek, Schoderbek & Kefalas, 1990). With this view of systems, the interrelations and the communication between the parts of the system are important for the system; the whole system is bigger than the sum of its constituent parts. A characteristic of living systems, being natural as human beings or constructed as organizations or IT-systems that include users, is self-regulation. "Their subsystems are integrated together to form, actively self-regulating, developing, reproducing unitary systems, with purposes and goals." (Miller, 1971, p. 60). Another feature of living systems is their ability to change and to adapt to new circumstances and demands from the environment. This is also referred to as the openness and viability of a system.

A System of Different Actors' Knowledge and Experiences

In a holistic stress management system, different actors are brought together to contribute with diverse knowledge and experiences. More optimized models of healthy lifestyles are mainly developed through the knowledge of health experts and factual knowledge, while the individual models are created and recreated by people with stress symptoms who experience different life situations, breakdowns, obstacles and issues of motivation. As illustrated in Figure 1, learning a new lifestyle can be regarded as a cogwheel of interrelated parts, combining factual knowledge, expert knowledge and reflections on personal stories and practical habits.

System Principles

In this section, the underlying design principles of the stress management system are presented. These principles together contribute to the design of a holistic and communication-based system. The principles are grouped according to their support of human-, communication- and continuous improvement-centered system design.

Human-Centered System Design

Integration of Different Actors and their Contributions: The stress management system must enable different actors to contribute with their knowledge and experiences. If letting the diversity meet in one system instead of having different types of actors and contributions kept separated, new understanding can be produced. To have direct communication with others who are in the same situation and also with health professionals can create a turning point for people who try to manage stressful situations. This also embraces the idea of users as both consumers and producers of health information and services.

Variety Management in Stressful Situations: People end up in different stressful situations that they struggle to manage; the system should help the users to increase their variety in these situations. Advice on how to approach different stressful situations and how to filter environmental signals and experienced demands, and illustrations of how to perform physical exercises to ease tension, are examples of support that can help the users to manage stressful situations.

System Diversity and Variety: Since people experience different stressful situations, react differently and have different needs, the system should be able to meet this with diversity and variety. Different stress-related areas can enable people with different experiences and needs to navigate between relevant stressful situations, information, exercises and conversations. It should be easy to navigate and to combine different parts of the system.

Multimedia for Virtual and Real Life Integration: In order to narrow the gap between the virtual world and real life, the system needs to consider not only text-based contents and services but also multimedia ditto. Different physical exercises and instructions, such as breathing exercises, could more easily be understood if demonstrated through online video clips, for example. Also online conversations could be made richer if supported by multimedia applications.

Extended Relations: With different health experts invited to the online conversations, new health topics and ideas can easily be introduced. Also people who have managed to recover from difficult and stressful life situations can contribute with their insights. These extended relations allow the system to be more in contact with the environment. The system thereby offers the users both strong and weak tie relations, i.e., the different types of relations that Haythornthwaite (2007) relates to.

Figure 1. Learning new lifestyle as an ongoing cogwheel of interrelated parts (Smedberg, 2011, p. 213)

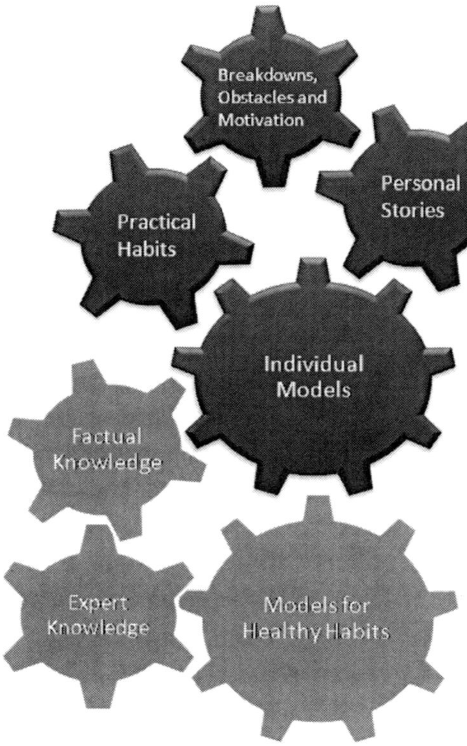

Communication-Centered System Design

Social and Learning Activities: It is essential that the system supports both social and learning activities. Well-functioning web communities foster social and empathical communication (Preece, 1999; 2000). At the same time, learning about stress and stress management has to be the focus of attention. The two – social and learning activities – need to exist in parallel. Assigned health moderators can encourage the users to express different and opposing ideas without jeopardizing social bonds.

Learning Conversations on Stress: Online conversations play an important role in changing unhealthy behaviors. For the users to be aware of and enhance their learning processes, it is important that there are questions and conversations about practical situations, experienced and foreseen difficulties as well as motivational issues (Smedberg, 2008a-b).

Tagged Conversational Topics and Acts: With the posted topics and answers tagged according to their contents and types of response, the conversations can more easily be navigated by the users. If the users tag their own topics and speech acts, it can also help them to reflect upon stress-related issues, and also make them more aware of how they communicate and learn together.

Continuous Learning: To change unhealthy behaviors and patterns of thinking demands for continuous interventions. The system should therefore offer ongoing support in everyday life situations.

Feedback Mechanisms (Health status): The platform should include stress measurements such as physiological markers and self-reports in questionnaires. If done at different times, this feedback helps measure progress in learning.

Continuous Improvement-Centered System Design

Viable Platform through User Patterns: The platform should learn from the users. Through patterns of conversational topics and requests from the users, involved health professionals can get feedback on what goes on in the users' lives and adopt and change the system accordingly. For example, exercises can be added and adjusted as to better suit current stress symptoms of the users.

Feedback Mechanisms (Health status and user needs): As mentioned previously, the platform should include stress measurements such as physiological markers and self-reports in questionnaires. Results from these tests could also be useful for identifying needs that the online intervention system should be able to meet. Also, experiences from using the system need to be made explicit through questionnaires. The users' experiences constitute a valuable source for improvements of the system design.

Help Services/Functionality of the System

In this section, the different help services, or functions, of the stress management system are described.

Ask-the-Expert

Ask-the-expert offers help and advice in various stress-related problems. This help service can be used for asking questions and browsing previously asked questions and answers. This part of the system is based on communication between a user and a medical expert and also the storage of questions and answers that are considered to be of interest to other users of the system.

Counseling Room

The counseling room is a chat where users and professionals meet in small group sessions. The counseling room is based on simultaneous communication between the participants. A time frame is allocated when users and health professionals can meet online. Current stress-related topics for these sessions are announced in advance. Cognitive behavioral therapy for stress management includes such topics as heavy workload, low self-esteem, lack of recovery, imbalance between work and family, labor mobility and skills matching.

Community Forum

Communication between peers is also important to deal with upcoming stressful situations. The community forum allows users to have conversations together about current events in their daily lives, on sleep, work situations or the balance between work and family, for example. Communication can take place anytime, as the need arises. Support from peers can help to gain insights and encouragement to develop new habits.

Practical Tools, Exercises

This help service provides the user with practical tools to use in stressful life situations. Depending on the stress area, there are different exercises that the users can perform on their own at anytime. Reflection exercises, practical relaxation exercises and breathing exercises to reduce physical tension are examples of exercises. The exercises are illustrated in text, audio and video, depending on the purpose of the exercise.

Stories Told and Research Results

This help service is about giving users access to stress-related research and real life stories from others who are or have been in stressful life situations. This part of the system is based primarily on the storage of texts. By allowing users to read about other people's stories together with comments from professionals, users can learn to see their own situation more clearly. It also helps to reduce stigma.

The different help services are summarized in Table 1.

Stress Intervention Areas

This section presents the different stress intervention areas of the web-based system.

Sleep

Sleep is a period of active recovery for the head and body. If you experience a high level of activity during the day the need to sleep increases. During sleep the body builds up new energy, brain and body get the recovery that is needed. The wear from the day before disappears. The immune system and ability to concentrate are promoted by sufficient and good sleep. There are many reasons why some people have insomnia or other sleeping disorders. Here we take up the

Table 1. Types of help services and support in the stress management system

Help Service	Technical Feature	Stress Management Support
Community forum	Asynchronous communication for groups of users	Continuous interactions among peers; exchange of knowledge, experiences and support.
Counseling room	Chat room for synchronous communication	Group learning sessions on stress management themes guided by an expert
Ask-the-expert	Questions posted by users and answered by experts. Selections of anonymous questions and their answers are presented and accessible to all users (Q&As).	Expert knowledge presented in answers to specific stress-related questions from users
Practical tools, exercises	Interactive text-, audio- and video-based exercises accessible to users	Stress management exercises as practical tools for users to do on their own, to ease stress symptoms, e.g.
Stories told & Research results	Text-based personal stories with accompanying expert comments and tips, and research results presented as popular science	Personal stories and stress management information to inspire, guide and educate users

tricks and techniques for people to sleep better if there is stress and anxiety that interfere with a good night's sleep.

Balance in Life

To have balance in life is being able to cope with demands, which enhance ability to manage work, leisure time activities and time spent with family and friends without asking too much. It is also related to being satisfied with what you have chosen to do and what you have not chosen to do.

Balance in life is to set limits and not to say "yes" too often. It is important to realize that it is ok to make demands on the environment. This is something that almost everyone needs to practice. It is possible to achieve better strategies that are health promoting and also prevent stress-induced disorders.

Physical Wellbeing

There is a strong link between physical wellbeing and mental state as body and mind are inseparable. Health promotion and prevention of stress related disorders can be achieved through a combination of physical and mental measures and exercises. Man is an indivisible creature when it comes to harmful stress, there is much people can do by themselves to enhance their health and wellbeing. People need to work regularly to strengthen themselves and make sure they get some time for themselves and for recovery. It need not be for long spells but they must occur frequently.

Work and Studies

The jobs have become more volatile and efficiency requirements in all sectors of the labor market are higher. Work organizations have become "borderless". We are no longer tied to our jobs and there are not clear boundaries for how to work. It has come to include more of autonomy and personal responsibility. Meanwhile, labor markets, such as the Swedish, for example, have become much more international. All this requires more of people as co-workers, to stay healthy and whistle on their way to work.

Structure of the Stress Management System

The web-based stress management system is structured in accordance with the different help services and stress intervention areas presented in the previous sections. In Figure 2, the system structure is illustrated. For each of the four stress intervention areas, the five help services contribute with different knowledge and experiences to the area. In the figure, the stress intervention area called "Sleep" has been expanded and the five help services related to this area are revealed. Indents in the figure illustrate subclasses or related help services. The user can move between the areas and services in a way that suits his or her needs. This means that the user creates his or her own path through the system, and chooses to do exercises, post questions to experts, participate in conversations, contribute with own experiences, reflect together with the others, etc. Web links assist the users to move between related areas and complementary contents and support. Stress intervention becomes dynamic since it is based on the participation of all the actors – both the users with stress symptoms and the experts.

Figure 2. Structure of the stress management system

- Start page
    - Stress Intervention Areas
        - Sleep
            - Ask-the-Expert
            - Practical tools, exercises
            - Forum
            - Counseling room
            - Stories told & Research results
        - Balance in life
        - Physical wellbeing
        - Work & studies
    - About
        - Contact
        - Site map

Example of System Use Scenario

In order to illustrate how the stress management system works, the following is a system use scenario.

David is a 35-year-old man who works with systems analysis at a large IT company in Sweden. He works very long hours at his computer. His back has started to hurt, and his body is stiff and his eyes dry. Recently, sleep has also been affected. He has trouble falling asleep and he also suffers from the fact that he wakes up frequently at night. The first thing David does when he enters the Stress Management System is to open the stress intervention area for issues related to sleep. He begins to search for stories from others who have been in similar situations, and he also posts a question in the Ask-the-expert service to find out what he can do to facilitate his sleep problems. The medical expert who answers the question from David presents some practical advice on how to relax before bedtime. But because David has several problems, the expert recommends also some physical exercises that David can do at work, both to increase the physical activity of the body while sitting in front of the computer and to reduce eyestrain. These exercises are presented in the stress intervention area of work-related issues. The medical expert also recommends David to visit the stress intervention area that deals with creating and maintaining balance in life, i.e., the balance between work, family and friends. Some research results on balance in life are recommended, and David is also encouraged to join the conversations with others about how to make room for activities outside work. In the community conversations, the members share different experiences including some positive experiences of various physical activities. David is curious about some of the activities presented by the others, and therefore he goes into the system's area focused on physical wellbeing. In the conversations on physical wellbeing, he connects with others who are proposing a local race for beginners and to meet IRL, in real life.

The scenario path can be seen in Figure 3.

EVALUATION OF A HOLISTIC LIVING STRESS MANAGEMENT SYSTEM

The stress management system described in this chapter allows for the users to get customized intervention based on their personal needs, and the intervention can also differ a lot from time to time dependent on the present participants, i.e., it is related to the dynamic characteristic of the system. Both health experts and the ones suffering from stressful lives contribute through their active participation in the intervention process.

Various types of health models for measuring stress interventions have been adopted by researchers. These models often assume that psychosocial stressors adversely affect both physical health and mental wellbeing. The experience of stress exposure and its consequences can be measured at the levels of the individual, the group and the organization. The scientific development of methodology measuring different self-rated issues have made it possible to map out the current status, and also before — after measurements regarding interventions.

A stress management system built on communication and interaction among the participants needs to be evaluated in accordance with its characteristics. The system differs from a health intervention program having a predefined step-by-step program and strict path for the user to enter. Although indicators of physical health and mental wellbeing need to be included as in other types of interventions, the online participation from different actors, working individually and in group to learn and develop new lifestyle patterns need also to be evaluated. This is important in order to better understand the value of the intervention systems. An important question is then what indicators or measurements should be used to assess the value of this type of intervention system, how to measure effectiveness of a web-based intervention. In Table 2, measurements of health status and expected outcomes from the interventions, and the communicative and learning activities in the stress management system are displayed. Questionnaires for self-evaluation of health status and also for the users to express their experiences from using the system are part of the evaluation process. In addition, the system user logs and observations of user patterns are also important sources of information for evaluating the stress management system.

Figure 3. Illustration of a fictive user's path through the stress management system

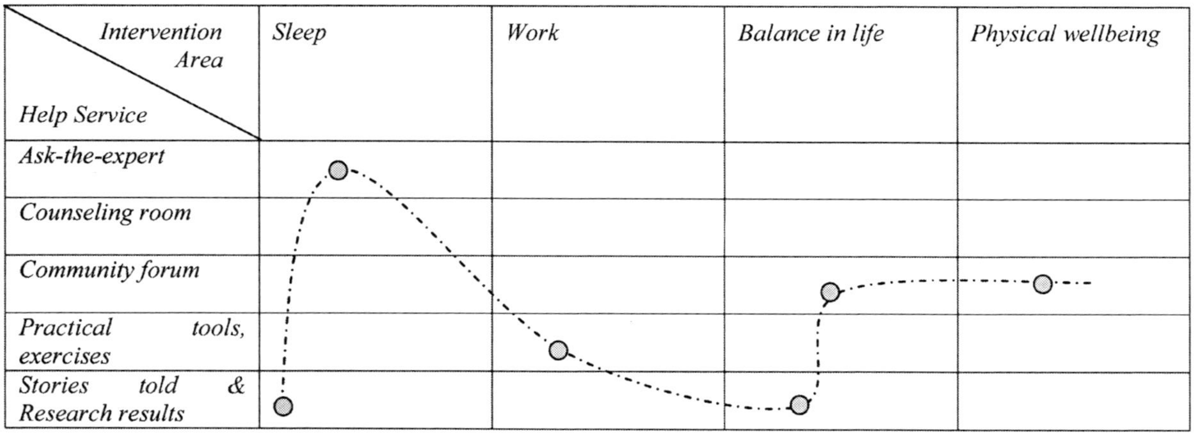

Table 2. What to measure in a holistic communicative stress management system

Type of outcome	Examples of measurement criteria
Stress related symptoms [1]	Irritation or rage, difficulty to control emotions, feeling anxious, anxiety, sadness, being depressed
Sleeping qualities [2]	Quality of sleep, insomnia, waking up in the night, difficulty staying asleep, fatigue during the day
Work –family balance [3]	Interaction between work and private life
Work organization and workplace psychosocial measures [4-5]	Job demands and role expectations, social support, organizational culture, predictability at work
Understanding stress problems	Semi-structured interviews with qualitative analyses
Online learning conversations [6]	Patterns of posted questions, advice, facts, experiences and opposing/reflective answers
Online social support [7]	Number of answers to posted questions, answers expressing empathy
Complementary service and contents [6]	Number of web links and manual references between services and contents, user experiences of the system
Help service/function use	Number of users accessing help service, user experiences of help service

1) Karolinska fatigue questionnaire
2) Åkerstedt, Knutsson, Westerholm, Theorell, Alfredsson & Kecklund, 2002
3) Sandmark, 2007
4) General Nordic Questionnaire
5) Dallner, Elo,Gamberale, Hottinen, Knardahl, Linstrom, Skogstad & Orhede, 2000
6) Smedberg, 2008a-b
7) Preece, 1999; 2000

FUTURE RESEARCH DIRECTIONS

The web-based stress management system presented in this chapter has resulted from previous research studies of web-based solutions for learning new lifestyles, stress management and clinical trials. The next step is to make the system available to a group of employees who experience stressful lives. The focus will be on white-collar workers: office workers and in middle management positions. Implementation and evaluation will follow.

The next technical step is to 'go mobile' and to investigate how the web-based system can be complemented by mobile applications. To integrate new technical features will further increase the system flexibility, and to let the users get help in their everyday lives, whenever and wherever they need support from peers, experts and information contents.

CONCLUSION

To develop and maintain health promotion in working life and balancing work-family; prevention of work related stress disorders is not always an easy task to achieve. In fact, the number of people who suffer from stressful lifestyles has increased in recent years. To manage stress includes learning how to balance the perceived demands of work and personal lives, and to question underlying thoughts and beliefs. E-health communities can contribute to this process through continuous interactions between people who are in similar situations. Studies have also shown that knowledge of health experts and experiences from peers can be complementary for people who look to develop and maintain healthy lifestyles. In this chapter we have presented a holistic approach to web-based stress management that addresses these previous research findings. A web-based stress management system was presented that includes different actors and support, and it was also discussed how to make use of these in a complementary way. In addition, the chapter showed how this kind of web-based stress management system needs to be evaluated in a way that considers both health outcomes and dynamic online learning activities.

REFERENCES

Åkerstedt, T., Knutsson, A., Westerholm, P., Theorell, T., Alfredsson, L., & Kecklund, G. (2002). Sleep disturbances, work stress and work hours—A cross-sectional study. *Journal of Psychosomatic Research*, *53*, 741–748. doi:10.1016/S0022-3999(02)00333-1

Austin, J. L. (1962). *How to do things with words*. Cambridge, MA: Harvard University Press.

Beecham, B., Dammers, J., & van Zwanenberg, T. (2004). Leadership coaching for general practitioners. *Education for Primary Care*, *15*, 579–583.

Benson, B. (2001). *The relaxation response*. New York, NY: Harper Collins.

Bergström, J. (2010). *Internet-based treatment for depression and panic disorder - From development to deployment.* Doctoral thesis, Karolinska Institute.

Budzik, J., & Hammond, K. (1999). Q&A: A system for the capture, organization and reuse of expertise. *Proceedings of the Sixty-Second Annual Meeting of the American Society for Information Science*, Information Today, Inc.

Churchman, C. W. (1968). *The systems approach*. Delacorte Press.

Cooper, C., Dewe, P., & O'Driscoll, M. (2001). *Organizational stress: A review and critique of theory, research, and applications*. Thousand Oaks, CA & London, UK: Sage Publications.

Dallner, A., Elo, A.-L., Gamberale, F., Hottinen, V., Knardahl, S., & Linstrom, K. (2000). *Validation of the general Nordic questionnaire for psychological and social factors at work.* Nordic Council of Ministers Copenhagen, DK. *Nord*, *2000*, 12.

Dekkers-Sánchez, P. M., Hoving, J. L., Sluiter, J. K., & Frings-Dresen, M. H. (2008). Factors associated with long-term sick leave in sick-listed employees: A systematic review. *Occupational and Environmental Medicine*, *65*, 153–157. doi:10.1136/oem.2007.034983

Ellis, J. B., & Bruckman, A. S. (2001). Designing palaver tree online: Supporting social roles in a community of oral history. *CHI*, *3*(1), 474–481.

Fox, N. J., Ward, K. J., & O'Rourke, A. J. (2005). The expert patient: Empowerment or medical dominance? The case of weight loss, pharmaceutical drugs and the Internet. *Social Science & Medicine*, *60*(6), 1299–1309. doi:10.1016/j.socscimed.2004.07.005

Gottwald, M. (2006). Health promotion models. In Davis, S. (Ed.), *Rehabilitation: The use of theories and models in practice*. London, UK: Churchill Livingstone.

Hannah, C. (2004). Improving intermediate skills through workplace coaching: A case study within the UK rail industry. *International Journal of Evidence Based Coaching and Mentoring*, *2*(1), 17–40.

Hasson, D., Anderberg, U. M., Theorell, T., & Arnetz, B. B. (2005). Psychophysiological effects of a web-based stress management system: A prospective, randomized controlled intervention study of IT and media workers. *BMC Public Health*, *5*, 78..doi:10.1186/1471-2458-5-78

Hasson, D., Arnetz, B. B., Theorell, T., & Anderberg, U. M. (2006). Predictors of self-rated health: A 12-month prospective study of IT and media workers. *Population Health Metrics*, *4*, 8..doi:10.1186/1478-7954-4-8

Haythornthwaite, C. (2007). Social networks and online community. In Joinson, A., McKenna, K., Postmes, T., & Reips, U.-D. (Eds.), *The Oxford handbook of Internet psychology* (pp. 121–137). New York, NY: Oxford University Press.

Henderson, M., Glozier, N., & Holland, E. K. (2005). Long term sickness absence is caused by common conditions and needs managing. *BMJ (Clinical Research Ed.)*, *330*, 802–803. doi:10.1136/bmj.330.7495.802

Holmgren, K., Dahlin-Ivanoff, S., Björkelund, C., & Hensing, G. (2009). The prevalence of work-related stress, and its association with self-perceived health and sick-leave, in a population of employed Swedish women. *BMC Public Health*, *2*(9), 73. doi:10.1186/1471-2458-9-73

Jacobson, E. (1938). *Progressive relaxation* (2nd ed.). Chicago, IL: University of Chicago.

Jones, M. C., & Johnston, D. W. (2000). Reducing distress in first level and student nurses: A review of the applied stress management literature. *Journal of Advanced Nursing*, *32*, 66–74. doi:10.1046/j.1365-2648.2000.01421.x

Josefsson, U. (2007). *Coping online – Patients' use of the Internet.* Doctoral thesis, 37, Dep. of Applied Information Technology, IT-University of Göteborg, Sweden.

Karasek, R., & Theorell, T. (1990). *Healthy work: Stress, productivity, and the reconstruction of working life*. New York, NY: Basic Books.

Karolinska. (n.d.). *Karolinska fatigue questionnaire* [Karolinska utmattingsformulär]. Retrieved from http://www.stressmottagningen.nu/ wp-content/ uploads/dokument/ utmattningsform.pdf

Kling, R. (2000). Learning about information technologies and social change: The contribution of social informatics. *The Information Society*, *16*(3), 217–232. doi:10.1080/01972240050133661

Lazarus, R. S., & Folkman, S. (1984). *Stress, appraisal and coping*. New York, NY: Springer Publishing.

Maloney-Krichmar, D., & Preece, J. (2005). A multilevel analysis of sociability, usability and community dynamics in an online health community. *ACM Transactions on Computer-Human Interaction*, *12*(2), 201–232. doi:10.1145/1067860.1067864

Marco, J., Barba, R., Losa, J. E., de la Serna, C. M., Sainz, M., Lantigua, I. F., & de la Serna, J. L. (2006). Advice from a medical expert through the Internet on queries about AIDS and hepatitis: Analysis of a pilot experiment. *PLoS Medicine*, *3*(7), 1041–1047. doi:10.1371/journal.pmed.0030256

Marine, S., Embi, P. J., McCuistion, M., Haag, D., & Guard, J. R. (2005). NetWellness 1995-2005: Ten years of experience and growth as a non-profit consumer health information and Ask-an-Expert service. In *AMIA 2005 Symposium Proceedings,* 22-26 October 2005. Washington DC, USA.

Mayo, C. S. R. (2005). Anxiety disorders: Taking control of persistent worries, fears, and phobias. *Mayo Clinic Women's Healthsource*, (July): 1–8.

Mehra, B., Merkel, C., & Bishop, A. P. (2004). The internet for empowerment of minority and marginalized users. *New Media & Society*, *6*(6), 781–802. doi:10.1177/146144804047513

Miller, J. G. (1971). Living systems. [North-Holland Publishing Company.]. *Currents in Modern Biology*, 55–77.

Murphy, L. R. (1996). Stress management in work settings: A critical review of the health effects. *American Journal of Health Promotion*, *11*, 112–135.

Pollak Eisen, K., Allen, G. J., Bollash, M., & Pescatello, L. S. (2008). Stress management in the workplace: A comparison of a computer-based and an in-person stress-management intervention. [Elsevier.]. *Computers in Human Behavior*, *24*, 486–496. doi:10.1016/j.chb.2007.02.003

Preece, J. (1999). Empathic communities: Balancing emotional and factual communication. *Interacting with Computers, 12*, 63–77. doi:10.1016/S0953-5438(98)00056-3

Preece, J. (2000). *Online communities – Designing usability, supporting sociability*. Chichester, UK: Wiley & Sons, Ltd.

Questionnaire, G. N. (2000). *QPS Nordic*. Retrieved from http://www2a.cdc.gov/ nioshworkorg/ detail.asp?id=84

Rootman, I., Goodstadt, M., Potvin, L., & Springett, J. (2001). A framework for health promotion evaluation. In Rootman, I. (Ed.), *Evaluation in health promotion: Principles and perspectives*. Copenhagen: WHO, Regional Office for Europe.

Sandmark, H. (2007). Work and family: Associations with long term sick-listing in Swedish women. *BMC Public Health, 7*, 287. doi:10.1186/1471-2458-7-287

Sandmark, H. (2009). Job mismatching, unequal opportunities and long-term sickness absence in female white collar workers in Sweden. *Scandinavian Journal of Public Health, 37*, 43–49. doi:10.1177/1403494808098916

Schoderbek, P. P., Schoderbek, C. G., & Kefalas, A. G. (1990). *Management systems – Conceptual considerations*. Richard D. Irwin, Inc.

Seaward, B. (2002). *Managing stress*. Boston, MA: Jones and Bartlett.

Siegrist, J. (1996). Adverse health effects of high effort – low reward conditions at work. *Journal of Occupational Health Psychology, 1*, 27–43. doi:10.1037/1076-8998.1.1.27

Smedberg, Å. (2008a). Learning conversations for people with established bad habits: A study of four health-communities. *International Journal of Healthcare Technology and Management, 9*(2), 143–154. doi:10.1504/IJHTM.2008.017369

Smedberg, Å. (2008b). *Online communities and learning for health – The use of online health-communities and online expertise for people with established bad habits*. Doctoral thesis, Stockholm University.

Smedberg, Å. (2011). E-health communities for learning healthy habits: How to consider quality and usability. In Moumtzoglou, A., & Kastania, A. (Eds.), *E-health systems quality and reliability: Models and standards* (pp. 204–219). Hershey, PA: IGI Global.

Sproull, L., & Kiesler, S. (1991). *Connections: New ways of working in the networked organization*. Cambridge, MA: The MIT Press.

The Swedish Social Insurance Agency. (2010). Social insurance statistics. Försäkringskassan. Retrieved October 10, 2010, from http://statistik.forsakringskassan.se/ portal/ page?_pageid=93,1&_dad=portal& _schema=PORTAL

Tones, K., & Green, J. (2003). *Health promotion: Planning and strategies*. Sage Publications.

Vaartjes, V. (2005). Integrating action learning practices into executive coaching to enhance business. *International Journal of Evidence Based Coaching and Mentoring, 3*(1), 1–17.

von Schéele, I., von Schéele, B., Hansson, G., Winman, A., & Theorell, T. (2005). Psychosocial factors and respiratory and cardiovascular parameters during psychophysiological stress profiling in working men and women. *Applied Psychophysiology and Biofeedback, 30*(2), 125–136. doi:10.1007/s10484-005-4309-6

Walther, J. B., Pingree, S., Hawkins, R. P., & Buller, D. B. (2005). Attributes of interactive online health information systems. *Journal of Medical Internet Research, 7*(3). doi:10.2196/jmir.7.3.e33

Wenger, E. (2004). Communities of practice and social learning systems. In Starkey, K., Tempest, S., & McKinlay, A. (Eds.), *How organizations learn: Managing the search for knowledge* (2nd ed., pp. 238–258). London, UK: Thomson Learning.

WHO. (1986). *Ottawa charter for health promotion*. Copenhagen, Denmark: WHO Europe.

Winograd, T., & Flores, F. (1987). *Understanding computers and cognition: A new foundation for design*. Boston, MA: Addison-Wesley Publishing Company.

ADDITIONAL READING

Andriessen, J., Baker, M. J., & Dan Suthers, D. (2003). Argumentation, computer support, and the educational context of confronting cognitions. In Andriessen, J., Baker, M. J., & Suthers, D. (Eds.), *Arguing to learn: Confronting cognitions in computer-supported collaborative learning Environments* (pp. 1–25). Dordrecht, The Netherlands: Kluwer Academic Publishers.

Bishop, J. (2005).The role of mediating artefacts in the design of persuasive e-learning systems. *Proceedings of the internet technology & applications 2005 conference*, North East Wales Institute of Higher Education, Wrexham.

Bishop, J. (2007). Increasing participation in online communities: A framework for human–computer interaction. *Computers in Human Behavior*, *23*(4), 1881–1893. doi:10.1016/j.chb.2005.11.004

Boyd, D. M., & Ellison, N. B. (2008). Social network sites: Definition, history, and scholarship. *Journal of Computer-Mediated Communication*, *13*, 210–230. doi:10.1111/j.1083-6101.2007.00393.x

Bradley, G. (2006). *Social and community informatics: Humans on the Net*. London: Routledge.

Dannecker, A., & Lechner, U. (2007). Online and offline integration in virtual communities of patients – An empirical analysis. In Steinfield, Pentland, Ackerman & Contractor (Eds.), *Communities and Technologies 2007: Proceedings of the Third Communities and Technologies Conference*, Michigan State University. London: Springer, 151-170.

De Cindio, F., Gentile, O., Grew, P., & Redolfi, D. (2003). Community networks: Rules of behavior and social structure. *The Information Society*, *19*, 395–406. doi:10.1080/714044686

Figallo, C. (1998). *Hosting web communities*. New York: John Wiley & Sons.

Johnson, G. J., & Ambrose, P. J. (2006). Neo-tribes: The power and potential of online communities in health care. *Communications of the ACM*, *49*(1), 107–113. doi:10.1145/1107458.1107463

Kling, R. (1999). What is social informatics and why does it matter? *D-Lib Magazine*, *5*(1). doi:10.1045/january99-kling

Noar, S. M., & Zimmerman, R. S. (2004). Health behavior theory and cumulative knowledge regarding health behaviors: Are we moving in the right direction? *Health Education Research*, *20*(3), 275–290. doi:10.1093/her/cyg113

Preece, J. (1998). Empathic communities: Reaching out across the Web. *Interaction*, *5*(2), 32–43. doi:10.1145/274430.274435

Preece, J. (2001). Sociability and usability in online communities: Determining and measuring success. *Behaviour & Information Technology*, *20*(5). doi:10.1080/01449290110084683

Preece, J., Nonnecke, B., & Andrews, D. (2004). The top 5 reasons for lurking: Improving community experiences for everyone. *Computers in Human Behavior*, 2.

Smedberg, Å. (2009). The use of an online health community on overweight: A member perspective, *Proceedings of IADIS International Conference Web Based Communities 2009 (WBC 2009), 21-23 June 2009* (51-58).

Wright, K. B., & Bell, S. B. (2003). Health-related support groups on the Internet: Linking empirical findings to social support and computer-mediated communication theory. *Journal of Health Psychology*, *8*(1), 39–54. doi:10.1177/1359105303008001429

Chapter 10
Living a Healthier Life Online:
On Blending Professional and Experiential Knowledge in Online Self-Help Groups

Roar Stokken
Norwegian University of Science and Technology, Norway & Sunnmøre Hospital Trust, Norway

Gjermund Eikli
Norwegian Net School, Norway

ABSTRACT

The chapter explores how organizations can facilitate online self-help initiatives in a manner that allows mutual aid to flourish between the participants. It takes a theoretical approach on the basis of pedagogy and self-help/mutual-aid research. It first develops an educational model, and then turns to practical aspects and investigates the Norwegian course "Living a healthier life – online." The initiative is transformed from face-to-face to online as a design-based research project. The two most important elements to pay attention to in the facilitation of online self-help initiatives are found to be socialization and overall assignments: the former to prepare for mutual exchange of knowledge, and the latter to make content relevant to daily life.

INTRODUCTION

In self-help groups, people who share the same or similar circumstances or conditions discuss and share ways of coping as mutual aid (Borkman, 1999). Computer-mediated self-help groups suit those who for various reasons are prevented from attending face-to-face initiatives, and they have existed for several decades; nowadays as discussion boards on the Internet, earlier on bulletin board systems (BBS). For the most part, such online groups have arisen from the same premises as traditional face-to-face groups: from fiery souls and mutual need, and they have been moderated and maintained on a voluntary basis.

DOI: 10.4018/978-1-60960-866-8.ch010

Nowadays online self-help groups are more often provided as e-health services by organizations within the public, voluntary and private sectors. As opposed to mutual need as a driving force, these stem from a demand for services to the target group. Nevertheless, mutual aid is a driving force, and the organizations' motive is often to help people to help themselves. In this article we explore how organizations can facilitate such online initiatives in a manner that lets mutual aid flourish between the participants.

Sharing knowledge of one's own experience, what Borkman (1976) terms 'experiential knowledge', is of great importance in self-help/mutual-aid groups, but is often not sufficient. This is reflected in the significant body of literature that concerns the role of professionals and professional knowledge in self-help groups (e.g. Matzat, 1993; Powell, 1987; Wilson, 1995). This body concerns in the main face-to-face groups, and literature concerning professional and experiential knowledge in online initiatives is, even outside the self-help literature, virtually non-existant. Furthermore, organizations in general possess knowledge of a certain topic, like cancer, diabetes or anxiety that they desire to impart. Due to its nature, this knowledge is to be considered as professional knowledge.

On this basis we adopt a theoretical approach to investigate how both experiential and professional knowledge can flourish and be amalgamated within online self-help initiatives. On the basis of pedagogy and self-help/mutual-aid research, we first develop an educational model that facilitates the amalgamation of professional knowledge and experiential knowledge. We then turn practical, and investigate the course 'Living a healthier life – online'. In the discussion we relate our findings to other initiatives where the exchange of experiential knowledge is central. From this we deduce some aspects that are vital when experiential and professional knowledge in online self-help initiatives is to be amalgamated.

BACKGROUND

On the basis of Borkman's seminal article from 1976, the body of self-help literature distinguishes between three kinds of knowledge: professional, experiential and lay. (1) Professional knowledge is developed, applied, and transmitted by an established specialized occupation that has financial and career interest in the topic. (2) Experiential knowledge is learned from personal experience and acquired by living through a problem firsthand. The experientialist is often thought of as the one in possession of a problem, like breast cancer or anxiety. Significant others, such as spouses, siblings or close friends, may also obtain experiential knowledge. This knowledge is not the same as that developed by the one suffering from the condition, but it overlaps somewhat. (3) In contrast to professional and experiential knowledge, lay knowledge is acquired by a bystander that has second-hand information of the problem, often from a combination of rumours, the media, professionals and experientialists (Borkman, 1976, 1999).

Professional and experiential knowledge relate to two modes of thought (Borkman, 1999). Professional knowledge is, according to Bruner, constructed within the "paradigmatic or logico-scientific [mode, which] attempts to fulfil the ideal of a formal, mathematical system of description and explanation" (1986, p. 12). On the contrary, experiential knowledge is constructed within the narrative mode of thought, which leads "to good stories, gripping drama, believable (though not necessarily 'true') historical accounts" (1986, p. 13). "Unlike the professional knowledge that is generated by logical and scientific procedures that can be weeded out by falsification; experiential knowledge can only achieve 'verisimilitude'." (1991, p. 4) For, narratives are bound to the context and thus their verisimilitude depends upon them appearing true or real in the context where the narrator is a central part. This makes professional knowledge more or less universal and context-independent, while experiential knowledge is closely bound to person, context and experience.

Professional and experiential knowledge are not mutually exclusive. Both patients and professionals usually allow for a second source as legitimate input. On the other hand, the universal and context-independent nature of professional knowledge makes it possible for patients to develop expertise in professional terms, as demonstrated by Heldal and Tjora (2009). On the contrary, the professional is prevented from accessing experiential knowledge directly, due to it being tightly bound to personal experience of a condition or a situation. Still, a professional can develop experiential knowledge from experiencing a problem first hand; an oncologist will develop experiential knowledge of cancer – if she gets cancer herself.

When initiatives are provided by organizations, not only experiential knowledge, but also professional knowledge is in need of a legitimate role. To find the place of such a role, we now take a look at the learning that occurs in self-help groups.

The Concept of Learning in Self-Help Groups

The reason for attending a self-help group is to learn how to cope with the situation that is the focus of the group. Munn-Giddings et al. (2007) found that personal gains were empathy, emotional coping, sharing of experiential knowledge and practical information, peer-support and friendship. In sum, it appears that such groups offer something that cannot be replicated in professional-user relations, and thus concern a kind of outcome that is somewhat wider than the traditional understanding of knowledge and learning, even though it undoubtedly is learning that takes place in the group.

Knowledge and learning have traditionally been understood as a behaviouristic or cognitive process. During recent decades this view has been broadened (i.e. Bateson, 1972; Cole, 1996; Engeström, 1987; Greeno, Collins, & Resnick, 1996; Hutchins; Vygotsky, 1978). This makes Illeris (2004) claim that a coherent overall theory of learning should concern changes in three dimensions: (1) cognitive change, (2) psychodynamic change, and (3) social change (Figure 1). These dimensions are not independent. Theorists attend to these dimensions in various degrees, and also in the process of learning their significance varies.

In Illeris' three-dimensional approach to knowledge and learning, cognitive change is about the classic approach to learning, which for instance Piaget and Kolb represent. In this dimension, learning is a change of understanding or skills, taking place in the head of the learner. In this way learning becomes a means of achieving alignment between contexts and how the context is being understood. The focus that professional knowledge has upon rationality, universality and context-independence, makes learning of such knowledge mostly involve cognitive change.

The broadening of pedagogy toward psychodynamic change concerns which psychological processes that ought to be understood as learning. Freud and Rogers are two theorists from within the psychodynamic approach in psychology that this

Figure 1. Learning in three dimensions (Adapted from Illeris (2004))

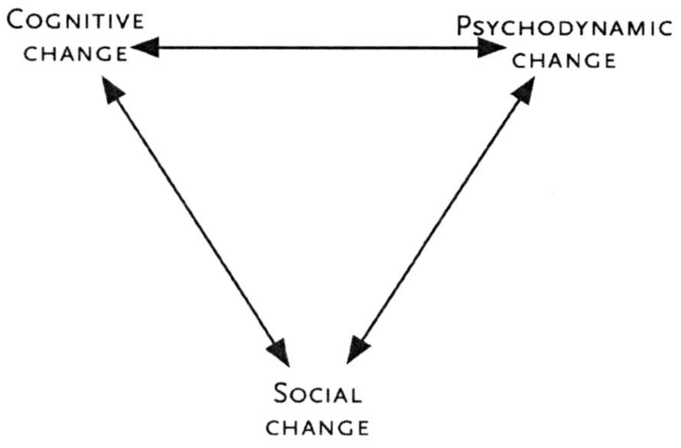

broadening has made relevant. The psychodynamic approach pays attention to how behaviour and feelings are affected by unconscious motives and forces within the person. Thus, in this dimension, learning is understood as changed psychic energy. Such change creates positive or negative energy that both can facilitate and obstruct learning. It usually concerns changed emotions, motivation or attitudes, and hence this change also is in the head of the learner. The nature of experiential knowledge, which belongs to the narrative mode of thought (Bruner, 1986), and is legitimized by verisimilitude rather than rationality, denotes that it is tightly bound to persons' emotions and daily life. Hence such learning mostly involves psychodynamic change.

The broadening towards social change has concerned to which extent recall, artefacts and practice are parts of the process of learning. This broadening has been connected to an approach where cognition is understood as being distributed between brain and context (i.e. Cole, 1996; Hutchins, 1995a; Lave & Wenger, 1991). This has made for instance Marx, Beck and Giddens relevant to the theories of learning. In this perspective, learning changes the premises for social interaction and becomes a societal process that involves artefacts used in social interaction (e.g. language, technology and political structures). In this dimension, changing such artefacts and/or related practices is understood as learning.

While cognitive and psychodynamic change goes on in the head of individuals, the social change takes place in the interaction between humans and between the humans and the contexts. In general, learning concerns change in all three dimensions, and even though to varying degrees, they influence each other in a reciprocal manner. Still it is important to pay attention to the fact that while the learning in the head is individual, the social learning is situated.

Self-Help Groups as an Arena for Learning

When attending a self-help group, one moves into a situation where certain challenges are common. In this situation one learns from and together with peers, to be able to cope in a better way with the challenges and integrate into a society where these challenges are not common. The self-help group can therefore be said to induce cognitive and psychodynamic changes in a person's head, by partaking in a social interaction. These are meant to alter the social interaction, e.g. in terms of changed ability for action in the situation one is *learning for*; whether it is daily life in general or more specific situations.

Self-help initiatives provided by organizations must, as pointed to above, often both facilitate the dissemination of professional knowledge and the exchange of experiential knowledge. The difference between how these two knowledge types mediate between the situation *one is learning in* and the situation *one is learning for* is illustrated by means of arrows in Figure 2.

Dissemination of professional knowledge means that the learning that is induced is meant to mediate from the situation one is *learning in* to the situation one is *learning for*. Due to the nature of professional knowledge, the mediation is mostly by means of cognitive change and is mainly one-directional.

With regard to experiential knowledge, the process demands that knowledge acquired in the situation *one is learning for* becomes a central vehicle for learning among the peers in the self-help group. Due to the characteristics of experiential knowledge, the mediation is mostly by means of psychodynamic change. The knowledge exchange must therefore be both bi-directional and qualitatively different from when the aim is the dissemination of professional knowledge. This demands facilitation of the close connection between experiential knowledge, the experimen-

Figure 2. Mediation of knowledge between the situation one is 'learning in' and the situation one is 'learning for'

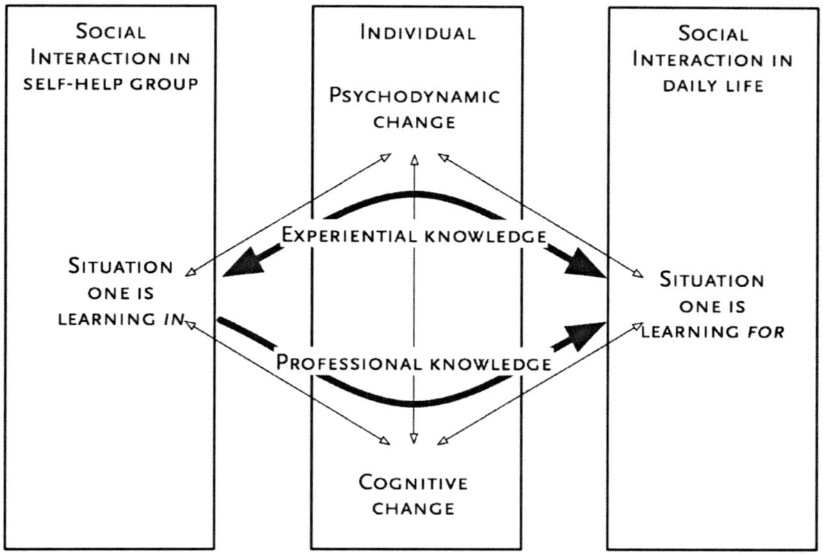

talist, emotions and the situation one is *learning for*, in order to give the experiential knowledge verisimilitude.

Techniques for making experiential knowledge into a vehicle for knowledge building are somewhat different from those used in the dissemination of professional knowledge, since the participants' thoughts in terms of reflections, stories and motivation must be given a central position. Thus it is not enough to facilitate individual learning when both professional knowledge and experiential knowledge are to be amalgamated in an initiative; the facilitation of social interaction and co-learning between the participants must also be included.

Learning as a Mutual Learning Process in Self-Help Groups

In our further development of an understanding of how both experiential and professional knowledge can flourish and be united within online self-help initiatives, we focus upon the social processes in the groups. We therefore make use of a social and context bound learning model developed by Nonaka et al. (e.g. Nonaka & Takeuchi, 1995; Nonaka, Toyama, & Konno, 2001). This approach focuses on how the surroundings must facilitate four types of transformation of knowledge in order to be optimal: (1) *Socialization*, which involves experiencing things together. (2) *Externalization,* which is the process by which tacit knowledge becomes explicit knowledge. (3) *Combination* where 'old' and 'new' knowledge is combined to form more complex knowledge structures. And (4) *Internalization* when what one thinks in the combination phase is translated into changed practice. Nonaka combines these transformations into what he calls the SECI-model. On the basis of this model, Stokken and Eikli (2010) discuss how technology can be designed to support these processes and propose an educational model for online courses (Figure 3). In the development of a methodology for blend experiential and professional knowledge in online self-help initiatives, we extend this model.

In the educational model we see in the lighter part of the diagram what can be included in the course, and in the darker part what the participants

Figure 3. Educational model for online learning (© 2010 Gyldendal Akademisk. Used with permission.)

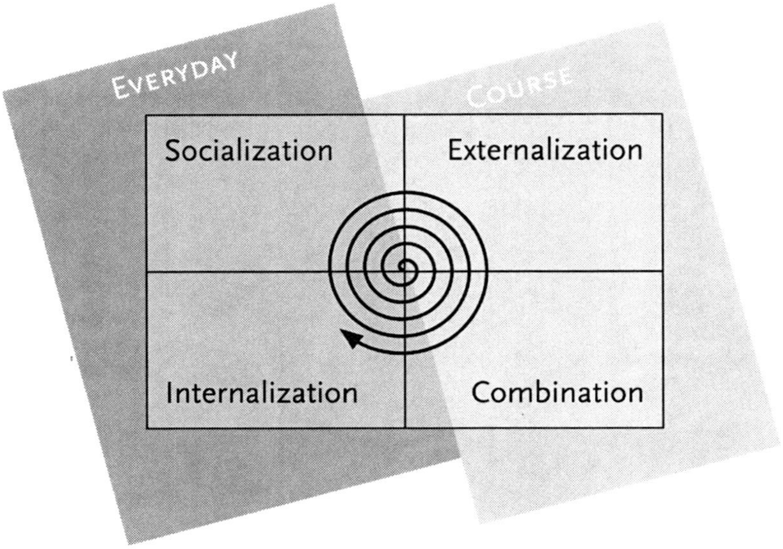

must do as part of their daily lives. In other words, the content of the darker part must take place in the participants' everyday lives, while the content of the lighter part can be studied on the course. With regard to self-help as social learning process, the darker part is where experiential knowledge originates, while the lighter part is where it is made explicit and exchanged. Reflection upon existing experiences is important in learning processes, and consequently one often oscillates between externalization and combination before entering the internalization phase (Yew & Karney, 2010). This is very relevant to the learning process in self-help groups due to the bi-directional exchange of experiential knowledge between the situation one is *learning in* and the situation one is *learning for*.

Avis et al. (2008) describe three main aspects of the value of partaking in mutual aid-groups. These are 1) *forming a sense of togetherness*, 2) *learning from one other,* and 3) *developing mutuality*. Relating to the educational model for online learning (Figure 3), *forming a sense of togetherness* (Avis, et al., 2008) takes place during the *socialization* process where individual tacit knowledge is shared, and becomes common tacit knowledge. In this process participants identify with one another and generate a foundation for empathy through shared experiences. This phase of the self-help group (the darker triangle of the socialization-rectangle) enables the verisimilitude that experiential knowledge is dependent upon.

In the *externalization phase* tacit knowledge becomes explicit knowledge. This is where the participants are *learning from each other* (Avis, et al., 2008). In traditional self-help groups, this for instance is facilitated by means of the 'round' where the participants tell stories and reflects upon their coping as part of daily life. This dynamic exchange of experiential knowledge between participants benefits both the provider and the receiver. Riessmann (1965) pinpointed this value of being of help to others in her seminal article where she introduced the term 'helper therapy principle'. In 12-step groups like AA and Al-Anon this dual value is embedded into the practices by means of sponsorship between newcomers and seniors.

In the *combination phase*, 'old' and 'new' knowledge is combined to form more complex knowledge structures. In this process reflection upon what is explicated by one self and other participants is essential in order to achieve this combination of 'new' and 'old' knowledge. This is where the *development of mutuality* (Avis, et al., 2008) takes place through co-learning between the participants. In daily life (the darker triangle of this light combination rectangle), the participants as part of their daily life activate and reflect upon knowledge acquired in the group.

In the *internalization phase*, what one thinks in the combination phase becomes practice. Thus it is here explicit knowledge forms the basis for tacit knowledge by becoming part of behaviour. This pinpoints the fact that the learning generated in the self-help group is not separate from the daily life of the participants, but is an ongoing and integrating part of the process of coping with own life and condition. This is why the bi-directional arrow between the situation *one is learning in* and the situation *one is learning for* in figure 2 is of great importance.

As discussed above, both professional knowledge and experiential knowledge must have a legitimate role in online self help initiatives provided by organizations. How both knowledge types can flourish and be amalgamated is our central point in the forthcoming text. If professional knowledge contributes to the process, this is added in the combination process. To make this type of knowledge distinct from experiential knowledge, we have added a fifth rectangle to the educational model (Figure 3). In this extended educational model (Figure 4) we make professional knowledge stand out as a second source of input to the combination phase, in addition to the externalization of experiential knowledge.

To understand the amalgamation of professional and experiential knowledge in online self-help initiatives, we now turn to an example where both professional and experiential knowledge occupy a legitimate and important position.

METHOD

Our main example is Stanford's Chronic Disease Self-Management Program (Lorig, Gonzalez, & Laurent, 1999; Lorig, et al., 2000). In the discussion, we also draw upon complimentary examples from the portfolio of the Norwegian Net School that unite professional and experiential knowledge. The self-management program aims both to impart professional knowledge from a set syllabus and to enable the participants to share their experiential knowledge. The course content and programme are set out in a detailed instructor handbook. The pedagogical foundation is to be found in the work of Albert Bandura (1997), in particular the concept of self-efficacy. The course has been translated into a number of languages and forms the basis of The Expert Patient Programme offered by the Department of Health in Britain.

The development of the Norwegian online version of Stanford's Chronic Disease Self-Management Program (CDSMP) was done at the Regional Patient Education Resource Centre in Central Norway, now part of the local Patient Education Resource Centre at Sunnmøre Hospital. The project was carried out in collaboration with the Norwegian Net School and the Norwegian Multiple Sclerosis Association. The project was motivated from judging it insufficient to translate the American online version, due to it being to individualistically focussed. The present American online version attunes to a similar pedagogic model as the Norwegian version.

The Norwegian online version was named 'Living a Healthier Life – online', and was transformed from classroom to online version within the framework of design-based research. Brown (1992) and Collins (1992) are regarded as portal figures for this type of research, but several directions exist, such as e.g. formative research (Reigeluth & Frick, 1999), design research (Edelson, 2002) and theory-based design (Hannafin, 1997; Land & Hannafin, 2000). It is theory-based design that is adopted in the development of 'Living a

Figure 4. Extended educational model

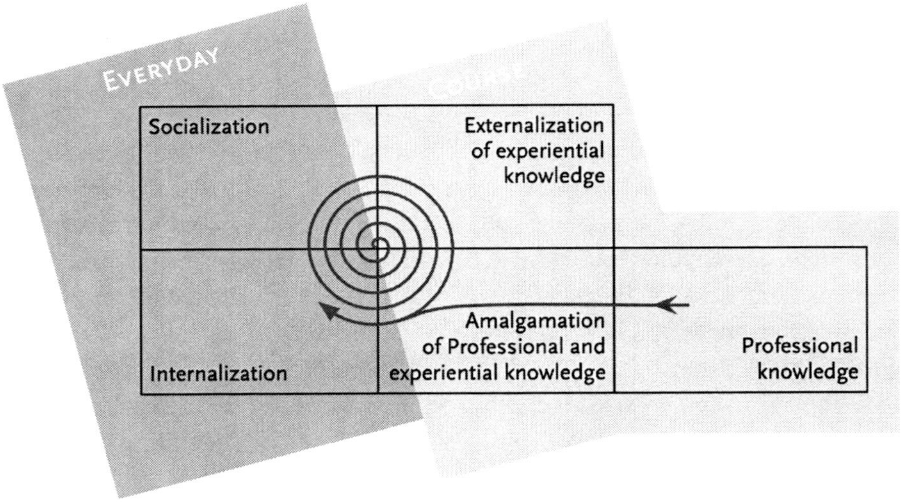

Healthier Life – online'. In design-based research the key feature is that the research aims and the developmental aims are closely interwoven (The Design-Based Research Collective, 2003). Moreover, it is essential that the development takes place in iterative development processes. Here this has been solved through so-called extreme programming (Beck, 2000).

Theory-based design (Hannafin, 1997; Land & Hannafin, 2000) is based on the assumption that all learning environments consist of five elements that stand in a dialectic relationship to each other. These are: (1) psychology, which forms how one understands learning and thinking, (2) pedagogy, which dictates how to organise learning environments, (3) culture, which reflects values appreciated, (4) technology, which supports, governs or makes for a richer learning environment, and (5) pragmatism with regard to the availability of resources. Thus the precondition for enacting a successful transformation from classroom to online version is knowledge about the course, combined with knowledge about e-learning. With the aid of this knowledge the course is built up pragmatically within the framework provided by the culture and the technology in accordance with the fundamental psychological and pedagogical principles.

The Norwegian Net School has developed PedIT, an online e-learning platform built on educational ideas well suited to the course. In May and June 2004 the course was run as a pilot using this platform. The pilot had 18 participants and four supervisors, all of whom were experienced instructors from classroom courses. In the autumn of 2004 a trial programme was run, consisting of 2 courses with a total of 78 participants in 8 separate groups. The material presented here originates from this trial. A similar model was tested in 2008 with 48 participants. From 2009 the project has been part of the regular portfolio of the Norwegian Study Organization for Disabled. At present, the organization runs 'Living a healthier life – online' two to four times a year. There are between ten and thirty participants on each run.

In the analysis of activity, e-learning has the advantage that the communication between the participants is visible to other people. We have therefore used information that is stored in the e-learning system as a 'black box', similar to the 'black boxes' that store records of what happens on board a plane. In this way we have re-created processes that took place in the past in order to understand how the various actors have interacted together. The material contains 3200 utterances. 75% of these are related to action plans. The authors were both central participants in the project.

LIVING A HEALTHIER LIFE – ONLINE

The Chronic Disease Self-Management Program is not linked to any specific diagnoses and is a supplement to normal treatment and education in managing specific illnesses/disabilities, both for people with chronic illnesses/disabilities and their families. The program intends to help participants manage their illness, carry out normal activities and tackle emotional challenges and rests upon cognitive psychology, in particular the concept of 'self-efficacy' (Bandura, 1997; Lorig, et al., 2000). Self-efficacy concerns the belief that one is capable of performing in a certain manner to achieve specific goals. Thus it is important to choose both realistic goals and adequate means to achieve these goals. By reaching these goals, one builds confidence in changing own life and thus also increases self-esteem, as a person's judgment of his or her capabilities is based on past experiences of mastery.

The Norwegian online version is an eight-week course (one week introduction, six weeks of content, and a week between session three and four with no new content). The course has two parallel tracks: (1) one track focussing upon dissemination of professional knowledge in terms of course content as in traditional educational initiatives, and (2) one track that facilitates exchange of experiential knowledge between peers. The course is partially synchronous. It is synchronous by all participants starting at the same time and following the same progress within the timeframe of a week; but within each week there is asynchronicity. This model has been chosen to facilitate interaction and co-learning between the participants while providing flexibility (within the timeframe of a week).

We structure our further investigation into how to facilitate online self-help initiatives along the main components in 'Living a Healthier Life – online'. In the investigation we pay special attention to how each of the means discussed contributes to cognitive, psychodynamic and/or social learning, and where the activities are to be found in our extended educational model (Figure 4).

Group

'Living a Healthier Life – online' is anchored in a self-help philosophy and emphasizes communication between equal parties, and thus the group of peers is important. Little communication is generated in a group with few members, while many participants might create an over-complex picture. Both extremes reduce the efficiency of the group (Preece, 2000). All the participants in the online version are therefore members of both a small and a large group. The large group numbers between thirty and fifty members and concerns for the most part the track concerning dissemination of professional knowledge. The small groups number from five to ten and concern the track that facilitates exchange of experiential knowledge between peers. Hence the small group can be said to equal a self-help group, while the large group is be considered more as an educational initiative. In this way it is possible to create intimacy, facilitate verisimilitude and establish trust with regard to sharing of action plans in the small group, and exploit the robustness that exists in a large group when it comes to contributions in activities like those on the 'discussion board' and in the 'brainstorms'.

In the programme, training in presenting yourself as a person with a problem is a key element. To achieve this goal, the course is based on a model where the group is not simply a gathering of individuals, but a unit to which activities are linked. Facilitating socialization is therefore an important feature. Parts of this function are taken care of by the computer system, and are thus independent of whether or not one of the participants is logged in.

When one meets in a room, one shares time and place. This is not the case when one meets online. Still the participants in 'Living a Healthier Life – online' explain that they have felt the sense of belonging to a group. Essential to this experience are the group pages, which are the first thing the participants meet when they log in (Figure 5). The group pages acting as an entry page is an important signal to participants that the group is a key component of the programme. On this page the group is presented as in the picture below.

In addition to presenting the small group, the group pages also serve as an entrance to action plans, course items, discussion board and the large group. The course programme and progress is also clearly introduced in terms of a progress bar at the top of the page embedding the number of assessments in each course-week and how many tasks the current user has completed. Each individual participant's symbol (or photo) is presented on the group-page. This symbol is also to be found on contributions made by that person other places in the computer system. In this way it is easier to link activity and person. Moreover, all the participants have their own personal pages where they can publish information about themselves.

When the presentation of the participants is taken care of by way of web pages, the participants cannot tailor their presentation to the recipients as one does in a face-to-face setting. This makes it important to state clearly who has access to what information and present a model for how one can present oneself. Such a model has been given by the way in which the supervisors have presented themselves.

In this aspect of the course the supervisor joins in on an equal basis. There is therefore no difference in principle between the system for a user and for a supervisor, apart from the fact that the supervisor is likely to be a member of several small groups and receives a little more information of an administrative nature. One example is that the supervisors are able to check how long it was since the various participants last logged into the website, which will allow them to get in touch by e-mail or phone with participants who are rather passive. Weeding out those who have signed up for the course but not joined from the start has an important contribution to make. This is taken care of by the system, which does not present to the group participants that have not logged into the system for the first time to avoid presenting non-participating peers to the group.

Together the group and personal pages cover that part of the SECI-model (Nonaka & Takeuchi, 1995) that involves socialization in the course (Figure 6), and provide a foundation for the other processes by creating an arena in which one can 'get to know' each other. This concerns sharing of experiences and thus builds a foundation for the verisimilitude needed in the exchange of experiential knowledge.

Discussion Board

The idea behind the discussion board is to provide a place where everyday experiences can be freely exchanged. Here it is possible to communicate in the same way as one would normally do during the breaks between classes on ordinary classroom courses. As such the discussion board creates a place for what does not fit in naturally elsewhere. The discussion board has little or no structure or control, with the exception of the desire for the supervisors to support good discussions and put a stop to or alter those that might seem unfortunate.

Our material shows the discussion board contains two different types of discussion: 1) those that concern the course and (2) those that concern the participants' everyday lives. Those concerning everyday life are founded upon experiential knowledge with some elements of what is to be considered as lay knowledge; second-hand

Figure 5. Front page of the course

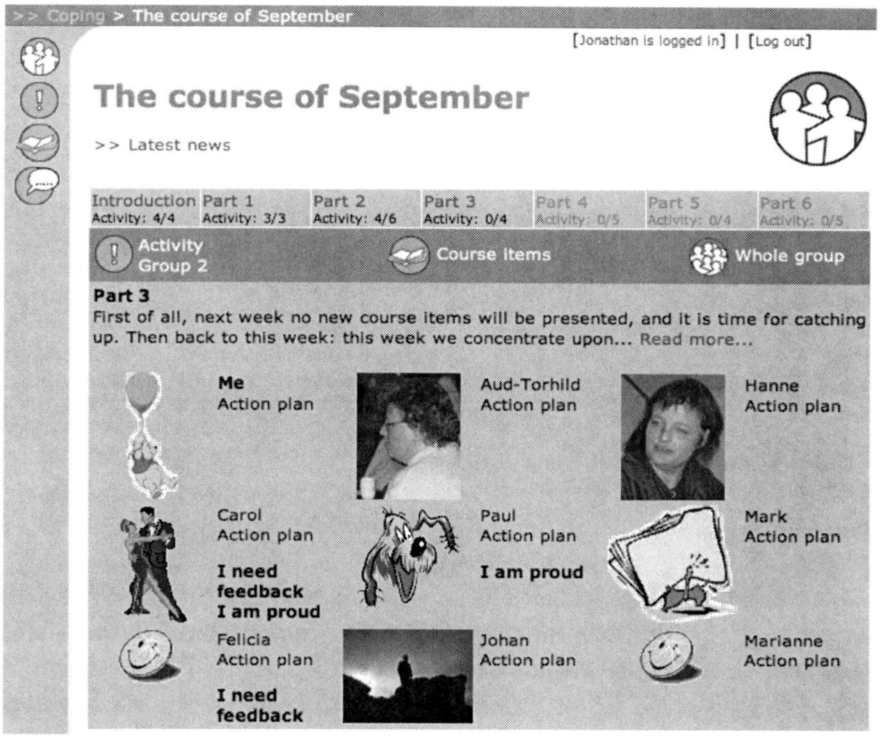

information from a combination of rumours, the media, professionals and other experientialists. Here the course leaders act as senior peers that possess the legitimacy to stop or alter contributions that they find inappropriate, like when one of the participants started to market a herbal product he was selling.

Discussions concerning the course are of two kinds: those where the topic is set by the participants, and those where the topic is set by the course leaders. The knowledge exchanged is for the most part learning in terms of cognitive change and rests upon knowledge of the professional kind.

When you click on 'Read more' under the first few lines of the message on the group page (Figure 5), you enter the discussion board, which offers you the chance to comment on the message. Lifting messages on the discussion board onto the group pages is in principle exactly the same as standing in front of the class and saying something. It provides a clear signal of this being part of the intention of the course and that it is meant to help to set the agenda.

The discussion board is an unstructured part of the externalization and combination in the extended educational model (cloud in Figure 7), taking care of co-learning between peers concerning those topics that the participants care for the most, and that is not taken care of by the curriculum and/or facilitated processes. It also triggers impartation of professional knowledge (arrow with exclamation mark in Figure 7) as answers to questions from the participants (arrow with question mark in Figure 7) rather than what the course consider as important. At the same time it serves as an arena for the facilitation of processes in the program, and thus contributes energy to the SECI-spiral (Nonaka & Takeuchi, 1995) (spiral in Figure 7). Most discussions lean towards learning as cognitive change. Thus it seems harder to initiate

Figure 6. Socialization on online courses

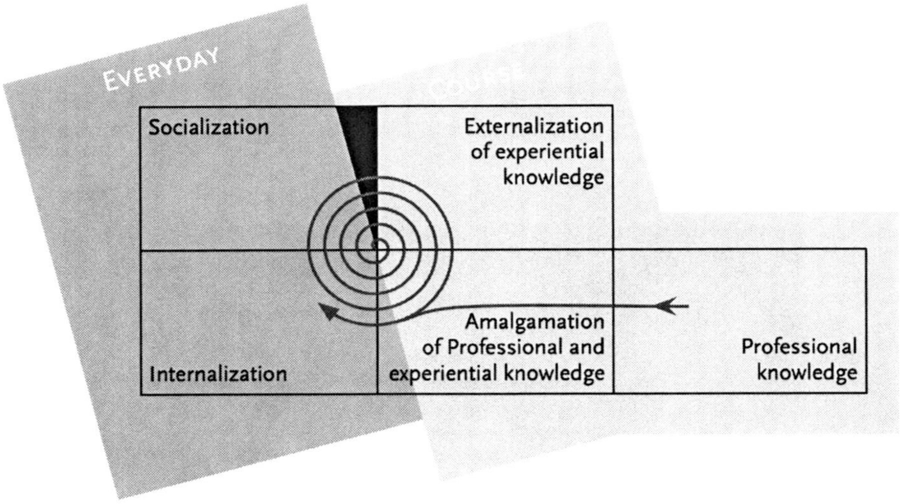

knowledge discussions founded upon learning as psychodynamic change, something that ought to be facilitated more directly if they are to flourish.

Course Items

In the face-to-face version the course content and programme are set out in a detailed instructor handbook (Lorig, et al., 1999). One important element in the programme is short lectures delivered by the instructors from a detailed manuscript called 'lecturettes'. A typical lecturette is quoted below, as it appears in the course leader manual. These lecturettes add either professional knowledge to the situation or concern how the course should progress, as in this case:

Lecturette (paraphrase the following): We have already discussed some of the ways of dealing with fatigue, such as exercise and muscle relaxation. During this workshop we also discuss others such as good nutrition, planning activity, and communication skills (Session 3, part 16).

In the online version the course items exist in the system when the course starts. Still they are opened one by one on each Monday as the course progresses. This is in order to keep the group together, so that the activity and reflections related to the course items are created at roughly the same time. This aims at keeping the group united and strengthens the socialization and co-learning processes, a prerequisite for experiential knowledge exchange.

In the extended educational model, the course items belong to the professional knowledge, and contribute to the combination phase as a second source of input, in addition to the externalization of experiential knowledge (arrow in Figure 8).

Contributions

On the traditional courses the lecturettes are followed up by questions and group exercises. These are meant to activate and integrate experiential knowledge in the content of the course. In the online version these have two different forms: brainstorming and problem-solving. In the brainstorming section the question is defined by the course programme, and the participants offer their thoughts in relation to this. It is not possible to comment upon each other's thoughts.

Figure 7. Activity on discussion board mapped in the extended educational model

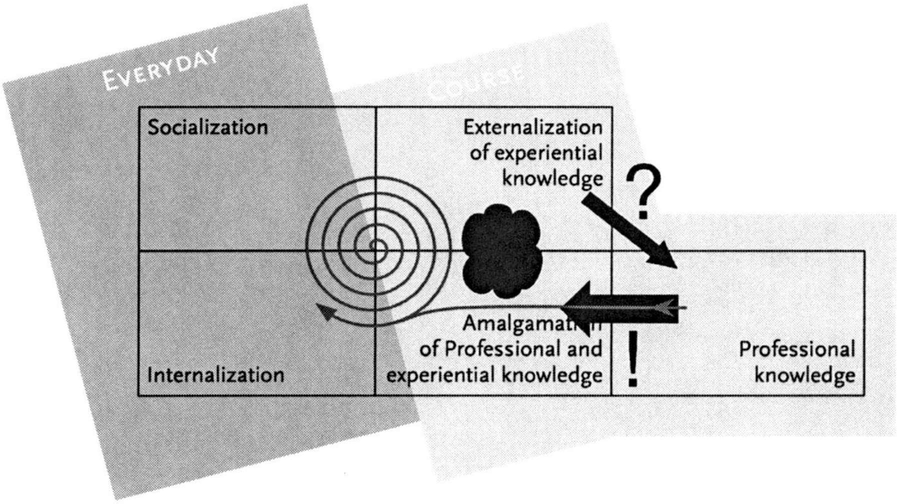

In problem-solving the participants are challenged to contribute by mentioning what they personally experience as difficult, and the other course members are challenged to help them find workable solutions. It is not possible to comment on responses to the initial problem, in order to avoid discussions developing and thus moving focus away from the initial problem. This is in accordance with the methodology presented in the classroom course where the course leaders are told to prevent such discussions from developing. The intention here is to let the one that owns the problem choose what (s)he believes is a good solution from experiences founded in own daily life and own coping strategies.

Both the brainstorming and problem-solving activities serve to incorporate the experiences of and suggestions from the participants in the course

Figure 8. Course items mapped in the extended educational model

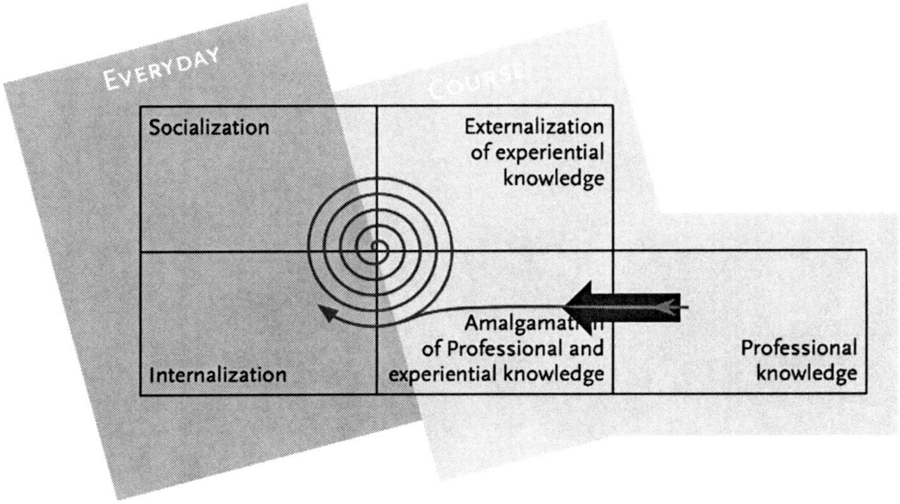

items. In this process, the supervisors are also important contributors, but most of all as equals as well as role models who demonstrate how one is expected to 'behave'.

In the extended educational model, brainstorming and problem-solving activities are placed in the transition between externalization and combination (cloud in Figure 9), while the course items feed professional knowledge into the combination phase (arrow in Figure 9) where experiential and professional knowledge are to be amalgamated.

Action Plans

Action plans are an important means of achieving increased self-efficacy in the chronic disease self-management program (CDSMP). An action plan can be described as a New Year's resolution that you keep for a week. The planning and evaluation of it is shared with the group. In 'Living a Healthier Life – online', 75% of the utterances in the trial run of the programme are related to action plans.

An action plan starts with a set of targets such as, e.g. that you plan to walk a kilometre three times a week. You tell the group that you intend to do this, and when you come back a week later, you tell them about your experiences. In a pedagogical perspective this guarantees that while you are on the course, you have to think about your daily routine, and think about the course as part of daily life.

Making use of the participants' experiences as a tool to make the content of the course relevant is not unusual, and it happens e.g. in the brainstorming and problem-solving activities. But what is less usual is that one to such a large extent obliges the participants to take the course with them into their everyday lives – something that is reported by the participants to be a positive experience.

As a rule the action plans cover a period from one Monday to the next. In the online version the action plan have four very distinct stages which are closely directed. The first step is that the participant draws up an action plan for the week ahead. The next step is that the action plan is commented on by the others in the group. Here small dialogues often develop. The third stage is that the owner of the action plan writes his or her own assessment of the plan. Finally, the owner's evaluation of the plan is commented on by the other group members.

Figure 9. Activity on discussion board mapped in the extended educational model

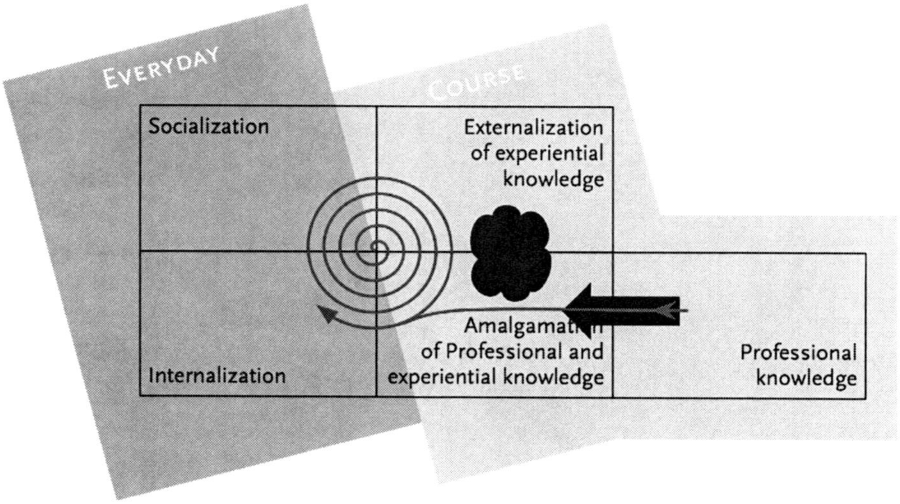

It is not possible to write your own evaluation of the action plan before it has been commented on by other people. This means that you cannot move on without the help of others. It is not possible for the participants to be the first ones to write comments during the first week. This has been done to ensure that the supervisors are given the chance to write the first comments, and thus establish the genre through modelling. These strong mechanical limitations help to facilitate peer-support, exchange of experiential knowledge and co-learning in the group.

Sharing the action plans in written form both emphasizes the obligatory nature of the task and offers the chance of a shared group experience. Here the technology makes a contribution in a number of ways. If the participant has written his or her action plan or their own evaluation without having received any feedback, the text 'I need comments' appears automatically on the group page (Figure 5). When you click on this sentence, you will be directed to the person's action plan. Moreover, 'I am proud of myself' appears if the participant checks this choice when he or she writes their own evaluation. This compensates for the reduced human presence, and replaces something of what is lost by the absence of body language and oral communication. Programming this into the system has a normalizing effect.

The action plan facilitates activity on all the four phases in the extended educational model (Figure 10). This is incorporated in the technology in a way which puts a focus on the group. The technology is here contributing energy to the spiral by both ensuring comments from peers and demanding reflections upon how things went when the plan was put into action in daily life.

DISCUSSION

The most crucial part to facilitate when experiential and professional knowledge is to be amalgamated in an online self-help initiative is the combination phase since it is here 'old' and 'new' knowledge is combined to form more complex knowledge structures. Still, the remaining four areas in the extended educational model (Figure 4) are prerequisites for this phase to flourish in a good manner. Without special attention, the learning will often take form of oscillation between externalization and combination only, since there are

Figure 10. Action plan activity mapped in the extended educational model

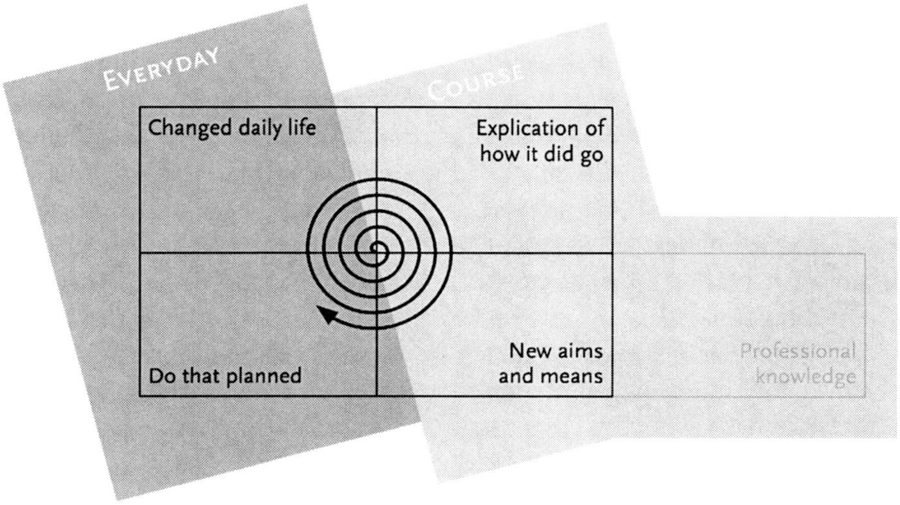

special challenges relating to internalization and socialization, since these are processes that take place in everyday life and not on the course. An important means of giving energy and momentum to the SECI-spiral (Nonaka & Takeuchi, 1995) is assignments that require the spiral to be repeated.

In the case of 'Living a Healthier Life – online' action plans serve this role. Comments from participants show that the action plans represent an important link between the course and everyday life. One commented: "Even though I have yet to follow a plan from A to Z, I always have it at the back of my mind. It makes me think more about the choices I make every day". Another commented that they "represent something concrete – it is easier to stick to them then". Another aspect that is mentioned a great deal is the way the action plans gave a feeling of shared experience. One comment said "both giving and receiving feedback meant a lot to me". The overall impression is that the action plans were regarded as useful because as one participant put it – "they give you a kick in the pants to make you get on with it". This sort of outcome is quite similar to that reported by participants in self-help groups, and relates to the 'helper therapy principle' (Riessman, 1965).

The background for the high level of activity and positive comments with regard to the action plan in 'Living a Healthier Life – online' is from our understanding that it facilitates activity on all the four contexts in the SECI-spiral (Nonaka & Takeuchi, 1995). This is incorporated in the technology in a way which puts a focus on the group and obliges the participants to take the course with them into their everyday lives. Furthermore, we observe that sharing the action plans in written form both emphasizes the obligatory nature of the task and offers the chance of a shared group experience. The technology makes a contribution in a number of ways. For instance it makes it impossible for the participants to be the first ones to write comments during the first week; to ensure that the supervisors are given the chance to establish the genre through modelling.

As part of their final reflections on the course, the participants are asked to say what they felt to be most useful. The reactions covered a wide spectre, but in general had to do with learning outcomes and shared experience among the participants. It is quite obvious from the participants' comments that they have felt that they have been part of a group. One of the participants writes: "Have met lots of nice, pleasant people, learned a great deal about myself, and have picked up loads of ideas and tips regarding my own process of coping." Another participant points out how important the contact with other people in the same situation was: "Got to know other people with the same problems. [...] Has been really useful to establish a network thanks to this course." Against this background we conclude that even though a great part of the facilitation is taken care of by the computer system in a machine-internalized manner, the participants feel that the system has supported relationship-building between humans. The system has therefore become quite transparent, and thus the participants do not feel that they are relating to a computer, but to the group.

The action plans push the content of the program into daily life, help make the content relevant, and provide energy and momentum to the SECI-spiral (Nonaka & Takeuchi, 1995). As a means to achieve momentum in the SECI-spiral, many of the online educative initiatives provided by the Norwegian Net School present an assignment that points towards the end of the course. This assignment embeds all or many of the topics covered in the course. In one course developed in cooperation with the Norwegian Study Organization for the Disabled concerning how to conduct 'board-work' in voluntary organizations, what is labelled 'the year-wheel' is the point of focus. This 'year-wheel' is a list of those topics that must be taken care of by the board at certain times of the year, like budget, audit report, yearly seminars, elections etc. Preparation, testing and revision of this 'year-wheel' serve as a hub for the activity, and put the content in the course into the place it belongs in the normal work schedule of the board. In a course for persons with diabetes that currently is under development, a training plan and a diet plan serve as overall-assignments. These are to be planned, carried out, reflected upon and revised several times during the course.

Socialization is a prerequisite for the exchange of experiential knowledge due to the need for this to have verisimilitude. In 'Living a Healthier Life – online', training in presenting yourself as a person with a problem is a key element. By this means, the group pages are important and serve as a place where the participants can present themselves as humans. This contributes to the verisimilitude needed in the exchange of experiential knowledge. In some of the educative initiatives provided online by the Norwegian Net School, participants commit their reflections to a blog that is shared between the participants. Here the participants can put forward thoughts as something more than answers to assignments given in the course program. This contributes to socialization, thus providing verisimilitude to the experiential knowledge exchanged between the peers.

The partially synchronous way of running the course provides both stability and flexibility. While the action plans on the ordinary course cover the period from gathering to gathering, not everyone's action plans run from one Monday to the next in the online version. The supervisors do it in this way, thus providing stability and a model activity, but there is considerable variation when it comes to how the participants carried out their action plans. This variation is a natural consequence of not getting together at the same time and same place. Furthermore, in the face-to-face version, the lecturettes tend to govern the action plans due to the proximity of these in time and place. In the online version this link is not as strong, and the action plans tend to lean more towards the long-term goal presented by each of the participants and the preceding action plan. Thus it seems harder to initiate knowledge discussions founded upon learning as psychodynamic change, and something that ought to be facilitated closely if they are to flourish.

FUTURE RESEARCH DIRECTIONS

There is a rather strong and growing body of research on how to gain from users' knowledge in the development of policies and professional knowledge, while the research on the amalgamation of professional and experiential knowledge in online self-help groups is virtually non-existant. As we have argued above, there is an important difference between professional and experiential knowledge. This difference poses great challenges if one seeks to apply knowledge gained from research on professional knowledge to what is going on in self-help groups. Thus it is important to develop a pedagogical philosophy that has experiential knowledge at its core.

We found that overall assessments is the most important way of making content relevant to daily life, thus such an approach should be embedded in the pedagogical philosophy. We also find that the facilitation of online self-help initiatives ought to be done in a firmer manner than in the case of processes taking place in a room. Further investigations into what kinds of methods that facilitate online experiential knowledge-building in good ways remain to be developed and implemented.

Furthermore, we found that the socialization of participants is important. How this process can best be facilitated needs to be further investigated. As long as self-help groups are facilitated online, technology will be an integrative part of the group's inner functioning, and thus investigation and development must concern both technology and methodology, and the interplay between them. It is, moreover, important that such research not only focuses on the course alone, but also on how it relates to the daily life of the participants.

CONCLUSION

When one meets in a room, one shares time and place. When one meets online, one attunes to a virtual place from various physical places at various times. Due to the dynamics of the group, meeting in a room commits the participants more, negotiations take place faster and the interaction is richer than in an online environment. This means that often less facilitation is needed in ordinary initiatives than in the online arena. Thus facilitation of online self-help initiatives ought to be done in a firmer manner than processes taking place in a room. Such facilitation is demanding because it calls for a more diverse set of educational tools than those used in traditional courses. In addition those chosen ought to suit the traits of the technology utilized.

Technology offers a systematic, rule-based approach, which is a great advantage over humans in some cases, and an equally great disadvantage in other cases. By transferring adequate parts of the role of the supervisor to the e-learning solution, it has in the case of 'Living a healthier life – online' been possible to make sure that the participants feel that they are both seen and respected by other participants, at the same time as they are learning from each other. This demands knowledge on the part of the supervisors so that they help to increase the effect of the technology and not work against it. Only then will the technology become an integrated part of a well-functioning course team.

From this we conclude that even though the combination phase in the SECI-model (Nonaka & Takeuchi, 1995) is where experiential and professional knowledge is amalgamated, the two most important elements to pay attention to in the facilitation of online self-help initiatives are: (1) socialization, since it contributes to the verisimilitude of experiential knowledge and (2) overall assignments, since they provide momentum and energy to the SECI-spiral. Both these can be focused upon in various ways, but there are some crucial elements that ought to be paid attention to. When it comes to socialization, providing a framework for how the participants should present themselves, by offering a model and by utilizing the technological facilitation of activity, is of great importance, due to the need for a framework and predictability when putting oneself forward as a human in the online initiative. With regard to overall assessments the most important part is to find meaningful tasks that fit naturally into the daily lives of the participants. Furthermore, in the process of making these relevant - engaged and smart supervisors are of great significance.

ACKNOWLEDGMENT

First of all, a debt of gratitude goes to all the participants and the colleagues in the project. Thanks are also owed to colleagues, friends, reviewers and editors who have read the text and passed on their comments. Finally, we would like to thank the Central Norway Regional Health Authority, The Norwegian Directorate for Health and Social Affairs, EXTRA funds from the Norwegian Foundation for Health and Rehabilitation and the Norwegian Net School that have financed the project.

REFERENCES

Avis, M., Elkan, R., Patel, S., Walker, B. A., Ankti, N., & Bell, C. (2008). Ethnicity and participation in cancer self-help groups. *Psycho-Oncology*, *17*(9), 940–947. doi:10.1002/pon.1284

Bandura, A. (1997). *Self-efficacy: The exercise of control*. New York, NY: Freeman.

Bateson, G. (1972). *Steps to an ecology of mind*. New York, NY: Ballantine Books.

Beck, K. (2000). *Extreme programming explained: Embrace change*. Reading, MA: Addison-Wesley.

Borkman, T. J. (1976). Experiential knowledge: A new concept for the analysis of self-help groups. *The Social Service Review*, *50*(3), 445–456. doi:10.1086/643401

Borkman, T. J. (1999). *Understanding self-help/mutual aid: Experiential learning in the commons*. New Brunswick, NJ: Rutgers University Press.

Brown, A. L. (1992). Design experiments: Theoretical and methodlogical challenges in creating complex interventions in classroom settings. *Journal of the Learning Sciences*, *2*, 141–178. doi:10.1207/s15327809jls0202_2

Bruner, J. S. (1986). *Actual minds, possible worlds (The Jerusalem-Harvard Lectures)*. Harvard University Press.

Bruner, J. S. (1991). The narrative construction of reality. *Critical Inquiry*, *18*(1), 1–21. doi:10.1086/448619

Cole, M. (1996). *Cultural psychology: A once and future discipline*. Cambridge, MA: The Belknap Press of Harvard University Press.

Collins, A. (1992). Towards a design science of education. In Scanlon, E., & O'Shea, T. (Eds.), *New Directions in Educational Technology*. Berlin, Germany: Springer Verlag.

Edelson, D. C. (2002). Design research: What we learn when we engage in design. *Journal of the Learning Sciences*, *11*(1), 105–121. doi:10.1207/S15327809JLS1101_4

Engeström, Y. (1987). *Learning by expanding - An activity-theoretical approach to developmental research*. Helsinki, Finland: Orienta-Konsultit Oy.

Greeno, J. G., Collins, A. M., & Resnick, L. B. (1996). Cognition and learning. In Berliner, D., & Calfee, R. (Eds.), *Handbook of educational psychology* (pp. 15–46). New York, NY: Macmillan.

Hannafin, M. J. (1997). *The case for grounded learning systems design: What the literature suggests about effective teaching, learning, and technology*. Paper presented at the ASCILITE'97, Perth Australia.

Heldal, F., & Tjora, A. H. (2009). Making sense of patient expertise. *Social Theory & Health*, *7*(1), 1–19. doi:10.1057/sth.2008.17

Hutchins, E. (1995a). *Cognition in the wild*. Cambridge, MA: MIT Press.

Hutchins, E. (1995b). How a cockpit remembers its speeds. *Cognitive Science*, *19*, 265–288. doi:10.1207/s15516709cog1903_1

Illeris, K. (2004). *The three dimensions of learning: Contemporary learning theory in the tension field between the cognitive, the emotional and the social. Frederiksberg, Denmark: Roskilde University Press*. Leicester, UK: Niace.

Land, S. M., & Hannafin, M. J. (2000). Student-centered learning environnments. In Jonassen, D. H., & Land, S. (Eds.), *Theoretical foundations of learning environments* (pp. 1–24). Mahwah, NJ: Lawrence Erlbaum Associates.

Lave, J., & Wenger, E. (1991). *Situated learning: Legitimate peripheral participation*. Cambridge, UK: Cambridge University Press.

Lorig, K., Gonzalez, V., & Laurent, D. D. (1999). *The Chronic Disease Self-Management Workshop - Leaders manual*. Stanford, CA: The Board of Trustees, Leland Stanford Junior University.

Lorig, K., Holman, H., Sobel, D., Laurent, D. D., Gonzalez, V., & Minor, M. A. (2000). *Living a healthy life with chronic conditions: Self-management of heart disease, arthritis, diabetes, asthma, bronchitis, emphysema & others* (2nd ed.). Palo Alto & Emeryville, CA: Bull Publishing Co., Publishers Group West.

Matzat, J. (1993). Away with the experts? Self-help groupwork in Germany. *Groupwork*, *6*(1), 30–42.

Munn-Giddings, C., & McVicar, A. (2007). Self-help groups as mutual support: What do carers value? *Health & Social Care in the Community, 15*(1), 26–34.

Nonaka, I., & Takeuchi, H. (1995). *The knowledge-creating company: How Japanese companies create the dynamics of innovation*. USA: Oxford University Press.

Nonaka, I., Toyama, R., & Konno, N. (2001). SECI, ba and leadership: A unified model of dynamic creation. In Nonaka, I., & Teece, D. J. (Eds.), *Managing industrial knowledge: Creation, transfer and utilization* (pp. 13–43). London, UK: Sage.

Powell, T. J. (1987). *Self-help organizations and professional practice*. Silver Spring, MD: National Association of Social Workers.

Preece, J. (2000). *Online communities: Designing usability, supporting sociability*. Chichester, UK: Wiley.

Reigeluth, C. M., & Frick, T. (1999). Formative research: A methodology for creating and improving design theories. In Reigeluth, C. M. (Ed.), *Instructional-design theories and models: A new paradigm of instructional theory* (pp. 633–652). Mahwah, NJ: Lawrence Erlbaum Associates.

Riessman, F. (1965). The helper therapy principle. *Social Work, 10*(2), 27–32.

Stokken, R., & Eikli, G. (2010). Den e-lærande pasienten. In Tjora, A. H., & Sandaunet, A. G. (Eds.), *Digitale pasienter. Oslo, Norway*. Gyldendal Norsk Forlag, AS.

The Design-Based Research Collective. (2003). Design-based research: An emerging paradigm for educational inquiry. *Educational Researcher, 32*(1), 5–8. doi:10.3102/0013189X032001005

Vygotsky, L. S. (1978). *Mind in society: The development of higher psychological processes*. Cambridge, MA: Harvard University Press.

Wilson, J. (1995). *Two worlds: Self help groups and professionals*. British Association of Social Workers.

Yew, T. M., & Karney, D. (2010). A framework and mental model to foster deep learning in the classroom. In Husain, A., & Idris, N. (Eds.), *Dimensions of education*. New Dehli, India: Gyan Publishing House.

ADDITIONAL READING

Borkman, T., & Munn-Giddings, C. (2008) The contribution of self-help groups and organizations to changing relations between patients/consumers and the health care system in the US and UK in Chambre, S and Goldner, M (Eds) *Patients, Consumers and Civil Society: US and International Perspectives*, Vol. 10 Advances in Medical Sociology, Bingley, UK: Emerald Group Publishing

Discusses self-help groups and organizations in relation to different health care systems and the voluntary sectors of society - discusses how health care systems shape and are shaped by self help activity.

Humphrey, K., & Rappaport, J. (1994). Researching Self Help/Mutual Aid Groups and Organisations: Many Roads. *One Journey in Applied and Preventive Psychology, 3*, 217–231. doi:10.1016/S0962-1849(05)80096-4

Good overview of the different ways in which self help groups are framed by researchers from 'therapeutic groups' to 'voluntary action groups'.

Hutchins, E. (1995). *Cognition in the wild*. Cambridge, Mass.: MIT Press.

In this groundbreaking book, Edwin Hutchins examines a set of phenomena that have fallen into the gap between the established disciplines of psychology and anthropology, bringing to light a new set of relationships between culture and cognition.

Illeris, K. (2004). *The three dimensions of learning: contemporary learning theory in the tension field between the cognitive, the emotional and the social. Frederiksberg: Roskilde University Press.* Leicester: Niace.

Deals with a new and comprehensive theory of learning, which is developed in the book. The theory is based on two fundamental assumptions: Firstly, that all learning is an external interaction process between the learner and environment, and an internal psychological process. Secondly, that all learning includes three dimensions, namely, the cognitive dimension, the psychodynamic dimension, and the social dimension.

Katz, A. H., & Bender, E. (1976). *The strength in US: Self help groups in the modern world.* New York: Franklin-Watts.

Katz' early definition of self help groups is widely used although it should be superceded by more contemporary definitions.

Kurtz, L. (1997). *Self-help and support groups: A handbook for practitioners*. Thousand Oaks, CA: Sage.

Excellent review of the North American research literature and issues on self help/mutual aid.

Lave, J., & Wenger, E. (1991). *Situated learning: legitimate peripheral participation*. Cambridge: Cambridge University Press.

In this important theoretical treatise, the authors put forward the notion of situated learning - that learning is fundamentally a social process and not solely in the learner's head.

Mol, A. (2002). *The body multiple: ontology in medical practice*. Durham: Duke University Press.

The book is an extraordinary ethnography of an ordinary disease: atherosclerosis. In this seminal and novel book, Mol demonstrates the multiplicity of a disease that does not imply fragmentation but cohesion. Mol draws on medical anthropology, sociology, feminist theory, philosophy, and science and technology studies to reframe the disease through vivid storytelling.

Mol, A. (2008). *The logic of care: health and the problem of patient choice*. London: Routledge.

Although it is possible to treat people who seek professional help as customers or citizens, Mol argues that this undermines ways of thinking and acting crucial to health care. She concludes that good care is not a matter of making well argued individual choices but is something that grows out of collaborative and continuing attempts to attune knowledge and technologies to diseased bodies and complex lives.

Rappaport, J. (1993). Narrative studies, personal stories, and identity transformation in the mutual help context. *The Journal of Applied Behavioral Science*, *29*(2), 239–256. doi:10.1177/0021886393292007

Major contribution in showing how stories and narratives of a group are major aspects of self-help groups.

Riessman, F., & Carroll, D. (1995). *Redefining self-help: Policy and practice*. San Francisco: Jossey-Bass.

A major contributor to self-help group concepts and research—Riessman's final and encompassing statement.

Wenger, E. (1998). *Communities of practice: learning, meaning, and identity*. Cambridge: Cambridge University Press.

This book presents a framework for thinking about how to foster learning in innovative ways. Wenger understands this from a social theory of learning that is both novel and easily accessible, and touches on issues from information and technology to those of human capabilities and the sources of motivation, creativity, and problem-solving skills.

KEY TERMS AND DEFINITIONS

Cognitive Change: Learning interpreted as changed understanding or skills. This takes place in the head of the learner and becomes a means of achieving alignment between contexts and how the context is being understood.

Combination: The process whereby 'old' and 'new' knowledge is combined to form more complex knowledge structures.

Experiential Knowledge: Knowledge learned from personal experience and acquired by living through a problem firsthand.

Externalisation: The process whereby tacit knowledge becomes explicit knowledge.

Internalization: The process whereby what one thinks in the combination phase is made into changed practice as foundation for tacit knowledge.

Lay Knowledge: Second-hand information from a combination of rumours, media, professionals and other experientialists.

Professional Knowledge: Knowledge developed, applied, and transmitted by an established specialized occupation that has financial and career interest in the topic.

Psychodynamic Change: Learning interpreted as changed psychic energy, usually in terms of changed emotions, motivation or attitudes. Such change creates positive or negative energy that both can facilitate and obstruct learning. This change also happens in the head of the learner.

SECI-Model: Pedagogical model developed by Nonaka et al. (e.g. Nonaka & Takeuchi, 1995; Nonaka, Toyama, & Konno, 2001). The model focuses on how the surroundings must facilitate four types of transformation of knowledge in order to be optimal: Socialization, Externalization, Combination, and Internalization. The most important contribution of the model is the focus upon the dialogic relationship between tacit and explicit knowledge.

SECI-Spiral: A repeated process in which learning goes through the four phases of the SECI-model: socialization, externalization, combination, and internalization.

Social Change: Learning interpreted as changed premises for social interaction. Thus learning is a societal process that involves artefacts used in social interaction (e.g. language, technology and political structures). This change takes place as an interaction between individual and context/society.

Socialisation: The process that lays the foundation for a social learning process by facilitating common experiences among the learners.

Chapter 11
The Amazing Impossibilities of Technology:
Factors that Inhibit Participation in Skype™ Based Self-Help Groups

Stein Conradsen
Sunnmøre Hospital Trust, Norway

ABSTRACT

A project in Norway attempting to start self-help groups based on Internet video conferencing experienced severe problems in recruiting participants. The chapter discusses how to interpret the project and compares it to other projects and trials. Theoretical perspectives on self-help and technology in a late modern context contribute to a tentative model of motivation for getting involved in Electronic Self-help Groups (ESGs). Anthony Giddens' contribution on the high modern society is central for our model of motivation. Also, the relationship between technology and social practice discussed by Ian Hutchby plays an important role. Both constrainers and enablers of such practices are considered in the theoretical model.

Using this model of motivation, five factors are suggested which may either enable or constrain engagement. These factors are (1) synchronicity, (2) identification, (3) specified diagnosis, (4) organizational trust, and (5) accessibility.

DOI: 10.4018/978-1-60960-866-8.ch011

INTRODUCTION

Electronic Self-help Groups (ESGs) seem to attract a substantial number of persons and the background for the rising number of such groups varies: practical convenience, social anxiety, health condition (Bjerke, 2010). Such groups also seem to be suitable for discussing matters believed to be of a private and shameful character (ibid.). The project "Self-help on Internet based Video Conference" (SIVC) was carried out over a period of two years. One of the main objectives was to make use of Skype™ for self-help purposes and to investigate the experiences of the participants. This kind of technology has grown more affordable and widespread recently. Another developmental trait in recent decades is the self-help groups that have emerged as an increasingly more vital part in many people's lives. However, perhaps especially in rural districts and for very busy people, opportunities to take part in groups like these are limited. Hence, one of the objectives was to find out whether these sorts of groups could be beneficial for the participants and what they would require with regard to technical support, organizational structure and group starting/leadership, information etc. How do these groups form themselves? The main objective of this chapter is: *What are the preconditions for recruiting persons to Electronic Self-help Groups? What factors enable such practice and what have a constraining effect?* By looking into the experience of the SIVC and other projects/trials the matter will be discussed and a tentative model of motivation for engaging in ESGs is suggested.

BACKGROUND

The SIVC project was initiated by a resource group associated with the National Center of Patient Education (NCPE) in Norway. NCPE received a grant from the Norwegian Directorate of Health to carry out the work and the Patient Education Resource Center (of Central Norway) was given the project management (The final report "Selvhjelp på videokonferanse", henceforth: SPV 2009). The project itself was carried out in cooperation between a number of partners; The National Center of Patient Education, The Norwegian Center for Integrated Care and Telemedicine, Volda University College, The National Union of Organizations for Disabled in Norway and The Norwegian Self-help Center (Selvhjelp Norge). It was managed through the Patient Education Resource Center of Helse Sunnmøre.

A number of patient organizations, hospitals, rehab centers and others cooperated to recruit persons for the groups. An Internet site provided the necessary information for both learning how the groups were supposed to work, how to sign up, how to use the technology and other information. For those who did make contact a package of information, data software, other necessary items, instructions and an agreement for signing was prepared (SPV, 2009). Despite the efforts made to contact people assumed to be interested, very few signed up and no groups were initiated.

The final report identifies three major challenges during the project process. The first one concerns practical and technological issues. Originally this was intended to be based on groups meeting on Internet-based video conference. After testing the existing applications that could be considered useful, the project group concluded that none of them was suitable for this purpose. Both freeware and commercial applications were considered. The commercial ones were not really suitable as they required high-quality broadband for all users; furthermore, a certain financial support is needed to put them into use and there are organizational challenges associated with this. As a central point in the project was to develop methods and solutions that user organizations and "techno-lay people" may benefit from, technological, financial and organizational obstacles needed to be as few and low as possible. After a while the free data applications proved to have their weaknesses. The most important one was lack of stability, and the quality of live images also was very vulnerable, especially on home broadband connections. A decision was made to leave the live picture out of the project and run the groups as audio communication only. The project group considered this as an important "result", though a disappointing one. Skype™ was chosen, as this solution was considered to be user friendly and one of the most widespread ones available. Considerable time and resources were spent on reaching this conclusion, which affected the project as a whole (SPV, 2009).

The second challenge described in the report is related to matters of privacy. Neither in the application nor in the letter of grant from the directorate this was mentioned, but during the planning process it became clear that there were substantial legal concerns involved. Investigating what departments that needed to be applied to for approval made it clear that the project strictly speaking only had to be registered by the Sunnmøre Hospital Trust and they sent it to the Data Inspectorate of Norway. There were a number of details that needed to be outlined, such as how to handle lists of names, confidentiality for the professionals, design of the web-based evaluation form, information security – especially challenging due to the fact that a number of private computers are involved. Organizations involved in self-help are partly obliged to follow the same or similar guidelines when organizing groups. They should be aware of both formal rules of privacy and concerned about effective and practical arrangements to protect information about participators. The Data Inspectorate stressed that the main concern is *what kind of information* is collected and *how it is used* (SPV, 2009).

Thirdly, perhaps the most obviously troubling experience in SIVC concerned recruitment to the self-help groups. Very few signed up and the project group decided after a series of attempts over a number of months, to conclude the project without having been able to run a Skype™ based self-help group. In addition to the project partners, one worked together with 15-16 other units and organizations to recruit members for the online self-help groups. These were regional offices for patient organizations, diverse other units in these organizations, a rehabilitation center for brain damage etc. (SPV, 2009). A rather great deal of work was spent on the "marketing" part of the project; a website including all information needed for understanding how the groups and the technology worked, flyers – both in paper and web versions. Both the flyers and the web were resources the cooperating organizations used for distributing information to potential participants. A "package" was also prepared for those who signed up with a step-by-step instructions on both the use of Skype™ and how the groups were intended to work. A headset and CD-ROM with the necessary software were also included. Those who wanted to join in were asked to sign and return an agreement, privacy concerns were described to assure them that the information they supplied would be treated in proper ways. They were not obliged to be a part of a group if they signed up, but were invited to the first meeting to receive information and share their expectations and needs.

The SIVC worked along two approaches: (1) to start self-help groups "from scratch" and *2) groups as a follow-up opportunity for patients "knowing each other" from a rehabilitation center. The "from scratch" groups were meant to be cross-diagnostic. A formal diagnosis was not – and could not for legal reasons be – a criterion for taking part. There have been positive experiences from some other groups of persons with a variety of challenges (Oral information from The Self-help Center of Norway). After extensive attempts to include persons on this basis and having received very few replies, the project opened for an alternative way, cooperation with a rehabilitation center for persons suffering from acquired brain damage. Many of these seemed interested in this opportunity of forming a follow-up group, but only two registered, which obviously provided too small a basis for forming a group.

So, the results of both the "from scratch" strategy and the "follow up" were quite poor and the final report compares this result with the "Women with eating disorders" project (WED 2003) which had several similarities, but a few and obviously decisive differences. This organization for women suffering from eating disorders arranged self-help groups based on *email* and another category of groups on *chatrooms* communication. The recruiting to the email based groups was significantly easier in this project than in the SIVC, despite this being a rather small organization and focusing on a very limited diagnostic category. The results from this project, the Women with Eating Disorder (WED), may provide an opportunity for understanding some of the mechanisms of self-help, technology and motivation. The final report points out a few crucial differences: WED used a well-known technology (email). WED also had far less formal and practical/bureaucratic procedures for registering. Finally, WED was based in an organization with which the participators were familiar, possibly with personal relationships between the facilitators and numerous members. For legal reasons SIVC did not have the opportunity to make the registering and evaluating system more user friendly. Neither was it an option in this case to situate the project in a user organization.

SIVC did produce several documents they found useful for others wanting to try to establish self-help groups on digital/technological platforms, like procedures for starting a group, evaluation of a number of digital applications, agreement between participant and facilitator and other documents.

METHOD

By using the SIVC project as a case and comparing it to other trials we will discuss why people did or did not become involved in self-help based on different technological platforms. In the SIVC the most striking finding was the paucity of the response, while others have been far more successful in recruiting.

The SIVC project serves as a case by which to study self-help and technology, and the main methods are *action research* and *design based research*. This chapter is also in part a comparative analysis, as we investigate other projects and trials as well. The idea of an action research project in general is that a good way of understanding problems and phenomena is for the researcher to be directly involved in the processes, and not only to observe them from the outside (Reason, 1994). This closeness provides the opportunity for a very high validity, as the researcher will be deeply involved in (all) aspects of the work. Reason (1994) describes this as one of the *participative inquiry research methods,* among others. Partly, these research traditions are based on a critical view of traditional empirical work as one finds it problematic to place the researcher *outside* the subject of his or her research. Participative inquiry – and action research being one possible method – is based on a worldview being "more holistic, pluralist, and egalitarian, that is essentially participative." (ibid. p 324). Still, the present project is hardly of the nature of classic action research, as this usually has a more explicit social agenda. The background of this tradition is, as mentioned, a critical view of distanced and presumably objective research and one intends to involve underprivileged social groups in the research, starting e.g. educational programs and studying the effect of these in society (Hellevik, 1999). Trondsen and Sandaunet (2009) argue that action research designs are very suitable for exploring online self-help groups, demonstrated by two studies in Norway. The method can contribute to knowledge in a way not possible using other approaches. They point out some potential conflicts, especially between the researcher's pursuit of data and ethical considerations regarding the informant's integrity (ibid.).

Design-based research emphasizes how knowledge is developed in a cooperative process between researchers, practitioners and designers (or *design*). This work is to be conducted within the framework of ordinary work – meaning not in a "laboratory" setting. The experienced *practice* is then analyzed and an attempt is made to develop a *theory*. From this there is potentially a basis for *knowledge* (Stokken & Eikli, 2010; The Design-Based Research Collective 2003).

The most important problem concerning a method like this is the lack of critical distance. In the case of SIVC the researcher and project manager were one and the same person, even more blurring the borders than in a traditional action research design where the researcher usually works closely together with the project and takes part in it. In this particular case there are a number of questions that will not be asked and therefore not answered because as an "insider" it is not possible to take a credible outside perspective. Critical reflection is necessary and possible, but not in the same way as an external researcher may have. Some aspects that seem hard to assess from an inside perspective are, for instance, internal organization and external presentation.

An important part of the SIVC was to investigate technological platforms useful for self-help purposes of this kind (SPV 2009). Originally the idea was the utilization of videoconference freeware like Skype™ combined with the Festoon plug-in application. This was tested over a period of time and proved not to be satisfactorily stable. Other solutions were also considered, but the project group decided to run the groups on an audio-only basis. The video freeware seemed too vulnerable. An evaluation program aiming at documenting the experiences of the groups was also developed, based on both qualitative and quantitative methods. Besides this, the methods of how to run the groups were thoroughly discussed and a manual for advising "group starters" was drawn up. (ibid.).

A general framework for interpreting electronic self-help data is needed. Some categories of relevance are outlined in this chapter, and these define what data that can be regarded as useful and a starting point for how to interpret them. When it comes to data: in addition to reflecting on the experience of the SIVC project this chapter discusses findings and discussions from other relevant trials, based on a literature search in PubMed and other sources. No publications reporting from exactly similar tests as in the SIVC project seem to have been published, but a number of trials have studied ESGs, most of them Internet-based. Finally this chapter will suggest a model for understanding the preconditions necessary for Electronic Self-help Groups.

THEORETICAL PERSPECTIVES: SELF-HELP IN A LATE MODERN CONTEXT

It seems a lot easier to explain why a phenomenon is taking place than to analyze why certain (desired) actions do *not* happen. Nevertheless, we will make an attempt to reflect on this point. How did this opportunity, which to the organizers looked accessible and useful, obviously not tempt the potential participants very much? This is a key question in the SIVC case – and other less successful ESG projects.

First, we will attempt to describe a cultural and social stage – or perhaps a theatre – where the play of self-help is performed. Societies of high modernity are considered to sustain interpersonal relations of other characteristics than traditional societies. In a traditional setting, such as a society dominated by natural household and agriculture, the *primary* relations are likely to be of great importance. Family and relatives provide the economic basis for the individual and also meet social and emotional needs and provide necessary training for adult life. As the socialization processes change and other institutions emerge and secondary agents of socialization increase their influence, especially school systems, primary relations tend to lose some of their earlier functions. As these tendencies accelerate into high modernity, the secondary relations become both increasingly fickle and increasingly important; doctors and therapists are distinct examples of such relations. The high modern culture is per se post-traditional, both in the sense that tradition as such does not direct everyday life, and also with regard to how interpersonal relations are formed and sustained. The individuals are in a context that demands making personal choices about how to live everyday life, including who to relate to. "*The more tradition loses its hold, and the more daily life is reconstructed in terms of the dialectical interplay of the local and the global, the more individuals are forced to negotiate lifestyle choices among a diversity of options* (Giddens, 1991, p. 5). Self-help groups may be understood as a typical phenomenon in the lifestyle choice situation, and perhaps ESGs in particular. As Giddens points out, the self is more or less constantly altering and this demands that the self needs to be explored and constructed as part of a reflexive process of connecting personal and social change (ibid.). On this basis, a greater occurrence of self-help groups is to be expected in societies of late modernity than in more traditional ones.

A distinct trait is also the "pure" relations (ibid.). Both as a part of and a reaction against the expert systems of high modernity, the self-help groups are typical of such societies; they are by definition not run (but often facilitated) by professionals, and the group members do not usually have any relations to each other prior to the group starting. In this sense the relationships in the groups are "pure" – their common life challenges are the factors bringing them together. This expectation should lead to a situation where in a society of late modernity the preconditions for self-help groups are present; likewise a more traditionally oriented one will lack these and the basis for groups of this nature will be weak. In other words, in a setting of "fixed" or multidimensional relations the likelihood of being in a digital self-help group is lower than in a setting of more "fickle" and pure relations. It should be underlined that this is not a normative assessment of which kind of relations is preferable. People in a traditional society may feel oppressed and even lonely despite the strong social relations, but they will also often feel free and safe due to the same conditions. And persons living in late modern societies are likely to experience what Giddens describes as "existential anxiety". Nevertheless, the level of anxiety does not necessarily rise and the sense of individual freedom is experienced as preferable by a great majority. In the context of self-help, this will for many be the most adequate and responsible strategy for coping with their situation in a high modern context.

A matter of current research is whether self-help groups based on technology are likely to be helpful or not. Several problems may be mentioned with regard to the validity and reliability of this approach; we will return to these questions later. Trials made in the field do not give a very clear picture of the "effect". A literature search did not succeed in finding other projects using Skype™ or similar technologies.

The issue of diagnosis-specific or cross-diagnostic groups is a question of how *relevant* the invitation is experienced by potential participants. In Collie, Kreshka, Ferrier, Parsons, Graddy, Avram, Mannell, Chen, Perkins and Koopman (2006) the informants report that the aspect of information is important, as also was the emotional support. Griffith, Cathleen, Calear, Banfield (2009) found in their systematic review work indications of the best outcome of Internet support groups for women with breast cancer, but they emphasize the general lack of high quality research in the field.

There might be a methodological problem as they also suggest a relationship between the nature of trial design and outcome. What they see as a confounding design gives the most positive result. So, there are possible – but uncertain – benefits for these particular people from engaging in support groups on the web.

The work by Hoey, Ieropoli, White and Jefford (2008), Collie et al. (2006) and Griffith, Cathleen, Calear and Banfield (2009) is based on trials of a quantitative nature, and psychometric methods like the Center for Epidemiologic Studies Depression Scale (CES-D) and others are the main methods adopted. Used in a proper way, scales like these are relevant and may provide data of great validity and reliability. Methodology of this kind also has limitations, especially regarding the concept of validity. And a key question in the field of self-help is why do people care about engaging in these groups and forums? Hoey et al. (2008) and Griffith et al. (2009) suggest an uncertain and possibly low *outcome* for people with various issues, but a significant part of the population still take part in them. In short: why keep posting messages if you feel just as bad as you did a month ago? A crucial question might be whether there is any reason why one should study self-help analogously with medical/pharmacological studies, as the nature of the objects studied vary greatly. It seems difficult to grasp the motivational elements in electronic self-help involvement using psychometric methods. At least with the tools available today the research seems to have problems explaining the vast growth of ESG. Why would all these persons engage in the forums and groups if it felt completely meaningless? Still, if the object is to reduce depression, post-traumatic stress and other psychological sufferings – especially following a serious somatic disease – being a member of groups like the one Collie et al. (2006) refers to would appear to be fruitful.

This phenomenon of "Why" is interesting, as the SIVC failed to convince people to become involved in their groups. The problems of explaining the "why" in other groups by using psychometric approaches might lead to a non-functionalistic approach. Self-help is more fruitful to assess in "relational" terms. Participators do not necessarily come with an agenda for reducing distress, but seek a community capable of providing emotional support and of giving them the opportunity to contribute to the well-being of others in similar situations. The borders of being a "gainer" and "giver" might be fluent. Hence, looking for "function" and "effect" is not always what will lead to the best explanations; exploring the nature of the relationship and the meaning and interpretation the participants could better tell why groups emerge and are sustained. The aspect of "similar situation" might be of importance, both as a motivational element for joining a group one identifies oneself with, but as Collie et al. (2006) demonstrate, the informational aspect plays a role for the way the outcome is experienced.

Borkmann (1999) argues that self-help is a holistic way of coping with demanding life situations. Other helpers, like physicians, therapists and priests may be helpful, but in a fragmentary way. They take care of certain specific aspects of life; even friends and family may not be able to see the situation as a whole, as they have a preset understanding of the individual and his or her nature. Following this view, there would seem to be little meaning in measuring the outcome of self-help in psychometric or other ways, especially if this is suggested as the only relevant value of the groups and forums.

When signing up for a self-help forum or group, the individual brings his or her expectations. These expectations may vary greatly for different persons in the same group, and they may also not be very well articulated and clear, at least when they are asked to explain the "effect" they count on gaining.

THEORETICAL PERSPECTIVES: AFFORDANCES

Tjora and Sandaunet (2010) outline three traits of development in the digitalization process: Objectification, activating and involvement. The growing use of ICT in health care offers increasing opportunities to represent the patient's situation in figures and numbers, this being the *objectification* trait. *Activation* refers to how patients are becoming more able to be an active part of their own health by communicating with medical staff. These processes are usually initiated by the health authorities and are often motivated by greater cost effectiveness. Finally, *involvement* describes how people utilize technological platforms to interact with others to exchange their experiences and look for information on the Internet. The latter point is of special interest in self-help.

Andreassen and Trondsen (2008) point out how technological solutions not only provide practical opportunities, but also determine or at least set frames for how we act. Ian Hutchby (2001) describes these phenomena as *affordances* and he provides an explanation of the relationship between technology and social practice. He emphasizes that technology both *constrains* and *enables* such practice. The concern is how technology influences social patterns, although he also recognizes technology being social constructions and interpretable. This two-sided view should be considered as useful in this case. Being an attempt to create a synthetic theory derived from a critique of both radical constructivist and a more deterministic "realist" or essentialist view, this represents a well-developed approach for studying how people use communication technology for self-help purposes.

Hutchby outlines the *functional* and the *relational* aspects that frame – not determine – relationships between people and objects. These concepts should not be confused with the earlier use of "functional" and "relational", as these referred to how self-help groups are assessed. Hutchby analyzes aspects of technological-human matters. *Functional* aspects of objects are properties that he argues are beyond interpretation. Let us use two objects as examples: a traditionally built wooden boat from the Amazonas and an iPhone. The handmade boat is rather useless for sending sms's, taking pictures and checking your e-mail. It cannot even make a phone call. Some are likely to claim that the iPhone is able to do "anything" – but then you have not tried to cross a 3 meter deep and 20 meter broad piranha-infested river on it. The boat also keeps all its properties regardless of access to electric power, while the iPhone soon loses some value after a few days in the same situation. These are functional aspects of these two objects.

The *relational* aspect deals with how objects have different affordances for different species – or even different people. Huchby uses the example of how water has the walk-on-ability for an insect waterboatman, but definitely not to a lion or a crocodile. Still; the walk-on-ability of fresh water *is* present, but it only becomes manifest when the insect walks on it. Likewise one may analyze the utilization of hi-tech communication to some people it seems like an endless sea of opportunities – possibly only limited by financial resources. To others it may be an endless sea of confusion, limited by the technology itself. In the relational aspect the constructivist perspective makes good sense, and Hutchby refers to Grint and Wooglar (1997) using the notion that technology should be treated as "text" which is written in certain ways with certain objectives. It is then "read", or interpreted, and the reader understands it and uses it in relation to the context in which he or she is. As Hutchby argues, this is an intriguing perspective, but as a universal view on the relationship between man and technology he advocates a more balanced theory. Still, as a useful metaphor "text" may work to describe the relational aspect of the affordances of technology, as it provides concepts for analyzing how objects are perceived differently by various individuals in different contexts. But by using the functional aspects in addition, we are able to identify properties of objects that are not subject to interpretation. There *are* differences between guns and roses.

In the following we will outline five concepts that are aspects of technologically supported self-help programs. The background is the SIVC project, but possibly these dimensions are relevant for further work in the field. They are in no way intended to be suggested as universal, but drawn out of this project and also viewed in the light of other trials. The attempt to define certain factors makes us able to investigate empirical work in other trials and the outcome is a model of constraining and enabling elements. The factors are aspects of the self-help design made by the facilitators, for instance in the SIVC the group was in "real-time", the members were identifiable (not anonymous) etc. Some of these factors are therefore of a functional nature, as they are not subject to interpretation by the participators. But whether these properties are interpreted as constraining or enabling will be a matter of relational kind. Or more precisely; *how* constraining or enabling they are.

Synchronicity

Flexibility seems to be a trait in late modernity; this might be understood as a part of the disembedding mechanisms (Giddens, 1991). Bjerke (2010) suggests that asynchronic forums are preferred among AA-members. The same groups also differed concerning content and character as the level of positive communicative content and the personal acceptance of others was significantly higher. We will look into other trials to see whether this expectation may be confirmed or falsified.

Identification

The possibility of anonymously expressing oneself in web forums and chatrooms is a typical trait of late modernity, as it enables communication without being fully responsible as a sender. This opportunity corresponds well with the need in late modernity to feel individual freedom. On the other hand, as individual reflexivity is a typical trait of this cultural situation, it encourages individuals to express themselves in public, also as identifiable persons. The world indicated in the famous Andy Warhol quote "In the future we all will be famous for 15 minutes" does not seem to be that far away, as anyone and everyone has their own blog or Facebook/Twitter site, publishing numerous pictures and letting the world know how we feel about any matter on our mind.

Specified Diagnosis

The SIVC was not exclusively dedicated to a single or specified diagnoses; one assumed there would be a number of benefits from arranging cross-diagnostic groups. Was this an approach that attracted potential participants? According to Philips (1996, Bjerke 2010) reaching a common base of identification is a crucial element in the success of self-help groups. This involves relating to each other's experiences, which in turn develops the "sense of we". We will return to this point to investigate whether empirical data supports or weakens the assumption that specific groups succeed better than general groups with regard to recruitment.

Organizational Trust

Anthony Giddens (1991) describes how *trust* and *mistrust* is a typical trait of late modern society. Individuals feel highly dependent on expert systems and trust them, but there is also a widespread mistrust of the same kind of systems. Both commercial organizations and public ones will find themselves in this situation. Health organizations are typical examples of this paradox, especially for chronically ill people. A person suffering from asthma for instance, will, to avoid unnecessary breathing problems, need a prescription for medicines. In this way he or she depends / is dependent on a number of systems: the doctor with a necessary education and licenses, the organization in which this doctor is employed (private or public), the pharmacy and not least the pharmacy industry that produces her medication, just to mention the most obvious ones. The paradox is striking; to live an independent and pleasant life, he or she is highly dependent on a great number of organizations. The individual independency of late modernity is therefore only possible by depending on numerous expert systems. Furthermore, these systems seem practically impossible for most people to "know" and understand. The matter of dependency is, of course, not solely restricted to the case in health matters; perhaps even more intricate items and systems are required to use computers, mobile phone payment services etc. These systems all depend heavily on a fair degree of user's trust. If the public suspects that the medication is harmful to their health in some way, if the telephones may be tapped or can break down, or the credit card system robs the card holders – these will be less used. Capitalism is one of the fundamental preconditions of late modernity and these systems are sustained by market interests and serve the purpose of making a profit for their owners. Hence, all kind of organizations do their best to keep the trust at an acceptable level by delivering products/services that meet the expectations and they constantly keep an eye on how they "look" from the customer's perspective. Thereby follows the focus of "image", "branding", "reputation" and such. Giddens describes these processes as organizational reflexivity. Despite the organizations' efforts to reduce it, the mistrust is still present at some level (ibid.).

Accessibility

One of the ways technology influences human behavior concerns the degree of accessibility. Computer users will interpret different programs and websites as more or less simple or complex to use. This is likely to be one of the aspects of the interaction man-computer that determines whether a program will be put into use or not. This is a part of the relational aspects of the design of the forums/programs using technology in self-help (Hutchby, 2001). Designs may be interpreted as easy to use or more demanding and difficult. Numerous elements determine what individuals find "easy" or "difficult" in this matter, and even a design that seems very understandable may be little used, simply because a competing design seems even more user friendly. Here the concept of technology as "text" seems relevant. It is "read", interpreted and (mis)understood in various ways (ibid.).

This leads to the following list of factors relevant to motivation for Electronic Self-help Groups:

- Synchronicity
- Identification
- Specified diagnosis
- Organizational trust
- Accessibility

In the next paragraphs these will be discussed in the light of experiences of the SIVC project and supplemented by other relevant empiric research. In the concluding section a model of motivational elements will be suggested.

SYNCHRONICITY: SHOW UP OR STAY AWAY!

Skype™ technology and the SIVC use of it provided the opportunity to talk to peers about personal experiences at meetings at certain times – but at a place of the user's choice. Participation required the signing of an agreement and returning it by (snail)mail to the project. Within this model lie a number of possibilities – and demands, like the need for signing up and revealing your identity. Another requirement is the need for making appointments and by that being obliged to meet at certain times of the week/month. Without arrangements like these Skype™ meetings cannot take place, as it is a synchronized platform. This is an example of affordance; the technology provides the opportunity of talking to each other – at no cost – in groups. But it also requires all the participants to be available at the same time. Self-help forums on an asynchronized basis recruit far more users – and these groups/forums also seem "helpful" with regard to measurable psychological aspects (Hoey et al., 2008). This would seem to indicate that asynchronic forums are more likely to attract people than synchronic ones.

An example of this is how people with rare diseases use digital forums; Lasker, Sogolow and Sharim (2005) have investigated how persons suffering from primary biliary cirrhosis communicate in an online community. The asynchronic design is highly valued among the participators, as it gives a feeling of freedom with relation to when and how much they engage in the forum. Furthermore, the sense of a 24-hour opportunity both to learn from, get support and contribute to others has great importance (Lasker et al., 2005).

In general, self-help groups/ peer-support programs do not always show very clear outcomes. Hoey et.al (2008) have in their review article examined how different forms of peer support affect people with cancer. In short, their conclusion is that the lack of research does not provide a good basis for deciding what kinds of support are the most beneficial for the patients. However, on the basis of the 43 research papers they find that the two forms of self-help that provide the best support are (1) one-on-one face-to-face and (2) group Internet. These latter groups are asynchronic and based on written messages. None of the reviewed papers are based on trials synchronic internet groups (ibid.). The authors emphasize the uncertainty of the findings due to weaknesses in many of the trials and the general need for more research in the field.

An example of an asynchronic system that did attract participants is the earlier mentioned groups for women with eating disorders – WED (SPV 2009). They communicated by email, which enabled them to write and answer messages whenever they liked – but they were obliged to maintain a certain level of activity to ensure that everybody got replies and that they all contributed. This opportunity attracted more than 30 persons. In a small country like Norway and for a small organization with limited resources this may be considered to be a fairly large number.

IDENTIFICATION: TO BE OR NOT TO BE

It does not appear to be easy to find clear answers regarding this aspect of attending self-help groups or forums. This may be partly because the question is not asked very often in the research, but also due to the fact that some self-help forums attract large numbers of participants regardless of whether they are required to identify themselves or not. Another point is that there are *degrees* of identification. An example is the social forum tudiabetes.com where members may display their name, picture, hometown and a great deal of personal information in their profile. But it is also fully possible to leave out most of this information and in reality be practically anonymous, with just an alias name and no picture – or a South Park character image.

Obviously being identified is not an absolute obstacle to taking part in ESGs, as for instance shown by Collie et al. (2006); being a part of a support group based on video conferencing presented with full names and clearly identifying information does not keep participators away. On the other hand, anonymity is clearly preferred by a number of persons taking part in these groups and possibly considered as a necessity. Takahashi et.al (2009) point to the possibility of being anonymous as an advantage for depressed persons and hence a motivating factor.

A very tentative conclusion might be that the more the individuals interpret their suffering as socially demanding, the more motivating an anonymous support service may be. Hence the cultural context and properties of the individual determine how weighty this factor is.

SPECIFIED DIAGNOSIS OR ANYONE? WHY SHOULD I TALK TO THESE PEOPLE?

In the SIVC project there were only a few criteria that limited participation; one did not include persons that primarily had psychiatric issues and not persons that primarily were relatives. Otherwise, people with all kinds of somatic chronic sufferings were invited and having a formal diagnosis was not necessary either (this would anyway be difficult to control). This choice was partly made in order to recruit as many as possible, but also because face-to-face groups put together this way seem to work very well, as the participants tend to be more focused on coping issues than on illness and diagnoses (SPV 2009).

But; the paradox may be that an invitation like this is not "tempting" enough – it may simply be *too* open. A possible indication is the website "healthboards.com" that hosts a vast number of online support forums relevant to all kinds of health conditions. On this site it does not seem to be easy to find any groups or threads announcing themselves as "cross-diagnostic" or anything similar. It is rather the opposite, some of them are indeed very specific on what conditions the groups are aiming to offer support to. There is a "General health" category, but this one is not by far the largest, and the discussions here do not seem to be really "general". This raises the question of motivation for joining groups of cross-diagnostic nature.

Let us return again to the WED project; they succeeded in recruiting a number of women with eating disorders to their email-based support groups. Perhaps the very specific group and diagnosis is a part of the explanation for the relatively large number of participants.

This touches upon the notion of *involvement* as a central trait in technology and health (Tjora and Sandaunet, 2010). It seems likely that an opportunity for communicating with persons in a situation similar to one's own stimulates a person to take part. A cross-diagnostic group may be perceived as too vague and therefore less motivating to become involved in. There is little empirical evidence on which to draw a conclusion on this subject, but SIVC compared to WED and the great number of diagnostic-specific groups and the rather few cross-diagnostic ones may point in this direction.

ORGANIZATIONAL TRUST: IMPOSSIBILITIES OF BUREAUCRACY

The project was embedded in a public health trust and not in an independent / volunteer organization, which was necessary for formal reasons. This unit was not even one that treats patients; the Patient Education Resource Center of Central Norway works primarily towards health staff in its region and therefore the average patient is not acquainted with it.

The general level of trust between the Norwegian population and the health service providers seems to be high. A survey from 2008 indicates that 87% of the population claims that they "absolutely agree" or "partly agree" with the statement: "I have full confidence in the treatment the doctor provides." (Ramm, 2010). The same survey reveals that the users of alternative treatment are more frequent users of the common health service than others. This may be because this group feels that they need health- related services more than the average population, but still the finding could indicate a rather high level of trust even among users of alternative therapy. However, this is probably primarily an expression of the informants' attitude towards their personal experience with doctors. The health authorities as a *system* do not necessarily benefit directly from these largely positive findings; other trials indicate that the further the distance from the user – the less trust, which seems demonstrated by the pharmacy company Pfizer's study from 2008. A kind of opposite hierarchy seems to exist on the dimensions of power and trust in the following order: Doctor/nurse – pharmacists – public hospitals – patient organizations – private hospitals – pharmacy companies – health politicians (pfizer.no). The primary doctors are trusted by 71%, politicians by 6%. The trust of all these actors in the health field has actually increased over recent years (till 2008), but this seems to depend partly on the design of the study. Other variables in the same study indicate a decreasing trust in politicians.

Even if the degree of mistrust has not necessarily been great, it represents one of the obstacles the participators had to pass in order to become part of the self-help group.

The SIVC was organized as a project run by the Patient Education Resource Center, a part of Central Norway Regional Health Authority. Contact info, website and logo on the flyers made this obvious to the public. The project was aware of the risk that this might lead to a more skeptical attitude from participants than if they were invited to a group run by a patient organization or someone else they felt more related to. But, for formal reasons it was not possible to let anybody else store the names of those who signed up. The research regulations do not allow names or other personal information be known by anyone else than the researcher.

Trust issues like this are, as we have discussed, a complex phenomenon. It therefore seems reasonable to suggest that a self-help group like this would be easier to establish if the possible participants did not have to sign up to a "faceless" bureaucratic unit. One of the attempts that was made in the SIVC was to let patients from a rehabilitation clinic for brain-injured persons use the method as a follow-up after having been together in the clinic. They therefore knew each other, they knew the group starter and they lived far away from each other, partly in rural areas. These patients who had been introduced to the idea of keeping in touch through Skype™ as a part of the SIVC had been largely positive to this. Yet, when they were formally invited and given the opportunity to return the form necessary for taking part, very few replied. The Giddens concept of mistrust enables a possible explanation for why recruiting turned out to be a major challenge in the project. In contrast, the WED project situated in a small organization with quite close relationships between the facilitators and the members recruited far better. This may also be explained as a matter of trust.

The experience described by Collie et al. (2006) raises the issue of trust and mistrust; what factors in their project enabled them to succeed in recruiting members to the groups? This will not be discussed broadly here, but the group leader may well play a determining role, given that a video conference talk requires even more of the participators as they need to show up at a "strange" location at certain times to be a part of the group, and that most likely several of them were not very familiar with the technology in advance. The article (ibid.) does not describe these practical details much, but it is most likely that some mechanisms must have been at work to reduce the effects of mistrust and technological alienation. This might have been "agents" of the systems who had the necessary confidence of the users, such as doctors, nurses, social workers or others who recommended the project and were actively supportive towards potential participators.

ACCESSIBILITY: HOW HARD CAN IT BE?

The idea of SIVC was to explore the use of a relatively new technological platform for self-help purposes – Internet-based video conferences. The project group decided to use the Skype™ application because it was free, seemed easy to use and was already one of the most widespread applications of its kind. Even so, this way of communication is far less common than the telephone, Internet or e-mail. Other trials using the more established platforms show higher attendance. There are a number of trials which confirm that Electronic Self-help Groups are extremely helpful – though not under elaborate conditions (Andreassen & Trondsen, 2008).

Collie et al. (2006) report from a trial using video conferences (VC) in studios to offer a support group to breast cancer patients living in rural areas. This was not a "true" self-help group as the sessions were lead by a professional oncology social worker. According to reports from the members they felt comfortable using the VC and also reported positively about both the informational aspect and the opportunity for emotional bonds with other women in this situation. They further emphasized the importance of having a professional facilitator. In this trial pretests and posttests measuring various psychological aspects were used and data from these seem to indicate a decrease in depression and posttraumatic stress disorder symptoms. So, in this case the videoconference group seems to have been beneficial to the patients, but this design demands substantial efforts on the part of the facilitator to compensate for the little-known technology.

The SIVC final report suggests that projects using established technology like telephone, e-mail and the Internet seem to recruit members far more easily than the Skype™ based (SPV 2009). The fact that a great number of ESGs exist, and very few groups based on video conference, is an indicator in itself that this is felt to be a less accessible technology and is therefore a constraining factor.

A MODEL OF MOTIVATION FOR ELECTRONIC SELF-HELP GROUPS

In an attempt to sum up the discussion made here, a model of motivational elements is suggested (see Table 1). The left-hand column indicates the factor described, the middle one traits of the factor that reduce motivation for taking part in a group, and finally, the right-hand column contains elements supporting motivation for self-help group participation. The first two factors are rather clearly of a functional nature, to use Hutchby's terminology. This also partly is the case for the third one, "diagnostic" factor, as this one is more open to the interpretation of the participants. The last two, concerning organizational trust and accessibility, have clear relational and interpretive dimensions (Hutchby, 2001). All the affordances are to be understood as scales and not typological.

The following interpretation seems reasonable: even if one or two factors of a self-help program are on the "reducing" side, this may be compensated by other, supporting elements. Likewise this works the other way. The factors are not equally strong, and the relationship between them is determined by the situation.

As for the SIVC project, too many of the factors ended up as reducing motivational factors. The organizational trust was questionable, it was cross-diagnostic, participants had to identify themselves, and access was more complicated

Table 1. A model of motivation for engaging in electronic self-help groups (ESGs)

Factors	*Affordances*	
	Constraining	*Enabling*
Synchronicity	High	Low
Identification	High*	Low*
Specified diagnosis	Low	High
Organizational trust	Low	High
Accessibility	Low	High

*Findings are diverse on this factor.

than with other digital forums. Furthermore, even if the Skype™ technology is quite widespread and must be considered as user friendly, for a large part of the population it is less well-known than communication technology like the telephone, mobile phone, Internet and e-mail. In addition, it was a synchronous technology, requiring the participators to be active at specific hours. So, this factor also drew the SIVC in a negative, constraining direction. Hence, a few potential users signed up, but not many and far fewer than were necessary to establish a group.

The model provides a tentative theoretical explanation of the dynamic interplay between motivation, factors and affordances in the field of Electronic Self-help Groups. Further research is needed to develop knowledge on the topic. As ESG is a growing and increasingly significant element for a large number of people, researchers, health professionals, health leaders and politicians should take greater interest in understanding it.

The model should be read in an interpretive and not literal way. The five factors are far from being a comprehensive list; it may be modified both in regard of the number of factors and for the individual factors. There is also a constant need for empirical work to determine which affordances that actually *are* constraining and enabling when it comes to motivation for self-help.

FUTURE RESEARCH DIRECTIONS

The suggested model is built on a limited empirical basis and therefore more research seems necessary in order to evaluate and develop it further. Reports on both successful and less successful projects may be helpful, but other designs are relevant, such as interviews with chronically ill persons regarding whether they find self-help groups and forums adequate for their situations or not, and what design or form they might prefer in these groups or forums.

The outlined factors in the model are modifiable and must not to be understood as fixed. Some of the concepts may not prove to be fruitful and others certainly may be added, and this requires more empirical work. Another element is the *significance* of each factor, which is not discussed here.

One of the factors is less clear than other, the matter of identification. One might expect that a number of participators in ESGs would prefer to be as anonymous as possible, but this is not by far the situation. However, many do *not* reveal names, pictures or other traces making identification possible. This field seems to be little investigated, and both qualitative and quantitative studies should be considered in future work.

CONCLUSION

In this chapter we have attempted to develop a model that aims at explaining in part why one would or would not take part in Electronic Self-help Groups. As it is based primarily on one project in particular – although including a look at others – the empirical basis is sparse. However, the suggested model may serve as a tool for institutions that want to offer self-help opportunities and it may hopefully contribute to further research. It suggests these five factors may possibly determine whether a person is motivated or not to become a member of a group or a forum: synchronicity, identification, specified diagnosis, organizational trust and accessibility.

REFERENCES

Alemi, F., Mosavel, M., Stephens, R. C., Chadiri, A., Krishnaswamy, J., & Thakkar, H. (1996). Electronic self-help and support groups. *Medical Care*, *34*, OS32–OS44. doi:10.1097/00005650-199610003-00004

Andreassen, H. K., & Trondsen, M. (2008). Pasient på e-post. I: Tjora, Aksel: *Den moderne pasienten*. Gyldendal akademisk. ("Patients by E-mail").

Berger, P. L., & Luckmann, T. (1966). *The social construction of reality*. London, UK: Penguin.

Bjerke, T. N. (2010). Fra kirkekjeller til Internett: En kvalitativ studie av to internasjonale internettbaserte AA-grupper. In: Tjora og Sandaunet: *Digitale pasienter*. Gyldendal akademisk. ("From the Church Cellar to the Internet: A Qualitative Trail of two International Internetbased AA-groups")

Borkmann, T. (1999). *Understanding self-help/ mutual aid. Experimental learning in the commons*. Rutgers University Press.

Collie, K., Kreshka, M. A., Ferrier, S., Parsons, R., Graddy, K., & Avram, S. (2006). Videoconferencing for delivery of breast cancer support groups to women living in rural communities: A pilot study. *Psycho-Oncology*, 16.

Giddens, A. (1991). *Modernity and self-identity. Self and society in the late modern age*. Polity.

Griffith, C., Calear, A., & Banfield, M. (2009). Systematic review on internet support groups (ISGs) and depression (vol. 1): Do ISGs reduce depressive symptoms? *Journal of Medical Internet Research*, *11*(3).

Hellevik, O. (1999). *Forskningsmetode i sosiologi og statsvitenskap. Universitetsforlaget*. Methods of Research in Sociology and Political Science.

Hoey, L. M., Ieropoli, S. C., White, V. M., & Jefford, M. (2008). Systematic review of peer-support programs for people with cancer. *Patient Education and Counseling*, 70.

Hutchby, I. (2001). *Technologies, texts and affordances*. Cambridge, UK: Cambridge University Press.

Interessegruppa for kvinner med spiseforstyrrelser. (2001). *Selvhjelpsgrupper via telekom*. ("Women with Eating Disorders" – WED)

Lasker, J. N., Sogolow, E. D., & Sharim, R. R. (2005). The role of an online community for people with a rare disease: Content analysis of message posted on a primary biliary cirrhosis mailing list. *Journal of Medical Internet Research*, *7*(1). doi:10.2196/jmir.7.1.e10

Ramm, J. (2010). *Helse – flere velger alternativt*. ("Health – rising numbers of alternative treatment users"). Retrieved from www.ssb.no/ samfunnss-peilet/ utg/201002/05/ art-2010-05-03-01.htmlUH

Reason, P. (1994). Three approaches to participative inquiry. In Denzin, N. K., & Lincoln, Y. S. (Eds.), *Handbook of qualitative research*. Sage.

Sluttrapport. (2009). *Selvhjelp på videokonferanse,* 2009. NK-LMS og LMS Helse Sunnmøre HF – regional. ("Self-help on Internet based Video Conference 2009. Final report")

Stokken, R., & Eikli, G. (2010). Den e-lærande pasienten. In Tjora, A., & Sandaunet, A. G. (Eds.), *Digitale pasienter. Gyldendal akademisk ("The E-learning Patient").*

Takahashi, Y., Uchida, C., Miyaki, K., Sakai, M., Shimbo, T., & Nakayama, T. (2009). Potential benefits and harms of a peer support social network service on the Internet for people with depressive tendencies: Qualitative content analysis and social network analysis. *Journal of Medical Internet Research*, *11*(3), e29. doi:10.2196/jmir.1142

The Design-Based Research Collective. (2003). Design-based research: An emerging paradigm for educational inquiry. *Educational Researcher*, *32*(1), 5–8. doi:10.3102/0013189X032001005

Tjora, A., & Sandaunet, A.-G. (2010). Digitale pasienter: En introduksjon og leseanvisning. In Tjora, A., & Sandaunet, A.-G. (Eds.), *Digitale pasienter. Gyldendal akademisk. ("Digital Patients: An Introduction and Reader's note").*

Trondsen, M., & Sandaunet, A.-G. (2009). The dual role of the action researcher. *Evaluation and Program Planning*, *32*(1), 13–20. doi:10.1016/j.evalprogplan.2008.09.005

KEY TERMS AND DEFINITIONS

ESG: Electronic Self-help Group. The term Electronic Self-help Groups (ESGs) is here used in a broad meaning, including both "groups" and "forums" regardless of technological platform, number of participants and structure of the communication. "Electronic" is chosen to include not only Internet, but also platforms like video conference, telephone, mobile phone etc. "Group" should be understood as both a limited, defined groups and open forums. See for instance Alemi, Mosavel, Stephens, Chadiri, Krishnaswamy, & Thakkar (1996): Electronic self-help and support groups.

Self-Help: "An individual taking action to help him- or herself, often drawing on latent internal resources and healing powers within the context of his or her lived experience with an issue or predicament." (Borkmann, 1999, p. 4). In this chapter "mutual aid" (ibid.) will be included in the "self-help" concept as these concepts together expresses both the individual and the collective/communicative aspects.

SIVC: Self-help on Internet based Video Conference, a project initiated by a resource group associated with the National Center of Patient Education (NCPE) in Norway. One of the main objectives was to make use of Skype™ for self-help purposes and to investigate the experiences of the participants.

Skype™: A software application that allows users to make voice calls over the Internet. Video conferencing is also possible if an additional application is adopted. The service is free to download and install from skype.com. It requires a computer access with broadband internet connection (skype.com).

Chapter 12
E-Health and Digital Inclusion

Lorna Gibson[1]
University of Dundee, UK

David Sloan
University of Dundee, UK

Wendy Moncur
University of Aberdeen, UK

ABSTRACT

E-health resources can deliver demonstrable benefits for quality of care, for example through provision of public health information and access to online communities and self-help groups for those experiencing ill-health. Digitally excluded groups of health consumers such as older people and those with disabilities have much to gain from the social connectedness and social support offered through these digitally facilitated resources – yet at the same time are most vulnerable to continued exclusion due to inappropriate technology design and implementation.

In this chapter, we describe in detail the opportunities e-health can offer in the context of digital inclusion by reducing social exclusion and enhancing quality of life through thoughtful technology intervention. We highlight the problems that may emerge or persist if the design of e-health systems does not fully take into account the challenges of user access and adoption. We show how principles of user-centred and inclusive design can be used as a basis on which successful e-health systems can be developed and implemented and offer suggestions for how these principles can best influence design of future systems.

INTRODUCTION

In recent years, the concept of a digital economy has arisen that focuses on digital services and network technologies, with access enabled by low-cost consumer devices. While seen by industry and government as a means of providing improved quality and reach of services and products at lower cost, this move to digital interactions has created a situation in which a large number of people may find it difficult or impossible to access these e-services. Those at greater risk of being digitally excluded include older people, those with a disability, lower income groups, and people who are

DOI: 10.4018/978-1-60960-866-8.ch012

unemployed (Dutton, Helsper, & Gerber, 2009). Additional groups at risk of exclusion include those with language or cultural differences (McKay, 2005) and those in locations where limited or lack of broadband service provision or access to skills training causes exclusion (Warren, 2007).

There is a growing number of initiatives to promote digital inclusion. Many of these initiatives concentrate on the practicalities such as broadband provision which, while relevant, do not represent the whole picture. For example, in the UK the government has an action plan to attract and support the estimated 17 million people over the age of 15 who are not using computers and the Internet (HM Government, 2009). They also emphasize the correlation between social and digital exclusion (see also Warren, 2007), estimating that this affects more than six million adults. The digital divide can also be seen in relation to the 'participation gap' (Jenkins, 2006). Jenkins states "As long as the focus remains on access, reform remains focused on technologies; as soon as we begin to talk about participation, the emphasis shifts to cultural protocols and practices" (Jenkins, 2006, p. 23), highlighting the need for digital inclusion to be user-focused.

It would be difficult to argue that technology has not made an overall positive contribution to quality of healthcare provision. Computers have consistently increased in speed and capacity over the last 30 years, meaning more powerful computations can be made and greater quantities of data can be processed. Such developments have the potential to transform healthcare, for example through improving patient record management and supporting informed diagnosis and treatment identification. Information and communication technology (ICT) has also provided an opportunity and platform for a vast quantity of health-related information to be made available to consumers, opening up potential for improvements to general public health and to illness management.

Frustratingly, though, successful technological innovation requires more than powerful hardware and feature-rich software, particularly if the end user is a consumer or someone who is part of the care pathway. Effective technological innovation requires human-centred design approaches in order to ensure that the innovation is useful and usable, and at minimum risk of rejection due to inappropriate or insensitive design. The field of user-centred design (UCD), and a more specific focus on inclusive design, with its ultimate goal of technology that is as easy as possible to use by as many as possible of the target audience, is of critical importance to the success of e-health innovations, but is arguably not yet as influential as it could be. Ironically, those population groups who are most likely to experience digital exclusion are also more likely to experience health issues and co-morbidities. Online communities are likely to be very beneficial with these groups who may find it difficult to find and connect with other people in similar situations.

Digital exclusion from e-health may exist for many reasons; but fundamentally falls into two categories:

1. **Availability:** exclusion resulting from a lack of access to hardware (such as a PC, smartphone or interactive digital television), or software, or sufficiently capable network connection, necessary to use an e-health system.
2. **Accessibility:** given its availability, a lack of ability to use an e-health system effectively due to the way it is designed.

While the former is a more general challenge for digital inclusion that may require intervention from the state and from industry, the latter is very much a challenge that can be tackled by providers of e-health systems. We focus on the latter challenge.

This chapter will explore the relationship between e-health and the wider digital population specifically considering e-health communities and online self-help groups. It highlights the problems of inequitable access by the digital population which can counteract any potential benefits the e-health resource can have. Identifying key issues and considerations, the chapter provides some positive steps towards more inclusive e-health applications in the future.

THE POTENTIAL FOR E-HEALTH TO REDUCE EXCLUSION

Opportunities for E-Health

The potential for e-health applications to deliver cheaper, better services and products ensures their appeal to both government and industry, specifically those within the medical community. E-health applications also appeal to patients. In a move away from medical paternalism, patients and their supporters are increasingly acting as consumers, demanding more involvement in decisions relating to their care (such as Cawsey, Grasso & Paris, 2007). They are now far more likely to question a healthcare professional's diagnosis or treatment plan, and less likely to trust a healthcare professional without reservation (Chin, 2002). This can be seen in the increasing trend for individuals to seek out health information beyond the doctor's consulting room - most notably via the Internet (such as Bromme, Jucks, & Wagner, 2005). This change, coupled with spiralling healthcare costs, has seen a rise in patient-centred thinking (approaches such as Participatory Medicine, Patient Partnership, Collaborative Medicine and Patient Led Care) within the medical community. The use of e-health not only facilitates these approaches but is often a key aspect to them.

E-health has the potential to provide more dynamic, engaging and motivating systems than straightforward information provision. Initiatives such as the European Commission's eEurope Action Plan have promoted the creation of personalised e-health services to patients, in contrast to the majority of e-health services which have been created with the needs of healthcare professionals in mind (Bisson, 2005). While such patient-centred e-health services cannot replace personal contact with health professionals, they can serve a beneficial, complementary role (Bental, Cawsey, & Jones, 1999). Patients prefer the information provided by e-health systems to be delivered in a personalised format (Cawsey, Jones, & Pearson, 2000). Such personalisation may relate to any or all of information content, information presentation and human-computer interaction.

The *goals* of personalized, adaptive e-health systems for patients vary. For example, systems have been created to foster patient compliance or adherence; promote patient autonomy; save time for healthcare professionals; and improve wellbeing. Whatever the goal, health consumers are individuals, and are likely to have individual characteristics and requirements.

Advanced adaptivity also requires acquisition of information about the user. These *inputs* have varied, depending on what was available and useful, and have included basic facts, demographics, belief models, mental health attitudes and medical records (Bental et al., 1999). Perhaps surprisingly, the person's emotional state has rarely been used as a system input, although it has been used to evaluate the effectiveness of giving tailored information to patients about cancer (Cawsey et al., 2000).

E-Health and Excluded Groups

E-health has a particular potential to help hard to reach and expensive-to-care-for groups. More importantly, it provides the possibility and opportunity to provide social support which is often sidelined in the traditional care pathway in favour of fulfilling essential requirements of access to medical care, and basic needs of food, water and heat. By providing appropriate social support, patients can feel more empowered and take a more active role in their own healthcare.

Facilitating social connectedness and social support is particularly relevant for many of these groups, such as older people and people with disabilities, who tend to be digitally excluded. For example, reduced mobility may make it difficult to meet people (Morris, 2005). Reduced income may also be a constraint. Beyond this, for those experiencing difficult circumstances, sharing of personal information is also governed by the desire for privacy, and a wish not to worry loved ones unnecessarily (Moncur, Reiter, Masthoff, & Carmichael, 2010).

One important role e-health systems interfaces can play is to provide information and interactivity to consumers with visual, hearing, physical or cognitive impairments, in a way that overcomes or reduces barriers present in more traditional means of healthcare delivery. Access to online public health information and remote consultation systems can reduce the need for people with restricted mobility having to travel to a surgery or hospital; alternative communication systems can help non-speaking people communicate health issues more effectively. Appropriately-designed web content can, in conjunction with web browsers and assistive technology, allow people to receive and interact with digital content in a way that best suits their own needs. For example, with appropriately designed e-health content, the same content can be automatically adapted so that:

- people with low vision can receive it in large print,
- people without functional vision can receive it in audio or haptic format, with the aid of screen reading software or Braille display devices,
- people with dyslexia can receive it with text and background colours optimised to help on-screen reading.

APPROACHES TO DIGITAL INCLUSION AND ONLINE SOCIAL SUPPORT

User Centred and Inclusive Design

One key challenge in creating e-health systems that genuinely improve quality of care is ensuring that they are usable by and useful to the target audience, including members of traditionally excluded groups. The long-established field of Human-Computer Interaction (HCI) exists at the intersection of computing science, psychology and sociology with the aim of better understanding how computer systems can be designed to be as useful as possible to society. Of particular promise is the concept of User Centred Design (UCD), an approach to technology design and development that attempts to overcome problems emerging from approaches that may focus on achieving technical objectives or aesthetic values at the expense of supporting efficient and effective task completion.

The basic premise of user-centred design (UCD) is that end users of a technology should be considered central to all stages of the development of that technology. This includes three key principles of:

- **Extensive user research in advance**, in order to understand as much as possible about the target audience and the intended usage environment of the technology to be developed (context), and how best a technical innovation can improve the quality and efficiency of task completion without adversely affecting existing workflows and social relationships (purpose). Techniques such as focus groups, interviews, ethnographic observations, task analysis, and assessment of existing technology in use help to generate information that can lead to definition of more accurate and sensitive requirements of the technology to be developed.

- **Early and continual user evaluation** of the technology being developed. UCD encourages engaging users, exposing them to design ideas as early as possible and asking for feedback, and conducting empirical usability testing of designs as they evolve.
- **Iterative design:** the regular gathering of user feedback and data from usability evaluations naturally requires frequent iterations of designs that respond to the findings of these user evaluations. Techniques such as paper and electronic prototyping are encouraged, in order to gather as much information as possible as early as possible so that refinements to designs can be made with as minimum effort as possible. This reduces the chances of serious usability problems being discovered later on in the design lifecycle, when changes may be difficult or impossible to make, due to time pressures, budget constraints or technical limitations; or, worse, after the technology is released for general use.

Inclusive design extends user-centred design to consider at the heart of any design considerations the needs of people with particular access constraints, whether due to the presence of a disability or because of environmental constraints. Inclusive design seeks to avoid perpetuating social exclusion for people who experience difficulty accessing information, communicating, and receiving services through traditional means, by using technology to overcome accessibility barriers, rather than introducing new ones. In many countries, public and private organisations have legal obligations to avoid unjustified discrimination against disabled people, which are widely recognised as applying to digital service provision

Inclusive design, variously known as 'Universal Design' and 'Design For All' (Keates & Clarkson, 2003), also recognises that designing for accessibility not only supports people with visual, hearing, physical and cognitive impairments, but supports people constrained by environmental or economic situations. The ultimate goal of inclusive design is to produce, in a cost-effective manner, a technology that is available and usable by the widest possible proportion of the target audience. Often-quoted examples of inclusive design that have had unexpected benefits include:

- **kerb-cuts on pavements:** originally intended for wheelchair users, but also of use to people pushing prams and trolleys;
- **predictive text input algorithms:** originally developed for non-speaking people who use alternative/augmentative communication devices, but now appreciated by millions of mobile phone users;
- **captions for television programmes:** originally intended for people who are deaf or hard or hearing, but also appreciated by people watching TV in a noisy pub or cafe.

As a guide to fundamental principles for inclusive design, the World Wide Web Consortium (W3C) Web Content Accessibility Guidelines (WCAG)[2] provides a convenient summary, in the form of four principles:

1. **Perceivable:** can a user sense (through vision, hearing, or by touch) the digital content in question?
2. **Operable:** can a user navigate, input data, or otherwise interact with the digital content?
3. **Understandable:** can a user process and comprehend the digital content presented to them?
4. **Robust:** is the digital content available in the intended way across a suitably wide range of access technologies, platforms and operating systems, including legacy and emerging technologies?

A growing number of resources exist to support ICT development teams in adopting user centred, inclusive design approaches. These include a range of guidelines, standards and methodologies to aid designers and developers in adopting a user-centred design approach[3]; several tools exist to allow for the evaluation of ICT content for inclusivity (Chisholm & May, 2008).

User-centred and inclusive design is increasingly recognised in tertiary education as an influential component of computing science and computing science related curricula and the adoption of inclusive design as core to a Computing Science degree programme can equip students with the skills needed to avoid designing for oneself or one's immediate peers. A dedicated industry has emerged to providing usability support, from advising on or conducting user research activity to inform design, to usability evaluations of prototypes or completed interfaces.

Implications of Lack of Usability and Accessibility of E-Health Systems

Given the benefits of user-centred, inclusively designed e-health systems, it follows that a failure to consider user needs throughout the design and development process is likely to lead to systems that are difficult or impossible to use by the intended audience. The usage environment and circumstances of e-health systems, and nature of the target audience, make the existence of accessibility and usability problems a particularly significant concern.

Usability problems can place additional cognitive demands on an e-health consumer who may already be under extreme stress – whether they are someone looking for cancer-related information for a relative, or a busy and tired clinician on ward rounds trying to process an order to the hospital pharmacy. The result may be an inability to find essential information, a reduction in efficiency of use of the system in question, or an increased chance of erroneous data input – and thus significant risk to health of patients (Czaja, Sharit, & Nair, 2008). Since e-health systems are particularly likely to be used by people who may be in poor health, and may have the very impairments that lead to barriers introduced by poor ICT design, the negative implications of accessibility barriers are accentuated.

For many consumers, ICT adoption and use remains a challenge, and usability and accessibility problems that inhibit or prevent someone from being able to use an e-health resource may prolong a digital divide, the reduction of which should be a key purpose of e-health systems. There are also obvious economic shortcomings of e-health systems where investment is not rewarded with systems that meet objectives of supporting the greatest possible proportion of the target audience in successfully using the system for its intended purpose.

Barriers to Effective Adoption of UCD/Inclusive Design

Despite advances in arguments for, and support for a user-centred, inclusive ICT design process that results in a system accessible to and usable by the widest possible range of users, why might existing systems still contain design issues that limit or prevent use by members of the intended user group? User research and user engagement may be perceived as a luxury that time and resource-constrained projects cannot fully justify and may be sidelined in favour of technical development activities. For project stakeholders, a system's simplicity and ease of use may appear less attractive as quality markers than extensive functionality, so usability may be sacrificed in a desire to provide more features (Cooper 1999).

The arguments against inclusive design include a perception that the numbers of people who benefit are not significant enough to warrant investment, and a belief that accessibility can be addressed at a late stage of a project if there is time. Yet, as evidenced by the examples above, the beneficiaries of inclusive design go far beyond those whom official statistics categorise as disabled, while addressing accessibility is most cost-effectively achieved by considering it from the early stages of a design project.

Inclusive design has also been rejected as an approach that stifles creativity and functionality, although this is frequently a symptom of poorly understood and poorly applied best practice in accessible design. By contrast, inclusive design can encourage innovative approaches to problem solving that lead to unexpected benefits for additional user groups (Pullin 2009).

Another barrier can be the procurement process used in commissioning e-health systems. If requirements of usability and accessibility are poorly specified, or not specified at all, or if suppliers awareness of and adoption of UCD processes are not considered during assessment of tenders or candidate systems, then the chances of the delivered system meeting acceptable levels of usability and accessibility are likely to be reduced.

E-Health, Social Networks and Social Support

One key application of e-health is that of social networks and their related social support. During times of ill health, consumers tend to require support from their social network. There are times were consumers may wish to seek support from other consumers with similar experiences. This is sometimes difficult within their natural social network as they may be experiencing a rare condition. Furthermore, some groups of digitally excluded people may be socially isolated and therefore miss the benefits on offer through social networks.

There is much to be learnt from the existing research on social networks. Research shows there is a consistent structure to personal social networks (also described as natural social networks) that is common across cultural and socio-economic groups (Stiller & Dunbar, 2007). At the centre lies the ego (the individual). Closest to the ego, the innermost layer of this structure is the *support clique*. This consists of around 3-5 stalwart network members with strong ties that the ego feels emotionally closest to. They provide the ego with advice, support or help at times of acute distress. The next layer, the *sympathy group*, typically contains 12-20 individuals who constitute the ego's foremost friends and relatives. The *band* (30-50 members) is an unstable layer consisting of network members that the ego commonly associates with. The changing membership of the band is drawn from the *clan*, a grouping of around 150 individuals that the ego knows individually and has a personal relationship with. Two larger groupings are the *mega-band* (approximately 500 members), and the *tribe* (approximately 1000–2000 members). Tie strength between the ego and members of these two large groups is weak.

The total size of an individual's personal social network may vary, and is influenced by the characteristics and circumstances of the individual. For example, an affluent extrovert is likely to have a wider social network than an impoverished introvert. In non-industrial societies, network size is strongly influenced by the size of the community that an individual lives in, and proximity to other communities. If you live in a remote, mountainous region in a tribe of 30, it is hard to expand your social network, no matter how extrovert you are.

Throughout life, the size of an individual's network varies. The social network of someone under age 18 contains a higher number of weak ties and a greater degree of instability, when compared to the network of an adult. In adulthood, major life events such as going to university, getting married, having children, getting divorced cause fluctuations in network membership and size. In later life, network shrinkage may occur through the death of network members, relocation towards caregivers, or inability to meet people because of reduced mobility (Morris, 2005).

Each of us has our own unique personal social network, made up of the people that we know (such as relatives, friends, neighbours, colleagues and acquaintances). The practical, emotional and informational support ("social support") that is exchanged with others, and the companionship shared, have beneficial effects. For the *recipient*, there is a correlation between appropriate social support and better mental health (Kawachi & Berkman, 2001), reduced morbidity (Uchino, Cacioppo, & Kiecolt-Glaser, 1996) and increased longevity (Berkman, Glass, Brissette, & Seeman, 2000). It should be noted that the strength of this correlation varies: US studies show a strong correlation, but one cross-national study found only a weak, inconsistent correlation (Brown, Nesse, Vinokur, & Smith, 2003). Recipients also experience improved *stress buffering* (the ability to cope with stress) when they feel that others in their network will give them appropriate support (Cohen, 2004). A network member can provide a reduction in the perceived importance of the problem, a distraction or solution to it, or even encourage healthy behaviour that was previously omitted (e.g. eating and sleeping, smoking less) (Ferlander, 2007). Emotional support can remind the recipient to care for themselves despite the problem being faced. Survival rates of those suffering a stroke or myocardial infarction are higher amongst those with plentiful emotional support (Berkman et al., 2000; Glass, Matchar, Belyea, & Feussner, 1993). Instrumental support may alleviate difficulty in undertaking routine practical tasks. Informational support may facilitate access to better healthcare or improved self-care, or just better understanding of a health condition. For older adults, the significance of maintaining diverse social networks is pronounced, as it staves off cognitive decline, depression and isolation. Additionally, frequent social interactions create an increased sense of well-being (Czaja, Guerrier, Nair, & Laudauer, 1993).

There are also benefits for *donors* in providing appropriate social support, beyond the 'virtuous circle' of building up social support credit. Donors experience positive effects on their mental health, morbidity and longevity (Brown et al., 2003). Other potential benefits include improved social integration, greater purpose in life, distraction from one's own problems and improved self-esteem (Post, 2005). When the support need arises out of distressing circumstances, for example a new parent having a seriously ill baby in NICU (Neonatal Intensive Care Unit), being able to help may make the supporter feel less upset about the situation (Penner, Dovidio, Piliavin, & Schroeder, 2005). The benefits described here are contingent upon the donor not being overwhelmed by support needs, a factor more likely to occur amongst the economically disadvantaged (Ferlander, 2007). Being swamped by demands for support can raise a donor's stress levels and place excessive demands on their own resources.

Implications of Lack of Appropriately Designed Social Networks

Social networks pre-date current online trends in social mediating technologies such as FaceBook and LinkedIn. Articulation of the concept of the social network originates in anthropological and sociometric studies from the 1930s onwards (Churchill & Halverson, 2005). The study of social networks has grown and branched since then, stretching across the domains of computing, psychology, anthropology, statistics, ethnography and sociology. Ambitious claims have been made for these on-line communities: that they are "neo-tribes" that "satisfy fundamental social needs" in an age of "social isolation and extreme individualism" (Johnson & Ambrose, 2006). Yet the friendships made on-line tend to be shallow and short-lived compared to those made in the real world (Churchill & Halverson, 2005). Their effectiveness in fostering mutual help and support is debatable (Sutcliffe, Gonzalez, & Kraut, 2009). Greater emotional proximity comes from face-to-face contact and telephone conversations than from electronic communications such as email (Cummings, Butler, & Kraut, 2002). However, in terms of digital inclusion there are groups of people where offline friendships are difficult to develop and where social mediating technologies could provide a significant boost.

The majority of these social networking sites fail to take into account known human behaviours and abilities relating to relationships. They do not arrange contacts by degree of intimacy. Nor do they automatically filter the information that users send out to members of their network - you either send information or you do not. This is even true for the *CarePages* website (CarePages.com, 2008), which claims to help people to "stay in touch with family and friends during times of illness or injury". CarePages are not secure – anyone can sign up to an individual's CarePage, receive updates about the individual's reported health status, and post messages, without even being known to the subject of the CarePage or those closest to them. We believe that there is room for improvement in social networking tools, to encourage deeper friendships embedded with greater network capital, and greater privacy.

A common intervention in health care is to try to generate social support through the creation of artificial social networks founded on common circumstances. However, artificially created support groups are not as effective in delivering support as an individual's real friends and family (Cohen, 2004). Emotional support is most effective when it comes from an individual's own pre-existing social network: delivering demonstrably positive physiological and psychological benefits (Uchino et al., 1996). Informational support may be effective when delivered by members of an on-line support group (Johnson & Ambrose, 2006), but even this outcome is dubious. Misinformation, violation of privacy, and inappropriate support can all arise when a social network consists of faceless 'friends' we have never met in the real world.

Artificial social networks have their good points. They link patients with others experiencing similar health problems, facilitating the sharing of experiences. This can result in the provision of informational and emotional support, and also online companionship. Patients may feel more comfortable disclosing information about their health problem to members of an online support group than they would to their closest family and friends. Anonymity is possible through many social mediating technologies and provides some protection and comfort for the consumer. There are also negatives. Without careful moderation by a health expert, medical information circulated around the group may be incorrect. Participants may conceal their real identity with the intention to misinform. Inappropriate support can arise when a social network consists of faceless 'friends' we have never met in the real world. It is also unlikely that online support group members will be in a position to provide practical support. Arguably, artificial social networks may deliver fewer benefits to the patient than those offered by a patient's pre-existing *natural* personal social network (Cohen, 2004).

It is also easier for groups to form without social approval online. One such example is pro-anorexia web sites (often termed as Pro-Ana) which facilitate individuals to gather together on a level not previously possible. Such a change has spurred lots of concern from society as a whole, particularly as the perception was that it was facilitating the illness and rather than encouraging them to get better. Much to many people's surprise it turns out that the Pro-Ana movement is actually a self-help movement (Shirky, 2008, p. 208). Anorexia is often an isolating condition where an individuals' perception of their body image drastically conflicts with others in their life. There is also a high incidence of depression and anxiety as co-morbidities. Consequently, facilitating connections to other individuals experiencing similar feelings starts to change the isolation and provides them with support (at a level not previously experienced).

CURRENT SITUATION

While the principles of UCD and inclusive design are well documented, current research indicates that these principles are not widely adopted in e-health developments. There are only a few documented examples of inclusive design being included within the development of e-health resources (for example Morrell, Dailey, & Rousseau, 2003). There is a wider collection of articles reporting evaluations of e-health materials (for example, Hinchliffe & Kerry, 2008; Czaja et al., 2008) with a significant subset looking at the older population (for example, Nahm, Preece, Resnick, & Mills, 2004) or people with disabilities (for example, Lüchtenberg, Kuhli-Hattenbach, Sinangin, Ohrloff, & Schalnus, 2008). However, many report poor usability or clear demonstrations where the end-user was not considered in the design of the application.

FUTURE RESEARCH DIRECTIONS

Integrating User Centred, Inclusive Design Approaches in E-Health Systems Design

We have argued that adopting a user-centred, inclusive approach to e-health system design and implementation gives the best possible chance that the system will be usable by the widest possible proportion of the intended target audience. Healthcare organizations may additionally have legal obligations to ensure that ICTs they procure and provide are accessible to and usable by people with disabilities.

Implementation of user-centred, inclusive design does, however, require awareness and action at all stages of an e-health project. Without an organization-wide accessibility strategy that is recognized by and adopted at all staffing and activity levels, Urban and Burks (2006) suggest that aspirations for implementing inclusive technology will be difficult if not impossible to meet, and sustain over time. Therefore, whether e-health systems are developed in-house or procured externally, appropriate measures need to be taken to ensure that a user-centred, inclusive design approach is adopted such that the delivered systems exceed acceptable levels of usability and accessibility (Nielsen, 1994; Cooper, 1999; Shneiderman, Plaisant, Cohen, & Jacobs, 2009).

This includes ensuring that UCD and inclusive design approaches are followed throughout the development of resources and, for outsourced development, expectations are clearly specified in any invitation to tender and contractual agreement with third-party suppliers[4]. Also, as is increasingly the case on a Web, where information-providing e-health resources are intended to be edited and maintained by healthcare professionals who were not responsible for the initial development and may not have advanced technical skills, there is a need to ensure that the information addition and maintenance procedure is not only as efficient and effective as possible, but that it preserves, rather than reduces, initial levels of usability and accessibility.

Enhancing Online Social Networks through E-Health Systems Design

Online and off, human social networks are imbued with network capital. These networks may be artificial or natural. It is instinctive for people to adapt the information that they share across their social networks, invoking their own inbuilt 'privacy protocols'. This holds true across genders, cultures, ages and (dis)abilities. Mobilisation of this network capital has a beneficial role to play in reducing spiralling healthcare costs, and in bringing quantifiable benefits to patients.

There is potential for e-health systems to tap into existing network capital, through the use of social network systems. However, they must adapt to reflect users' inbuilt privacy protocols. A divide exists at present between the 'confessional' nature of online support groups where patients with similar conditions unburden themselves and share information, and the practical and emotional support offered by those in a patient's natural social network. This division, we argue, is caused by poor granularity in privacy controls.

With better privacy control, membership of natural/ artificial social networks can blur into one, without causing concerns of over disclosure. For the vulnerable and the excluded, this is particularly important, as it can increase opportunities for friendship and support. We invite further research into the effects of online social support on morbidity and mental health which offer granular, usable privacy protocols.

CONCLUSION

E-health can potentially provide a solution to many of the problems faced by digitally excluded groups. All consumers, in particular digitally excluded groups of health consumers, have much to gain from social connectedness and social support on offer through artificial social networks. Yet at the same time these groups are most vulnerable to continued exclusion due to inappropriate technology design and implementation. It is vitally important to involve health information consumers as part of UCD or inclusive design in the development of information content for e-health systems.

For the future, e-health has the obligation to provide applications available for everyone irrespective of any impairment (visual, hearing, physical and cognitive) or constraint by environmental or economical situation. Furthermore, e-health has the opportunity to develop enhanced online social networks to support consumers in difficult health circumstances. Both of these activities would make considerable steps towards more effective applications in e-health that engage the widest possible audience.

REFERENCES

Bental, D., Cawsey, A., & Jones, R. (1999). Patient information systems that tailor to the individual. *Journal of Patient Education and Counselling*, *36*, 171–180. doi:10.1016/S0738-3991(98)00133-5

Berkman, L. F., Glass, T., Brissette, I., & Seeman, T. E. (2000). From social integration to health: Durkheim in the new millennium. *Social Science & Medicine*, *51*(6), 843–857. doi:10.1016/S0277-9536(00)00065-4

Bisson, G. (2005).E-health portal and SNOMED for a more personalized integrated EHR. *Proceedings of the 1st International Workshop on Personalisation for e-Health,* Aberdeen, Scotland.

Bromme, R., Jucks, R., & Wagner, T. (2005). How to refer to 'diabetes'? Language in online health advice. *Applied Cognitive Psychology*, *19*, 569–586. doi:10.1002/acp.1099

Brown, S. L., Nesse, R. M., Vinokur, A. D., & Smith, D. M. (2003). Providing social support may be more beneficial than receiving it: Results from a prospective study of mortality. *Psychological Science*, *14*(4), 320–327. doi:10.1111/1467-9280.14461

CarePages.com. (2008). *Welcome to CarePages*. Retrieved July 4, 2008, from http://www.carepages.com/

Cawsey, A., Grasso, F., & Paris, C. (2007). Adaptive information for consumers of healthcare. In Brusilovsky, P., Kobsa, A., & Nejdl, W. (Eds.), *The adaptive web* (pp. 465–484). Heidelberg/ Berlin, Germany: Springer. doi:10.1007/978-3-540-72079-9_15

Cawsey, A., Jones, R., & Pearson, J. (2000). The evaluation of a personalised health information system for patients with cancer. *User Modeling and User-Adapted Interaction*, *10*(1), 47–72. doi:10.1023/A:1008350913145

Chin, J. J. (2002). Doctor-patient relationship: From medical paternalism to enhanced autonomy. *Singapore Medical Journal*, *43*(3), 152–155.

Chisholm, W., & May, M. (2008). *Universal design for Web applications: Web applications that reach everyone*. O'Reilly.

Churchill, E. F., & Halverson, C. A. (2005). Social networks and social networking. *IEEE Internet Computing*, *9*(5), 14–19. doi:10.1109/MIC.2005.103

Cohen, S. (2004). Social relationships and health. *The American Psychologist*, *59*(8), 676–684. doi:10.1037/0003-066X.59.8.676

Cooper, A. (1999). *The inmates are running the asylum: Why high-tech products drive us crazy and how to restore the sanity*. Sams.

Cummings, J. N., Butler, B., & Kraut, R. (2002). The quality of online social relationships. *Communications of the ACM*, *45*(7), 103–108. doi:10.1145/514236.514242

Czaja, S. J., Guerrier, J. H., Nair, S. N., & Laudauer, T. K. (1993). Computer communication as an aid to independence to older adults. *Behaviour & Information Technology*, *12*, 197–207. doi:10.1080/01449299308924382

Czaja, S. J., Sharit, J., & Nair, S. N. (2008). Usability of the Medicare health web site. *Journal of the American Medical Association*, *300*(7), 790–792. doi:10.1001/jama.300.7.790-b

Dutton, W. H., Helsper, E. J., & Gerber, M. M. (2009). *The Internet in Britain 2009*. Oxford Internet Institute, University of Oxford.

Ferlander, S. (2007). The importance of different forms of social capital for health. *Acta Sociologica*, *50*, 115–128. doi:10.1177/0001699307077654

Glass, T., Matchar, D., Belyea, M., & Feussner, J. (1993). Impact of social support on outcome in first stroke. *Stroke*, *24*(1), 64–70. doi:10.1161/01.STR.24.1.64

Government, H. M. (2009). *Delivering digital inclusion - An action plan for consultation*. Crown Copyright.

Hinchliffe, A., & Kerry, M. W. (2008). Applying usability testing techniques to improve a health promotion website. *Health Promotion Journal of Australia*, *19*, 29–35.

Jenkins, H. (2006). *Convergence culture: Where old and new media collide*. New York, NY: New York University Press.

Jones, S. (2009, April 24). The formula that felled Wall St. *Financial Times Magazine.*

Kawachi, I., & Berkman, L. (2001). Social ties and mental health. *Journal of Urban Health*, *78*(3), 458–467. doi:10.1093/jurban/78.3.458

Keates, S., & Clarkson, P. (2003). *Countering design exclusion: An introduction to inclusive design*. Springer. doi:10.1007/978-1-4471-0013-3

Lüchtenberg, M., Kuhli-Hattenbach, C., Sinangin, Y., Ohrloff, C., & Schalnus, R. (2008). Accessibility of health information on the internet to the visually impaired user. *Ophthalmologica: International Journal of Ophthalmology*, *222*(3), 187–193.

McKay, E. (2005). Human-computer interaction closes the digital divide: Aa multicultural, intergenerational ICT case study. *Proceedings of the 2005 South East Asia Regional Computer Science Confederation (SEARCC) Conference* (pp. 29-33). Darlinghurst, Australia: Australian Computer Society.

Moncur, W., Reiter, E., Masthoff, J., & Carmichael, A. (2010). Modelling the socially intelligent communication of health information. *IEEE Transactions on Information Technology in Biomedicine*, *14*(2), 319–325. doi:10.1109/TITB.2009.2035361

Morrell, R. W., Dailey, S. R., & Rousseau, G. K. (2003). Applying research: The NIHSeniorHealth.gov Project. In Charness, N., & Schaie, K. W. (Eds.), *Impact of technology on successful aging* (pp. 134–161). New York, NY: Springer.

Morris, M. E. (2005). Social networks as health feedback displays. *IEEE Internet Computing*, *9*(5), 29–37. doi:10.1109/MIC.2005.109

Nahm, E. S., Preece, J., Resnick, B., & Mills, M. E. (2004). Usability of health web sites for older adults: A preliminary study. *Computers, Informatics, Nursing*, *22*(6), 326–334. doi:10.1097/00024665-200411000-00007

Nielsen, J. (1994). *Usability engineering*. Morgan Kaufmann.

Penner, L., Dovidio, J., Piliavin, J., & Schroeder, D. (2005). Prosocial behavior: Multilevel perspectives. *Annual Review of Psychology*, *56*(1), 365–392. doi:10.1146/annurev.psych.56.091103.070141

Pullin, G. (2009). *Design meets disability*. MIT Press.

Shirky, C. (2008). *Here comes everyone*. Allen Lane.

Shneiderman, B., Plaisant, C., Cohen, M., & Jacobs, S. (2009). *Designing the user interface: Strategies for effective human-computer interaction*. Pearson Education.

Stiller, J., & Dunbar, R. I. M. (2007). Perspective-taking and memory capacity predict social network size. *Social Networks*, *29*(1), 93–104. doi:10.1016/j.socnet.2006.04.001

Sutcliffe, A., Gonzalez, V. M., & Kraut, R. (2009). Social mediating technologies: Developing the research agenda. *CHI EA '09. Proceedings of the 27th International Conference Extended Abstracts on Human Factors in Computing Systems,* Boston, MA, USA (pp. 4775-4778).

Uchino, B. N., Cacioppo, J. T., & Kiecolt-Glaser, J. K. (1996). The relationship between social support and physiological processes: A review with emphasis on underlying mechanisms and implications for health. *Psychological Bulletin*, *119*(3), 488–531. doi:10.1037/0033-2909.119.3.488

Urban, M., & Burks, M. (2006). Implementing accessibility in the enterprise. In Thatcher, J. (Eds.), *Web accessibility: Web standards and regulatory compliance*.

Waller, A., Hanson, V. L., & Sloan, D. (2009). Including accessibility within and beyond undergraduate computing courses. In *Proc. ACM SIGACCESS (ASSETS '09).*, (pp. 155-162). New York, NY: ACM Press.

Warren, M. (2007). The digital vicious cycle: Links between social disadvantage and digital exclusion in rural areas. *Telecommunications Policy*, *31*(6-7), 374–388. doi:10.1016/j.telpol.2007.04.001

ADDITIONAL READING

Alpay, L., Toussaint, P., & Zwetsloot-Schonk, B. (2004). Supporting healthcare communication enabled by information and communication technology: Can HCI and related cognitive aspects help? *Proceedings of the Conference on Dutch Directions in HCI,* Amsterdam, Holland., *65* 12-15.

Bickmore, T., & Giorgino, T. (2006). Health dialog systems for patients and consumers. *Journal of Biomedical Informatics*, *39*(5), 556–571. doi:10.1016/j.jbi.2005.12.004

Dunbar, R. I. M., & Spoors, M. (1995). Social networks, support cliques, and kinship. *Human Nature (Hawthorne, N.Y.)*, *6*(3), 273–290. doi:10.1007/BF02734142

Gloyd, D. (2003). Positive user experience and medical adherence. *DPPI '03: Proceedings of the 2003 International Conference on Designing Pleasurable Products and Interfaces,* Pittsburgh, PA, USA. 17-21.

Hill, R. A., & Dunbar, R. I. M. (2003). Social network size in humans. *Human Nature (Hawthorne, N.Y.)*, *14*(1), 53–72. doi:10.1007/s12110-003-1016-y

Post, S. G. (2005). Altruism, happiness, and health: It's good to be good. *International Journal of Behavioral Medicine*, *12*(2), 66–77. doi:10.1207/s15327558ijbm1202_4

Roberts, S. G. B., Wilson, R., Fedurek, P., & Dunbar, R. I. M. (2008). Individual differences and personal social network size and structure. *Personality and Individual Differences*, *44*(4), 954–964. doi:10.1016/j.paid.2007.10.033

Zhou, W. X., Sornette, D., Hill, R. A., & Dunbar, R. I. M. (2005). Discrete hierarchical organization of social group sizes. *Proceedings. Biological Sciences*, *272*(1561), 439–444. doi:10.1098/rspb.2004.2970

KEY TERMS AND DEFINITIONS

Adaptive Interface: An interface that (typically using a user model) changes behavior depending on the user's data, behavior and preferences.

Digital Inclusion: The incorporation of information technologies into the whole community, including those who might experience social exclusion due to factors such as age, disability, geographical location, ethnicity or economic status.

E-Health: The term used to describe the delivery of health services and information across the Internet and related technologies.

Inclusive Design: The process for designing products and technology to be flexible enough to serve the broadest possible range of users, including those with disabilities or those impaired by their environment.

Social Network (Natural and Artificial): A social network is a collection of ties between people and the strength of those ties. A natural social network is offline and includes relatives, friends and neighbours. An artificial social network is online and can include similar groups to the natural network as well as virtual friends met through online communities.

Social Support: The currency of social networks which comes in the form of emotional and practical support, information and companionship.

User-Centered Design: The process in which the needs, wants and constraints of the end user is considered and incorporated at every stage of the development lifecycle.

ENDNOTES

1 The author acknowledges support from RCUK Digital Economy Research Hub EP/G066019/1 "SIDE: Social Inclusion through the Digital Economy".

2 W3C Web Content Accessibility Guidelines (WCAG): http://www.w3.org/TR/WCAG20/

3 The Usability Professionals' Association (UPA) provides a useful web based collection of resources on user-centred design: http://www.upassoc.org/usability_resources/index.html

4 In the UK, the standard *BS8878: Web accessibility. Building accessible experiences for disabled people. Code of practice,* published in December 2010, supports organisations by codifying best practice in procurement of inclusive web technologies. A pan-European Union initiative, Mandate 376, aims to promote a co-ordinated approach to addressing accessibility in technology procurement and commissioning stage.

Chapter 13
Online Health Communities and Health Literacy:
Applying a Framework for Understanding Domains of Health Literacy

Erin Willis
University of Memphis, USA

Ye Wang
University of Missouri – Kansas City, USA

Shelly Rodgers
Missouri School of Journalism, USA

ABSTRACT

The purpose of the chapter is to define health literacy and e-health literacy in the context of online health communities (OHCs). The chapter has three sections. The first section defines and discusses features of OHCs. The second section defines health literacy and e-health literacy, including domains of health literacy, which, as the authors argue, is necessary for a greater understanding of health literacy and OHCs. The third section applies the health literacy domains using The Biggest Loser League weight-loss OHC as a case study. A content analysis of posts was conducted between September 1, 2009 and December 31, 2009. Domains of health literacy were coded. Results show that functional literacy and interactive literacy were present in the OHC discussions to a greater degree than any of the other health literacy domains examined. Results are discussed in light of health literacy and e-health literacy, and practical implications of OHCs are explored.

DOI: 10.4018/978-1-60960-866-8.ch013

INTRODUCTION

The Internet has become a valued part of managing consumers' health. For physicians and health care professionals, the Internet offers cost-effective communication for patients, including the potential for health education (Cline & Hayes, 2001; Stout, Ball, & Villegas, 2004). For consumers, the Internet offers virtually limitless information on health, multiple health perspectives, and the ability to communicate with others regarding health issues. Online health communities, or OHCs, are a popular source of health information online. Consumers join OHCs in search of specialized health information, social support, and psycho-social benefits (Cline & Hayes, 2001; Rodgers & Chen, 2005; Wright, 2000). It has been estimated that one in four consumers actively participates in an OHC (Raines, 2005). Initial studies suggest that basic health literacy skills and knowledge are needed to effectively communicate about a health problem and technology places greater demands on consumers' health literacy as well ability to effectively use technology, suggesting the need to examine e-health literacy in conjunction with health literacy in OHCs. However, compared with the growing popularity of OHCs among everyday health consumers, research has lagged regarding the examination of health and e-health literacy in OHCs. Additionally, while OHCs remain an untapped resource in which to examine health literacy, it is unclear as to the extent to which consumers use health literacy – the development of which can improve health behaviors - in online communication. Recent health literacy research shows a need to streamline the definition of health literacy and e-health literacy; multiple definitions of health literacy abound, necessitating consideration of both the context (setting) in which health literacy demands are made and the skills that people bring to the setting (Rudd, Moeykens, & Colton, 1999). The purpose of this chapter is to explore consumers' health literacy in OHCs using domains of health literacy, defined below. To develop a more robust view of health literacy and e-health literacy, it is important to look at the domains of health literacy in the capacity of OHCs; in addition to active exchange of information (Korp, 2006; White & Dorman, 2001) consumers provide emotional and psychological support to each other in OHCs (Rodgers & Chen, 2005; Wright, 2000; 2002). With consumer benefits such as psychological support, personal connection, and anonymity, health information provided in online discussions can influence consumers' health-related attitudes, decisions, and behaviors - more so than health information found on general health-related Websites (Wang, Walther, Pingree, et al., 2008). It is, therefore, crucial to examine domains of health literacy within an e-health literacy context to better understand the types of domains of health literacy being used, as well as extent of health literacy use, in OHCs. To orient the reader, the remainder of this chapter is outlined as follows. First, features of OHCs are discussed; second, health literacy and e-health literacy are defined. Multiple domains of health literacy are adopted in order to provide a multi-dimensional perspective of health literacy within OHCs. Last, the results of a case study are presented to demonstrate the use of domains of health literacy in OHCs, followed by a discussion to further explore the implication of OHCs in relation to health literacy and e-health literacy.

BACKGROUND

Online Health Communities

The Internet has become a widely used source for health information. According to the Centers for Disease Control and Prevention (CDC, 2010b), consumers search for information about specific diseases and treatments, doctors and hospitals, experimental treatments, health insurance, medicines, fitness, and nutrition online. Among many applications provided by the Internet, online communities have become increasingly popular and carry a unique capacity to facilitate interpersonal communication through online discussion (Raines, 2005).

Online communities have been defined as "groups of people with similar concerns who communicate via information technology" (du Pre', 2000, p. 182). Initial research on online health communities found that participation may lead to positive health outcomes (Finn, 1999; Wright, 1999; 2002). Online health communities (OHCs) provide referrals to other Websites through links containing information about the issue or information based on the experiences of other members (Wright, 2000), and this type of informational support empowers consumers to seek additional knowledge, change health behaviors, and manage chronic disease (Cline & Haynes, 2001; Eysenbach, 2000; Pecchioni & Sparks, 2007; White & Dorman, 2001). For example, an American survey of cancer patients showed that 92% of patients believe that Internet information empowers them to make health decisions and helps them talk to their physician (Eysenbach, 2003).

Participants of OHCs are more likely to adopt advice found in the online community rather than health-related Web sites because of its hyper-personal nature and capacity to connect people who have the same or similar health problems (Wang, Walther, Pingree, et al., 2008). Since peer-to-peer communities are public forums for communication, OHCs allow consumers with the same interests to network and form relationships through computer-mediated communication. Hyper-personal environments can facilitate the seeking and exchanging of information and making information more accessible to consumers (Cline & Hayes, 2001). Simply stated, these are peers discussing personal health topics online. Online communities eliminate many of the barriers that exist in "off-line" interpersonal communication like socioeconomic status, gender, race, and even disability (Berland, Elliott, Morales, et al., 2001; Carlson, Neal, Magwood, et al., 2006; Wellman, Salaff, Dimitrova, et al., 1996). However, a scarcity of research has examined online discussions about health within these OHCs to gain greater insights into the consumer's health literacy. Health policy reports such as *Healthy People 2010* recognize the link between poor education, low literacy, poor health, and early death in the United States. In 2003, 40 million Americans scored on the lowest of five levels (level 1) on the National Assessment of Adult Literacy survey, and another 50 million scored on level 2. These levels correspond to: having trouble finding pieces of information or numbers in a lengthy text, integrating multiple pieces of information, or finding numbers in a chart and performing simple calculations (Kutner, Greenberg, Jin, & Paulsen, 2006). The survey also showed that only 12% of U.S. adults were found to have proficient health literacy, where proficiency is the most advanced of four levels of literacy including below basic, basic, intermediate, and proficient. That means that over one-third of U.S. adults – about 77 million people – have difficulty with common health behaviors, such as following a doctor's orders or reading a prescription bottle label. Such low levels of health literacy cost the U.S. economy more than $69 billion in health care expenditures (Institute of Medicine, 2004). This reflects a lack of understanding of medical regimens such as improper use of medications, poor understanding of medical treatment options, and insufficient understanding of preventative care (Kutner et al., 2006).

Online health communities (OHCs) offer an opportunity to bridge the gap and increase consumers' health literacy skills through patient education. In order to improve consumers' understanding of health and health outcomes, we first have to know basic levels, or domains, of understanding of health and health literacy as it applies to the consumer's current health situation. Individual levels of health literacy are associated with individual health outcomes. In fact, poor health literacy is "a stronger predictor of a person's health than age, income, employment status, education level, and race" (Ad Hoc Committee on Health Literacy for the Council on Scientific Affairs, American Medical Association, 1999, p. 554). Health literacy assumes health and education intersect. DeWalt and his colleagues (2004) found that low levels of health literacy have a negative impact on consumers' health status, including disease knowledge. Likewise, Williams et al. (1998) found that half of their study's participants (either with hypertension or diabetes) had low levels of health literacy, including a lack of knowledge of how to properly manage their chronic disease. In short, consumers with low levels of health literacy usually have less disease-related knowledge, poor health status, less access to health services, but are more likely to be hospitalized (Gazmarian et al., 2003) than individuals with higher levels of health literacy.

Given that low levels of health literacy are associated with negative health outcomes, it is important for health communicators to seek effective tools to communicate and enhance health literacy. Since the majority of content found in OHCs are consumer conversations about health issues between everyday consumers, OHCs have the potential of being an effective channel for communicating and improving individuals' health literacy. Early studies show that OHCs can improve health literacy through interaction with others and with the exchange of health information (Kalichman, Weinhardt, Benotsch, et al., 2000). Research shows that greater use of the Internet for health information on HIV/AIDS positively correlates with greater use of coping strategies and social support (Kalichman, Weinhardt, Benotsch, et al., 2000) as well as health knowledge (Kalichman, Benotsch, Weinhardt, et al., 2002).

Related to this discussion, the advertising literature has shown that online communities can improve consumers' knowledge about the topic(s) under discussion (Baker, Parker, Williams, et al., 1998; Schillinger, Grumbach, Wang, et al., 2003; Williams, Baker, Parker, et al., 1998). These studies help to establish the importance of examining health literacy online since consumers' knowledge, attitudes, and behaviors are influenced by the content found within these OHCs. To explore this in more detail, we begin with a definition of health literacy and health literacy domains.

A Definition of Health Literacy

Early definitions conceptualized health literacy as a function of individual skills used to interpret and understand health information (Simonds, 1974; World Health Organization, 1998). Initial definitions of health literacy took a biomedical approach, which dominated the U.S. in the 1980s and 1990s, and assumed that individuals are *passive* in their reception and use of health literacy and, therefore, models of literacy and health literacy were believed to be neutral and universally applicable.

However, despite the numerous correlational studies that have come from the biomedical approach (Pleasant & Kuruvilla, 2008), early definitions of health literacy are not adequate for understanding health literacy in an Internet context since OHCs did not exist then, and early definitions did not account for the fact that consumers *actively* seek out and use health information online to make informed health choices, decrease health risks, and increase well being (Zarcadoolas, Pleasant, & Greer, 2006). Online health communities (OHCs) provide health information and also personal experience, psychological support, and empowerment (Rodgers & Chen, 2005; Wright, 2002) not accounted for in earlier definitions.

The benefits beyond health information provided by these communities indicate that OHCs have the capacity to develop health literacy above basic levels of numerical skills and understanding of medical facts. Recent definitions reflect this and define health literacy in terms of not only basic knowledge about health but also skills needed to obtain such information and the context in which health information is provided. The authors argue that an understanding of health literacy within OHCs requires a broader definition of health literacy to account for these unique features and capabilities of OHCs. Drawing on *Healthy People 2010* (CDC, 2010) report, health literacy is defined as "the degree to which individuals have the capacity to obtain, process, and understand basic health information and services needed to make appropriate health decisions" (section 11-2).

The present chapter, building on the Healthy People 2010 definition, adopts a definition of health literacy that arose from a public health perspective, and that views health literacy as a social determinant of health that can vary depending on a wide range of skills and competencies developed over a lifetime. The public health perspective broadened the range of skills and competencies needed for health literacy including the ability to: understand and read health content and health research; speak and write online and offline; interpret mass media messages; navigate complex health care systems; understand and use community capital and resources; use cultural and indigenous knowledge in making health decisions (Nutbeam, 2000; Ratzan, 2001; Zarcadoolas, Pleasant, & Greer, 2002). Hence, multiple perspectives and definitions of health literacy abound, in part because health literacy involves both a context in which health literacy demands are made *and* skills that consumers bring to a given situation (Rudd, Moeykens, & Colton, 1999). However, the perspective offered in this chapter differs from previous studies in that we "marry" two disciplines that have been, thus far, treated separately in health literacy, i.e., the public health discipline from which early definitions of health literacy have arisen, and the health communication discipline, which provides strategies in which to inform the public about health concerns and maintain important health issues on the public agenda (Turnock, 2009).

Based on this discussion, we drew on Nutbeam's (2000) three domains of health literacy and Zarcadoolas, Pleasant, and Greer's (2005) four domains of health literacy. Starting with Nutbeam's (2000) definition of health literacy that uses three domains: *basic/functional literacy*, *communicative/ interactive literacy*, and *critical literacy*. *Basic/functional literacy* refers to the basic skills (i.e. reading and writing) used to function effectively in everyday situations. *Communicative/interactive literacy* refers to more advanced cognitive or literacy skills necessary, as Nutbeam argues, to derive meaning from different forms of communication. *Critical literacy* refers to the most advanced cognitive skills used to critically analyze information and then even further, the ability to apply such information to personal situations. Nutbeam's definition of health literacy incorporates psychological, social, and environmental factors that influence health choices and the adoption of health-related behaviors.

Similarly, Zarcadoolas, Pleasant, and Greer (2005) identified four domains of health literacy, including *fundamental literacy*, *science literacy*, *civic literacy*, and *cultural literacy*. Here, *fundamental literacy* refers to basic skills like reading, writing, communicating, and numeracy. *Science literacy* refers to consumers' familiarity with scientific facts, including recognizing the uncertainty of science. *Civic literacy* describes consumers' knowledge of economic and political structures, also advocacy. Finally, *cultural literacy* recognizes that cultural differences can lead to different interpretation and understanding of a particular health message.

Both Nutbeam (2000) and Zarcadoolas, Pleasant, and Greer (2005) agree that health literacy should look beyond the level of language used in health content to the socio-cultural aspects of consumers' understanding of health; for example, the understanding of health issues as a social problem (*civic literacy*), the ability to use communication channels such as online communities to obtain health information and psychological support (*cultural literacy* and *interactive literacy*). Since OHCs are more than a source of health information and additionally satisfy members' diverse psychological and social needs, it is both logical and appropriate to use a combination of definitions to examine health literacy in OHCs.

E-Health Literacy

It is noted that mass communication plays an important role in shaping individuals' health literacy (Zarcadoolas, Pleasant, & Greer, 2005). As more consumers turn to the Internet for health information, researchers and health care professionals have begun to consider the implications of this popular form of health literacy – termed electronic health literacy, or "e-health literacy." Eng (2001) defines e-health as "the use of emerging information and communication technology, especially the Internet, to improve or enable health and health care" (p. 20).

Closely related to e-health is the concept of e-health literacy. Norman and Skinner (2006a, b) define e-health literacy as "the ability to seek, find, understand, and appraise health information from electronic sources and apply the knowledge gained to addressing or solving a health problem" (2006a, p. e9). This definition of e-health literacy also includes six core skills, or "literacies": *traditional literacy*, *health literacy*, *information literacy*, *scientific literacy*, *media literacy*, and *computer literacy*. E-health literacy "aims to empower individuals and enable them to fully participate in health decisions informed by e-health resources" (Norman & Skinner, 2006a, p. e11).

Comparing Norman and Skinner's (2006a) definition of e-health literacy and Nutbeam's (2000) and Zarcadoolas, Pleasant, and Greer's (2005) domains of health literacy, we can see that the definition of e-health literacy mainly focuses on basic levels of health literacy (*fundamental* and *science literacies*). Given the features of OHCs discussed in the first section (e.g., providing psychological support, anonymity, connecting with people sharing similar interests), the present chapter argues that OHCs could be a vehicle in which consumers' levels of health literacy may be examined, but that OHCs can also improve levels of health literacy domains (*civic*, *cultural*, and *interactive literacies*). The Internet is the context in which health literacy demands are made and consumers bring individual skills to the OHC.

A few studies have disclosed that online communities can serve as a source of health literacy in various ways. For example, Donelle and Hoffman-Goetz (2008) noted that OHCs are not only a venue for the dissemination of health information but also a voice of lifestyle coaching and advocacy. While Dollene and Hoffman-Goetz's (2008) study was based on OHCs with a comparatively narrow audience, i.e., the Canadian aboriginal population, the present chapter applies the health literacy domains using The Biggest Loser League weight-loss OHC as a case study. A content analysis of posts was conducted between September 1, 2009 and December 31, 2009. Domains of health literacy were coded, as denoted below. Online health discussions such as *The Biggest Loser League* provide rich and fertile content in which to examine domains of health literacy. Therefore, the purpose of the case study is to demonstrate that online discussions are comprised of various domains of health literacy and e-health literacy, and that domains of health literacy vary, accordingly. A discussion is presented after the case study to explore implications of the role of OHCs in the use and distribution of health and e-health literacy.

CASE STUDY: THE BIGGEST LOSER LEAGUE

Background

Obesity has become a national epidemic in the United States, and one that affects both children and adults in increasingly large proportions (Wang & Beydoun, 2007). It has been estimated that two out of every three adults, and more than one in six children, are overweight or obese (Flagel, Carroll, Ogden, & Curtin, 2010). Being overweight increases the risk for certain diseases such as type 2 diabetes, heart diseases, stroke, sleep apnea, respiratory problems, and some cancers (CDC,

2009). Being obese poses the greatest health risks for these same health conditions.

There are a number of factors that contribute to overweight and obesity, making it a complex health issue. According to the CDC (2010a), factors like lifestyle behaviors, environment, and genetics play a role in being overweight and obese. In 2003, Surgeon General Richard Carmona stated that low health literacy was "one of the biggest contributors to our nation's epidemic of overweight and obesity" (Carmona, 2003). Supporting this view, recent studies have found that low health literacy or numeracy is associated with difficulty in understanding food labels and portion sizes, and higher Body Mass Index (BMI) in adults and children (Pelletier, Chang, Delzell, et al., 2004; Rothman, Housam, Weiss, et al., 2006; Wardle, Parmenter, & Waller, 2004; Young & Nestle, 2000).

Many overweight and obese consumers are turning to the Internet for information and support (Eysenbach, Powell, Englesakis, et al., 2004). In fact, most adults prefer the Internet to face-to-face weight loss interventions (Tate, Wing, & Winnett, 2001). OHCs have become one of the most popular outlets for overweight and obese consumers for obtaining information and psychological support. As noted earlier, the major contents of OHCs are conversations about topically relevant health issues, including the sharing of knowledge concerning health conditions.

There are various motivations for participating in OHCs, but most people come in search of health information (Benigeri & Pluye, 2003; Fin, 1999; Han & Belcher, 2001; White & Dorman, 2000). People with chronic health conditions, like overweight and obese, share stories with each other, not just for emotional support, but for the medical knowledge they gain from participating with others in similar situations in the OHC (Eysenbach, Powell, Englesakis, et al., 2004; White & Dorman, 2001). However, people participating in OHCs have different experiences and different knowledge related to health (Frost & Massagli, 2008). For example, an overweight member will have different concerns and questions than a morbidly obese member. Likewise, a member who has had gastric bypass surgery will have a different experience to share than a member on a diet regimen.

Within the OHC, all members are welcome to participate regardless of their knowledge or experience related to being overweight and obese. By sharing ideas, discussing weight-loss strategies, and debating treatment options together, all OHC members potentially gain "knowledge" that can improve patient care (Frost & Massagli, 2008). In order to better communicate and educate the population with overweight and obesity problems within the United States, we must first understand consumers' knowledge – including health literacy knowledge, i.e., health literacy domains, with regard to fitness and nutrition.

Sampling

The Biggest Loser League is an online discussion board located on NBC's Website (http://tbll.nbc.com/). *The Biggest Loser League*, started in 2008, allows community members to create their own profile, join weight-management teams, and set and keep track of health and fitness goals. This consumer led, peer-to-peer OHC boasts more than 8,000 members and nearly 30,000 posts, demonstrating the breadth and depth of use of this particular OHC. We choose the OHC associated with *The Biggest Loser* because, as a popular "reality show" in the U.S., it attracts a lot of viewers, and consequently grows active membership in the online community. Thus, *The Biggest Loser League* Web site serves as an appropriate OHC since it offers – due to its active membership and association with the TV show – a diverse audience demographics who presumably also bring diverse health literacy knowledge and skills and that should enable determination of the presence and extent of use of health literacy domains in weight-management related OHC.

The method was a content analysis, which is one of the most prominent research methods in mass media studies (Berelson, 1952) due to its ability to analyze the content of media message (Wimmer & Dominick, 1983). The present study sampled individual posts of online discussions on *The Biggest Loser League* from September 1, 2009 to December 31, 2009, during which time Season 8 of *The Biggest Loser* was on television. The final sample yielded 100 posts from 52 different participants in the four constructed weeks, with an average of 1.9 posts from each participant. Since *The Biggest Loser* is a weekly TV show during its regular season, four constructed weeks were sampled to represent this period of time. Constructed weeks are an effective way of sampling media content with periodical features (Hester & Dougall, 2007).

The unit of analysis was the individual post, defined as each message written by a user and sent to an online discussion board of an online community. All instances of health literacy were coded. Posts that contained more than one domain of health literacy were coded for each domain. For instance, a post could identify scientific literacy and civic literacy, so both scientific literacy and civic literacy domains were coded.

Intercoder Reliability

There were two coders. An intercoder reliability was taken at the beginning (during the pre-test of the codebook) and, again, after the codebook was pretested. An intercoder reliability using Cohen's Kappa coefficient was calculated for each variable. Cohen's Kappa coefficients ranged from 0.816 to 1, confirming that every variable met the minimum 0.75 that is acceptable for two coders (Tinsley & Weiss, 2000). The overall average Cohen's Kappa coefficient for all variables was 0.92.

Variables Coded

Six variables representing five domains of health literacy were coded: *nutritional facts*, *health services*, *science literacy*, *interactive literacy*, *cultural literacy*, and *civic literacy*. *Nutritional facts* and *health services* constitute *functional literacy* since, by definition, *functional literacy* includes the basic skills necessary to read, write, analyze numbers, and communicate effectively (Zarcadoolas, Pleasant, & Greer, 2006). Specific to the issue of obesity, an important part of *functional literacy* is the ability to understand nutritional facts about food products, including portion sizes, and knowledge of health services that assist with weight-management.

All categories were coded as 1 (present) or 0 (not present), except for *cultural literacy*, which had five categories, where 1 = *making recommendations*, 2 = *seeking recommendations*, 3 = *cannot tell*, 4 = *either making or seeking recommendations*, and 5 = *both making and seeking recommendations*.

Nutritional facts were defined as macronutrients that can be commonly found in foods, such as low-fat or low-carbohydrate foods. For example, a post that mentions that soft drink contains 300 calories per serving is an example of a nutritional fact. Nutritional facts could consist of aspartame, caffeine, calories, protein, carbohydrates, fat, fiber, corn syrup, or gluten-free foods, among others.

Health services was defined as services that help people to manage their weight or treat weight-related problems, such as gyms, health clinics, or weight-loss programs. For example, one post may mention that the individual (doing the post) had a successful experience with a particular health clinic. Note: Exercise DVDs and video games were coded as health services given their goal of providing weight-management "services" to consumers.

Science literacy was defined as scientific facts about certain health issues, such as content about health risks, statistics, and citation of medical sources. For example, a post may provide a description of how to calculate BMI (Body Mass Index).

Interactive literacy was defined as the ability to derive meanings from health content, such as motivation, self-confidence or self-care behaviors from communication within OHCs (Nutbeam, 2000). In the content analysis, interactive literacy was operationalized as messages about one type of health-related content, i.e. self-care behaviors. Specifically, self-care manifests in content about any self-care efforts or methods to manage weight. For instance, a post may mention use of an online calendar to keep track of daily diet and exercise.

Civic literacy was defined as consumers' understanding of health issues as a social problem, which included any mention of health advocacy or actions taken on behalf of public health organizations. For example, a post may mention that obesity was a social problem, or that the food industry should practice more self-regulation in advertising food products. Both are examples of civic literacy.

Cultural literacy was defined as "the ability to recognize and use collective beliefs, customs, world-view and social identity in order to interpret and act on health information" (Zarcadoolas, Pleasant, & Greer, 2006, p. 197). *Cultural literacy* in online discussions is an understanding of this online culture, including its values, norms, and beliefs, as well as the ability of making use of this culture to help interpret health information. Additionally, part of the culture of online discussions is making and seeking recommendations in online communities. Therefore, *cultural literacy* was operationalized as the action of making or seeking recommendations.

Results

As shown in Figure 1, cultural literacy was present in nearly every post coded here and accounted for 99 out of the 100 posts. Specifically, the results showed that 30% of the posts (n=30) were making recommendation, and 12% of the posts (n=12) were seeking recommendations, and 3% (n=3) of the posts were both making *and* seeking recommendations. Fifty-four percent (n=54) of the posts did not make nor seek any recom-

Figure 1. Domains of health literacy present in the Biggest Loser League OHC

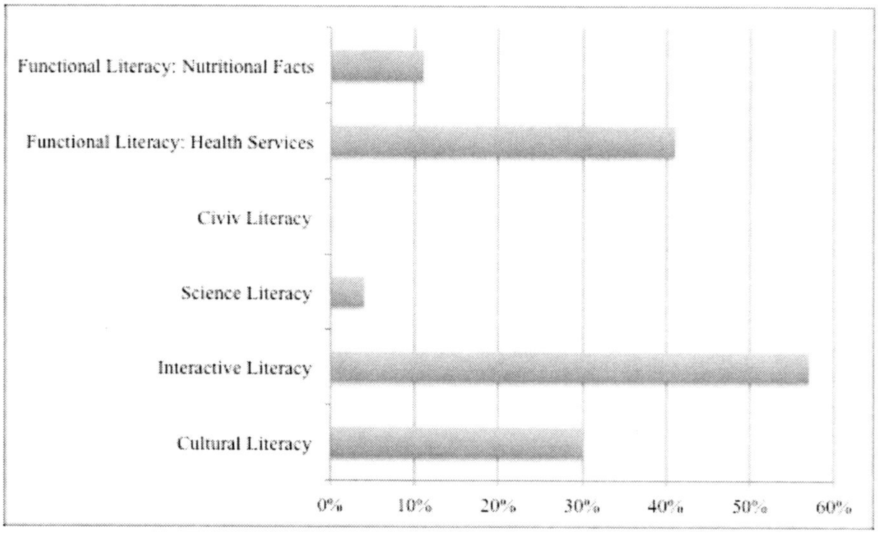

mendations. Interactive literacy, the second most frequent domain of heath literacy, was present in 57% of the posts (n=57), followed by functional literacy – which had two parts: health services (n=41) and nutritional facts (n=11), and science literacy was mentioned in 4% (n=4) of posts. No posts were about *civic literacy*.

DISCUSSION

This chapter seeks to develop a framework for understanding online health communities (OHCs) and health literacy. We began with a definition of online health communities (OHCs), which represents a unique type of online community that focuses discussion on a particular health topic. We presented features that make OHCs unique and argued that OHCs represent a viable outlet in which health literacy skills and competencies may be shared in the context of a health topic. Next, we defined health literacy and e-health literacy by drawing on definitions from the public health perspective that includes domains of health literacy. We argued that while such domains have been offered, few studies have examined the presence of these health literacy domains in new media environments, particularly OHCs, which serve as a rich and fertile context in which health literacy domains *should* be present given the active give-and-take of health information among members of OHCs. Last, we applied the health literacy domains using The Biggest Loser League weight-loss OHC as a case study. A content analysis of posts was conducted between September 1, 2009 and December 31, 2009. Domains of health literacy were coded. Results show that functional literacy and interactive literacy were present in the OHC discussions to a greater degree than any of the other health literacy domains coded.

The results of this case study indicate that consumers' health literacy knowledge regarding nutrition and fitness consist of lower-level domains. Our results support the exchange of health information within peer-to-peer OHCs. In this study, consumers discussed nutrition and fitness at basic levels of health literacy (*functional* and *science literacies*), showing that there is an interest in discussing these topics. Results indicate that consumers discussed topics related to self-care (*interactive literacy*). The opportunity to seek and exchange health information with like-individuals is important to consumers, as seen in this case study and other research (Jones, 1997; Korp, 2006; Lindsay, Smith, Bellaby, & Baker, 2009). The interactive component of online discussion allows consumers to infuse their own opinions, perceptions, and experience in these computer-mediated discussions.

As mentioned previously, both context and consumers' individual skills are important to the definition of health literacy. In fact, Vasanta, Gupta, and Devi (2002) note that health literacy is defined by the consumer's environment and that no one definition is sufficient because context is experienced differently by individual consumers within various timeframes of the lifespan. Within this online OHC, the online culture helped participants define their health knowledge related to topics on overweight and obesity. Participants of *The Biggest Loser League* took advantage of the online culture to make and seek recommendations regarding weight-management (*cultural literacy*). Online health communities create the opportunity and network for both seeking and sharing information related to a specific disease, offering a vehicle for improving disease-related knowledge. Culture within *The Biggest Loser League* refers to the OHC, but also to the health condition of overweight and obesity that links participants.

There was no discussion of *civic literacy* in any of the posts sampled here. The overall goal of *civic literacy* is to place a health issue within the context of a consumer's environment, including understanding national policy or ecological health related to overweight and obesity. Such skills enable consumers to become aware of public issues, to participate in discussion about them, and to become better involved in decision-related processes related to the issue (Zarcadoolas, Pleasant, & Greer, 2005). *Civic literacy* is also consumer knowledge that personal behaviors and lifestyle choices affect others in a larger community and society. Since consumers join *The Biggest Loser League* in order to manage their weight, *civic literacy* issues may not be seen as important in facilitating weight loss. Such acknowledgement of the broader implications of this chronic disease may not be necessary or overweight or obesity may be perceived as an individual problem versus one influenced by external factors, including an individual's environment or genetics.

In short, the evidence presented here from *The Biggest Loser League* shows that less sophisticated domains of health literacy (*functional* and *science literacies*) are being used more often than more sophisticated domains (*civic*, *interactive*, and *cultural literacies*). Less sophisticated domains of health literacy are associated with basic knowledge of nutrition and fitness. Consumers have to understand "the basics," like nutritional facts, including calories and fat intake, in order to successfully manage their weight. Since a major goal of *The Biggest Loser League* is to facilitate weight management among participants, it only makes sense that consumers would focus on these basic domains of health literacy. Through the application of multi-dimensional domains of health literacy framework to online health communication content, we see that consumers are not utilizing the more sophisticated domains of health literacy in online health communication. As defined by Nutbeam (2000) and Zarcadoolas, Pleasant, and Greer (2005), all of the identified domains of health literacy work together to shape individual's understanding of health. Thus, it stands to reason that if one domain is absent, an individual's health literacy is not complete. Perhaps this is evidence that consumers do not understand the complexity of the issue of being overweight and obese and suggests that media – the primary provider of health information - should seek to discuss and present health issues in different ways. This is an opportunity for the mass media to act as an educational tool, increasing audiences' levels of health literacy. Media frames are orientations toward information that shape the interpretation of events by audiences: what facts are used to report events, what words are used to describe events, and what options are presented to address the problem in the news story (Fiske & Taylor, 1991; Miller, 2002). If overweight and obesity were framed in such a way that included civic literacy components, consumers might participate more fully in the decision-making processes regarding weight-management and make educated decisions as to the solution of such problems.

For health communication researchers and health care professionals, it is important to know how consumers understand health based on the domains of health literacy. This includes e-health and the application of e-health literacy to consumers' health-related attitudes and behaviors. Our goal here was to establish a framework that could be used in future research of OHCs, specifically of health literacy domains within these online contexts. We applied such a framework to *The Biggest Loser League* in order to identify domains of health literacy used by consumers within OHCs. While the results of the case study are not generalizeable across chronic diseases, the framework presented may be applied to other OHCs in order to identify the domains of health literacy used by consumers. The results suggest that the framework is viable, at least to the extent that domains of health literacy were identified in OHC posts shown here. Application of these domains across other chronic disease like diabetes, arthritis, or heart disease would allow insight into consumers' health literacy of disease and its self-management behaviors. Chronic disease interventions might then be created to improve disease-related knowledge and target missing domains of health literacy.

Although both Nutbeam (2000) and Zarcadoolas, Pleasant, and Greer (2005) recognize the importance and influence of mass media in health literacy, none of their domains capture the specific skills necessary to participate in e-health. As Norman and Skinner (2006) point out, e-health literacy is different from these other health literacy definitions. E-health literacy as a domain of health literacy could potentially capture consumers' e-health use, including patient care, preventative medicine, and health promotion. We must understand the extent to which consumers are using domains of health literacy. Domains of health literacy that are missing from OHC must be targeted for improvement and these online OHCs provide the opportunity for education and promotion.

FUTURE RESEARCH DIRECTIONS

The future of e-health has already arrived. Consumers are ahead of the curve in regards to the use of the Internet to inform attitudes and behaviors regarding health. There is much to learn from these consumer-led online health communities (OHCs). Patient perspective of chronic disease is especially important to self-management behaviors (Monninkhof, van der Aa, van der Valk, et al., 2004). Examining peer-to-peer computer-mediated communication allows for insights into how people with chronic disease manage disease symptoms and ecological issues related to the disease. As Zarcadoolas, Pleasant, and Greer (2005) note, health literacy has less to do with the content of health information than with the context and individual skill related to the situation. Thus, future research should seek to explore consumers' levels of health literacy related to disease knowledge and self-management behaviors.

By examining computer-mediated communication within bulletin boards, blogs, and chat rooms, consumers' health literacy might be assessed. The Internet provides an opportunity to test the potential of improving these consumers' health literacy. It stands to reason that if these consumers are already motivated to seek health information or to participate in online groups, they have a desire for knowledge. Thus, health communicators may be able to improve consumers' health literacy in regards to specific diseases using OHCs as a viable channel in which to reach audiences who are at highest risk for the disease.

More research must be directed at assessing the health literacy knowledge being shared in OHCs, including the level of health literacy and "off-line" effects on consumers' health behaviors. Future studies may also explore how OHCs might be utilized to improve consumers' self-management behaviors. Increasingly large numbers of consumers are turning to the Internet for information, social support, and empowerment – all of which are influential in self-management. Thus, the Internet might be used as existing forums to improve consumers' health status through health literacy.

CONCLUSION

The concept of health literacy has evolved as a multi-dimensional concept that considers multiple domains and socio-cultural factors that influence individuals' understanding of health (Nutbeam, 2000; Zarcadoolas, Pleasant, & Greer, 2004). Here, we argue that online health communities (OHCs) must be considered as an important source of health information for consumers, contributing to participants' use of domains of health literacy. We have established a framework that is especially useful in identifying domains of health literacy within an OHC context. Health literacy evolves over an individual's life and is impacted by health status as well as demographic, sociopolitical, psychosocial, and cultural factors (Zarcadoolas, Pleasant, & Greer, 2006). In today's Information Era, OHCs must be included as part of the this also includes online health information, especially content within OHCs that have a loyal and active audience like *The Biggest Loser League*. We must consider the influence OHCs have on individuals' health literacy, both from informational support and interactive components that make these OHCs unique.

REFERENCES

American Medical Association Ad Hoc Committee on Health Literacy for the Council on Scientific Affairs. (1999). Health literacy: Report of the council on scientific affairs. *Journal of the American Medical Association, 281*, 552–557. doi:10.1001/jama.281.6.552

Baker, D. W., Parker, R. M., Williams, M. V., & Clark, W. S. (1998). Health literacy and the risk of hospital admission. *Journal of General Internal Medicine, 13*(12), 791–798. doi:10.1046/j.1525-1497.1998.00242.x

Benigeri, M., & Pluye, P. (2003). Shortcomings of health information on the Internet. *Health Promotion International, 18*(4), 381–386. doi:10.1093/heapro/dag409

Berland, G. K., Elliott, M. N., Morales, L. S., Algazy, J. I., Kravitz, R. L., & Broder, M. S. (2001). Health information on the Internet: Accessibility, quality, and readability in English and Spanish. *Journal of the American Medical Association, 285*, 2612–2621. doi:10.1001/jama.285.20.2612

Berleson, B. (1952). *Content analysis in communication research*. New York, NY: Free Press.

Carlson, B. A., Neal, D., Magwood, G., Jenkins, C., Givens King, M., & Hossler, C. L. (2006). A community-based participatory health information needs assessment to help eliminate diabetes information disparities. *Health Promotion Practice, 7*(3S), 213S–222S. doi:10.1177/1524839906288694

Carmona, R. H. (June 14, 2003). *Prepared remarks given at American Medical Association House of Delegates meeting,* Chicago. Retrieved from www.surgeongeneral.gov/ news/speeches/ama061403.htm

Centers for Disease Control and Prevention. (CDC). (2010). *Healthy People 2010*. Retrieved from http://www.healthypeople.gov/ document/html/volume1/ 11healthcom.htm

Centers for Disease Control and Prevention. (CDC). (2010a). *Data and statistics*. Retrieved from http://www.cdc.gov/ obesity/data/index.html

Centers for Disease Control and Prevention. (CDC) (2010b). *National health and nutrition examination survey data*. National Center for Health Statistics (NCHS). Hyattsville, MD: U.S. Department of Health and Human Services, Centers for Disease Control and Prevention.

Cline, R. J. W., & Haynes, K. M. (2001). Consumer health information seeking on the Internet: The state of the art. *Health Education Research, 16*(6), 671–692. doi:10.1093/her/16.6.671

DeWalt, D. A., Berkman, N. D., Sheridan, S., Lohr, K. N., & Pignone, M. P. (2004). Literacy and health outcomes. *Journal of General Internal Medicine, 19*(12), 1228–1239. doi:10.1111/j.1525-1497.2004.40153.x

Donelle, L., & Hoffman-Goetz, L. (2008). An exploratory study of Canadian aboriginal online health care forums. *Health Communication, 23*(3), 270–281. doi:10.1080/10410230802056388

du Pre'. A. (2000). *Communicating about health: Current issues and perspectives*. Mountain View, CA: Mayfield Publishing Company.

Eng, T. R. (2001). *The eHealth landscape: A terrain map of emerging information and communication technologies in health and health care*. Princeton, NJ: The Robert Wood Johnson Foundation.

Eysenbach, G. (2000). Recent advances: Consumer health informatics. *British Medical Journal, 320*, 1713–1716. doi:10.1136/bmj.320.7251.1713

Eysenbach, G. (2003). The impact of the Internet on cancer outcomes. *A Cancer Journal for Clinicians, 53*, 356-371.

Eysensbach, G., Powell, J., Englesakis, M., Rizo, C., & Stern, A. (2004). Health related virtual communities and electronic support groups: Systematic review of the effects of online peer to peer interactions. *British Medical Journal, 328*(7449), 1166. doi:10.1136/bmj.328.7449.1166

Finn, J. (1999). An exploration of helping processes in an online self-help group focusing on issues of disability. *Health & Social Work, 24*, 220–240.

Fiske, S. T., & Taylor, S. E. (1991). *Social cognition*. New York, NY: McGraw-Hill.

Flagel, K. M., Carroll, M. D., Ogden, C. L., & Lester, C. R. (2010). Prevalence and trends in obesity among US adults, 1999-2008. *Journal of the American Medical Association, 303*(3), 235–241. doi:10.1001/jama.2009.2014

Frost, J. H., & Massagli, M. P. (2008). Social uses of personal health information within PatientsLikeMe, an online patient community: What can happen when patients have access to one another's data. *Journal of Internet Medical Research, 10*(3), e15. doi:10.2196/jmir.1053

Gazmararian, J. A., Williams, M. V., Peel, J., & Baker, D. W. (2003). Health literacy and knowledge of chronic disease. *Patient Education and Counseling, 51*(3), 267–275. doi:10.1016/S0738-3991(02)00239-2

Han, H. R., & Belcher, A. E. (2001). Computer-mediated support group among parents of children with cancer – An exploratory study. *Computers, Informatics, Nursing, 19*(1), 27–33.

Hester, B., & Dougall, E. (2007). The efficiency of constructed week sampling for content analysis of online news. *Journalism & Mass Communication Quarterly, 84*(4), 811–824.

Institute of Medicine. (2004). Health literacy: A prescription to end confusion. In Nielsen-Bohlman, L. T., Panzer, A. M., & Kindig, D. A. (Eds.), *Committee on health literacy*. Washington, DC: National Academies Press.

Jones, Q. (1997). Virtual-communities, virtual-settlements and cyber-archaeology: A theoretical outline. *Journal of Computer-Mediated Communication, 3*(3). Retrieved from http://jcmc.indiana.edu/ vol3/issue3/ jones.html.

Kalichman, S. C., Benotsch, E. G., Weinhardt, L., Austin, J., & Luke, W. (2002). Internet use among people living with HIV/AIDS: Association of health information, health behavior, and health status. *AIDS Education and Prevention, 14*(1), 51–61. doi:10.1521/aeap.14.1.51.24335

Kalichman, S. C., Benotsch, E. G., Weinhardt, L., Austin, J., Luke, W., & Cherry, C. (2003). Health-related Internet use, coping, social support, and health indicators in people living with HIV/AIDS: Preliminary results from a community survey. *Health Psychology, 22*(1), 111–116. doi:10.1037/0278-6133.22.1.111

Kalichman, S. C., Weinhardt, L., Benotsch, E., DiFonzo, K., Luke, W., & Austin, J. (2000). Internet access and Internet use for health information among people living with HIV-AIDS. *Patient Education and Counseling, 46*(2), 109–116. doi:10.1016/S0738-3991(01)00134-3

Korp, P. (2006). Health on the Internet: Implications for health promotion. *Health Education Research, 21*(1), 78–86. doi:10.1093/her/cyh043

Kutner, M., Greenberg, E., Jin, Y., & Paulsen, C. (2006). *The health literacy of America's adults: Results from the 2003 National Assessment of Adult Literacy*. Washington, DC: National Center for Education Statistics, US Department of Education.

Lindsay, S., Smith, S., Bellaby, P., & Baker, R. (2009). The health impact of an online health disease support group: A comparison of moderated versus unmoderated support. *Health Education Research*, *24*(4), 646–654. doi:10.1093/her/cyp001

Miller, K. (2002). *Communication theories: Perspectives, processes, and contexts*. Boston, MA: McGraw Hill.

Monninkhof, E., van der Aa, M., van der Valk, P., van der Palen, V., Zielhuis, G., Koning, K., & Pieterse, M. (2004). A qualitative evaluation of a comprehensive self-management program for COPD patients: Effectiveness from the patients' perspective. *Patient Education and Counseling*, *55*(2), 177–184. doi:10.1016/j.pec.2003.09.001

Norman, C. D., & Skinner, H. A. (2006a). eHealth literacy: Essential skills for consumer health in a networked world. *Journal of Medical Internet Research*, *8*(2), e9f. doi:10.2196/jmir.8.2.e9

Norman, C. D., & Skinner, H. A. (2006b). eHEALS: The eHealth literacy scale. *Journal of Medical Internet Research*, *8*(4), e27f. doi:10.2196/jmir.8.4.e27

Nutbeam, D. (2000). Health literacy as a public health goal: A challenge for contemporary health education and communication strategies into the 21st century. *Health Promotion International*, *15*(3), 259–267. doi:10.1093/heapro/15.3.259

Pecchioni, L. L., & Sparks, L. (2007). Health information sources of individuals with cancer and their family members. *Health Communication*, *21*(2), 143–151. doi:10.1080/10410230701307162

Pelletier, A. L., Chang, W. W., Delzell, J. E., & McCall, J. W. (2004). Patients' understanding and use of snack food package nutrition labels. *The Journal of the American Board of Family Practice*, *17*, 319–323. doi:10.3122/jabfm.17.5.319

Piotrow, P. T., & Kincaid, D. L. (2001). Strategic communication for international health programs. In Rice, R. E., & Atkin, C. K. (Eds.), *Public communication campaigns* (3rd ed., pp. 249–266). London, UK: Sage Publications, Inc.

Raines, L. (2005). The average American Internet user is not sure what podcasting is, what an RSS feed does, or what the term "phishing" means. *Pew Internet Project Memo*. Retrieved from http://pewinternet.org

Ratzan, S. C. (2001). Health literacy: Communication for the public good. *Health Promotion International*, *16*(2), 207–214. doi:10.1093/heapro/16.2.207

Rodgers, S., & Chen, Q. (2005). Internet community group participation: Psychosocial benefits for women with breast cancer. *Journal of Computer-Mediated Communication, 10*(4), article 5. Retrieved from http://jcmc.indiana.edu/vol10/issue4/ rodgers.html

Rothman, R. L., Housam, R., Weiss, H., Davis, D., Gregory, R., & Gebretsadik, T. (2006). Patient understanding of food labels: The role of literacy and numeracy. *American Journal of Preventive Medicine*, *31*(5), 391–398. doi:10.1016/j.amepre.2006.07.025

Rudd, R., Moeykens, B., & Colton, T. C. (1999). Health and literacy: A review of medical and public health literature. In Comings, J., Garners, B., & Smith, C. (Eds.), *Annual review of adult learning and literacy* (*Vol. 1*). New York, NY: Jossey-Bass.

Schillinger, D., Grumbach, K., Wang, F., Wilson, C., Daher, C., & Leong-Grotz, K. (2003). Closing the loop: Physician communication with diabetic patients who have low health literacy. *Archives of Internal Medicine*, *163*(1), 83–90. doi:10.1001/archinte.163.1.83

Simonds, S. K. (1974). Health education as social policy. *Health Education Monographs*, *2*, 1–25.

Stout, P., Ball, J. G., & Villegas, J. (2004). Health marketing and the Internet. In Schumann, D. W., & Thorson, E. (Eds.), *Internet advertising: Theory and research*. New Jersey: Lawrence Erlbaum Associates, Publishers.

Tate, D. F., Wing, R. R., & Winett, R. A. (2001). Using Internet technology to deliver a behavioral weight loss program. *Journal of the American Medical Association*, *285*(9), 1172–1177. doi:10.1001/jama.285.9.1172

Tinsley, H. E. A., & Weiss, D. J. (2000). Interrater reliability and agreement. In Tinsley, H. E. A., & Brown, S. D. (Eds.), *Handbook of applied multivariate statistics and mathematical modeling*. San Diego, CA: Academic Press. doi:10.1016/B978-012691360-6/50005-7

Turnock, B. J. (2009). *Public health: What it is and how it works*. Sudbury, MA: Jones and Bartlett Publishers.

U.S. Department of Health and Human Services. (2000). *Healthy people 2010: Understanding and improving health*. Washington, DC: US Government Printing Office.

Vasanta, D., Gupta, S., & Devi, P. (2002). Evaluating the social impact of literacy: Some lessons from the literacy campaign. In Mukherjee, A., & Vasanta, D. (Eds.), *Practice and research in literacy* (pp. 154–186). New Dehli, India: Sage India.

Wang, Y., & Beydoun, M. A. (2007). The obesity epidemic in the United States – Gender, age, socioeconomic, racial/ethnic, and geographic characteristics: A systematic review and meta-regression analysis. *Epidemiologic Reviews*, *29*(1), 6–28. doi:10.1093/epirev/mxm007

Wang, Z., Walther, J., Pingree, S., & Hawkins, R. (2008). Health information, credibility, homophily, and influence via the Internet: Web sites versus discussion groups. *Health Communication*, *23*(4), 358–368. doi:10.1080/10410230802229738

Wardle, J., Parmenter, K., & Waller, J. (2000). Nutrition knowledge and food intake. *Appetite*, *34*, 269–275. doi:10.1006/appe.1999.0311

Wellman, B., Salaff, J., Dimitrova, D., Garton, L., Gulia, M., & Haythornthwaite, C. (1996). Computer networks as social networks: Collaborative work, telework, and virtual community. *Annual Review of Sociology*, *22*, 213–238. doi:10.1146/annurev.soc.22.1.213

White, M., & Dorman, S. (2000). Online support for caregivers: Analysis of an Internet Alzheimer mailgroup. *Computers, Informatics, Nursing*, *18*(4), 168–176.

White, M., & Dorman, S. M. (2001). Receiving social support online: Implications for health education. *Health Education Research*, *16*(6), 693–707. doi:10.1093/her/16.6.693

Williams, M. V., Baker, D. W., Parker, R. M., & Nurss, J. R. (1998). Relationship of functional health literacy to patients' knowledge of their chronic disease. A study of patients with hypertension and diabetes. *Archives of Internal Medicine*, *158*(2), 166–172. doi:10.1001/archinte.158.2.166

Wimmer, R. D., & Dominick, J. R. (1983). *Mass media research, an introduction*. Belmont, CA: Wadsworth, Inc.

World Health Organization. (1998). Health promotion glossary. *Health Promotion International*, *13*(4), 349–364. doi:10.1093/heapro/13.4.349

Wright, K. (1999). Computer-mediated support groups: An examination of relationships among social support, perceived stress, and coping strategies. *Communication Quarterly*, *47*, 402–414. doi:10.1080/01463379909385570

Wright, K. (2000). Computer-mediated social support, older adults and coping. *The Journal of Communication*, *50*(3), 100–118. doi:10.1111/j.1460-2466.2000.tb02855.x

Wright, K. (2002). Social support within an online cancer community: An assessment of emotional support, perceptions of advantages and disadvantages, and motives for using the community from a communication perspective. *Journal of Applied Communication Research*, *30*(3), 195–209. doi:10.1080/00909880216586

Young, L. R., & Nestle, M. (2002). The contribution of expanding portion sizes to the US obesity epidemic. *American Journal of Public Health*, *92*(2), 246–249. doi:10.2105/AJPH.92.2.246

Zarcadoolas, C. Pleasant, A., & Greer, D. (2006). *Advancing health literacy: A framework for understanding and action*. San Francisco, CA: Jossey-Bass.

Zarcadoolas, C., Pleasant, A., & Greer, D. (2005). Understanding health literacy: An expanded model. *Health Promotion International*, *20*(2), 195–203. doi:10.1093/heapro/dah609

ADDITIONAL READING

Nutbeam, D. (2000). Health literacy as a public health goal: A challenge for contemporary health education and communication strategies into the 21st century. *Health Promotion International*, *15*(3), 259–267. doi:10.1093/heapro/15.3.259

Rodgers, S., & Chen, Q. (2005). Internet community group participation: Psychosocial benefits for women with breast cancer. *Journal of Computer-Mediated Communication, 10*(4), article 5. Available from http://jcmc.indiana.edu/ vol10/issue4/ rodgers.html.

Zarcadoolas, C. Pleasant, A., & Greer, D. (2006). *Advancing health literacy: A framework for understanding and action*. San Francisco: Jossey-Bass.

Zarcadoolas, C., Pleasant, A., & Greer, D. (2005). Understanding health literacy: an expanded model. *Health Promotion International*, *20*(2), 195–203. doi:10.1093/heapro/dah609

Chapter 14
Identifying the Essential Design Requirements for Usable E-Health Communities in Mobile Devices

Ricardo Mendoza-González
Instituto Tecnológico de Aguascalientes, Mexico

Miguel Vargas Martin
University of Ontario Institute of Technology, Canada

Laura C. Rodríguez-Martínez
Instituto Tecnológico de Aguascalientes, Mexico

ABSTRACT

We believe that well-designed and usable user interface is critical, as the adequate use and the effectiveness of any application usually depend on it, especially when a specific system is oriented to play a key role into the process of patients' care (healthcare applications). Very good examples of healthcare applications are E-Health Communities, which are generally oriented to contribute in the process for improving the quality of life for members of a community suffering from chronic diseases. In order to contribute to previous efforts, we propose a set of 15 basic usability requirements specifically oriented to mobile interfaces for blog-based instant messaging e-health communities. We structured our set of usability requirements on two sources: Firstly we consider the survey-obtained feedback from 72 participants who regularly access social networks from mobile devices. Then we complemented this information with some ideas presented in previous research. We show the effectiveness of the proposal by using an illustrative example (designing an interface-prototype for a mobile e-health community) as a proof-of-concept together with a preliminary usability study. The prototype was entirely created by observing our usability requirements. The results of the study are encouraging and reflect a good correlation between

DOI: 10.4018/978-1-60960-866-8.ch014

the requirements proposed and the users' perception. This seems to indicate that although this research-work is focused on providing a starting point to developers with guidance in designing usable interfaces for e-health communities accessed by mobile devices, our findings could be easily adapted and applied to other mobile scenarios for blog-based instant messaging applications.

INTRODUCTION

According to Toyoda & Harrison (2002), and Vronay et al. (1999), a great deal of research has been conducted on computer-mediated communications (CMC) especially on computer-based communications, such as e-mail and chat. Chat applications are designed to allow the simultaneous type of messages by multiple participants "*Chatters*" who appear together on a channel of communication frequently known as "*Chat room*", "*room*", or "*channel*". Currently, the chat represents the most popular computer-based communication method in the Internet. Additionally this technology enables participants to exchange information, experiences, knowledge, and feelings, around the world with millions of people.

Nowadays many people are interested and involved in research and development of novel information technologies (IT) directly related to a number of specific topics. One of the most interesting is undoubtedly the application of IT to healthcare issues (e-health). According to Hesse & Shneiderman (2007), e-health applications must be based on joining best evidence from the user sciences, such as human factors engineering, human–computer interaction (c.f. Hewett et al., 1996), psychology, and usability (c.f. Nielsen, 1999), with best evidence in medicine to create transformational improvements in the quality of care that medical sciences offer. These improvements should follow recommendations from the Institute of Medicine to create a healthcare system that is: safe, effective (evidence-based), patient-centered (usable), and timely.

Ahern (2007) emphasize that advances in Internet and related communication technologies, such as mobile devices, contribute to the fast growth in e-health. In addition, emerging studies and experiments provide support for the beneficial effects of online interactive e-health applications and strategies, and the acceptance and popularity of these items between users (patients). An example of such advances is the *E-Health Communities*, which represents a relatively new strategy.

Grimes et al., (2010) and Welbourne et al., (2009) states that e-health communities emulate the motion of the Face to Face (FtF) support groups, widespread in Psychology and Psychiatry for the treatment of several disorders and psychological illnesses. Early in this decade it began using virtual communities as part of the treatment to improve the quality of life in patients suffering from chronic diseases (e.g. breast cancer) by means of a number of aspects including sharing experiences and information between individuals, professional orientation, and promoting the socialization, among others.

According to Welbourne et al. (2009), available on-line technologies for social networking allow e-health communities to increase the virtues of traditional FtF Support Groups, e.g.

- E-health communities can overcome temporal or geographic boundaries that FtF Support Groups cannot.
- The members of an e-health community may exchange information about treatments, symptoms, perspectives, or even feelings, and obtain support from others. Some members of offline networks may not be comfortable or even able to provide this support. This way, introversion in members of the group could be reduced.

- Individuals may feel more comfortable sharing personal information in an e-health community, where there is some degree of separation from their FtF Support Group.
- In e-health communities it is possible to establish open sessions between members. Additionally, private talks could be set between specific members using a private chat tool during the same session.
- Other members of their offline networks may not be comfortable or even able to provide this support.

Related with the above, Arunachalan & Light (2007) states that mobile healthcare and assisted living environments are becoming leaders in integration of IT into real-time applications. Also, the proliferation of mobile and portable devices, e.g. mobile phones, with increased storage and wireless communication capabilities has created a new networking environment for peer-to-peer applications. According to (Ioannidis & Chaintreau, 2009) mobile users can take advantage of encounters with other users to share information easily by means of these technological advantages.

In order to improve the quality of life by providing customized support to people in need of assistance, several initiatives have emerged recently, such as social networks and mobile technology that assist individuals members of a virtual communities (e.g. patients of mental illnesses (Chang et al., 2008; Ioannidis & Chaintreau, 2009; Kulkarni & Agrawal, 2008)). Although, this current healthcare systems and e-health approaches (e.g. e-health communities) are good enough at providing effective solutions for patients, several researches must be done to enhance this applications considering essential issues such as usability, security, privacy, and networking, among others (Kulkarni & Agrawal, 2008).

According to the standard ISO 9241-11 (ISO, 1998, p. 2), usability is the "*extent to which a product can be used by specified users to achieve specified goals with effectiveness, efficiency and satisfaction in a specified context of use.*" Besides the previous definition and primarily focusing on the design of user interfaces for mobile applications, it is also necessary to consider the processing and display limitations of mobile devices as PDA's and cell phones. In this way, the elements of generic interfaces must be re-interpreted and rendered according to the specific characteristics of different mobile devices (Sanchez et al., 2005). Similarly, some researchers (Burak & Sharon, 2004) believed that many web applications such as chats and blogs are not suitable for mobile phones due to hardware limited capabilities.

Furthermore, user interface designs that work effectively and efficiently in the context of stationary systems (specifically e-health applications) may not yield the same effect in the mobile systems. We try to reduce specific gaps by providing a set of basic usability requirements specifically oriented to mobile interfaces for blog-based e-health communities.

In order to complement and abridge the content of this section we propose a possible basic scenario for e-health communities, see Figure 1.

This chapter highlights the most important issues of our research work. We analyze, combine, and strengthen a number of previous efforts in designing adequate generic mobile interfaces to generate a new approach routed to enhance interfaces for e-health communities accessed by mobile devices.

The remaining of this chapter is organized as follows: *Background* section provides an overview of several previous approaches related to our proposal. Section *Design Requirements for Usable e-health Communities in Mobile Devices* represents the main section of the chapter and covered aspects such as: Problem, Mission, Solutions and Recommendations, and also include a wide description of the performed Case Study. Section *Future Research Directions* shows some motivational aspects for further research. Finally,

Figure 1. Our suggested scenario for mobile E-Health Communities

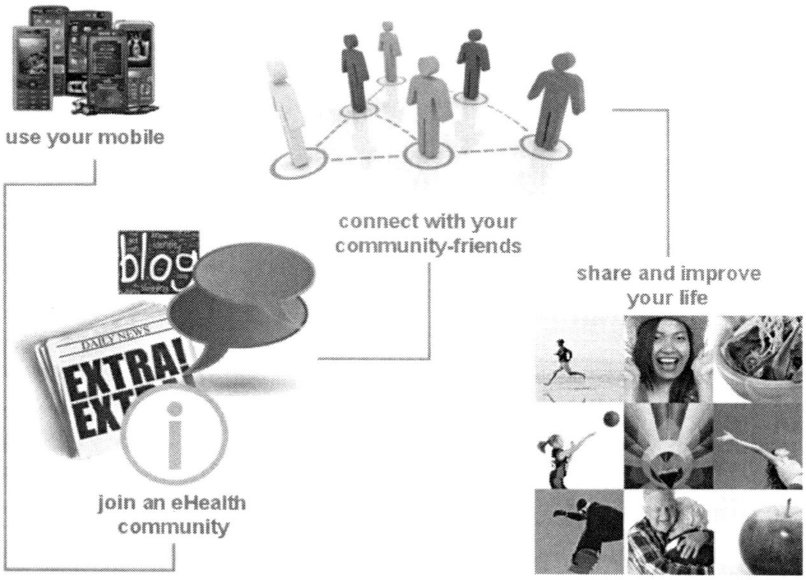

some concluding remarks and results are summarized in section *Conclusion*.

BACKGROUND

There are a number of studies that reflect certain incompatibilities between different web applications (e.g. blogging and instant messaging applications) and mobile devices. A good example is the long term study performed by Burak and Sharon (2004). The authors analyze the usage of mobile location-based community services involving 47,000 participants in a 21 month study. The study explores the relative usage of the different services offered, pattern changes over time, and the specific interaction style of users within instant message applications. Burak and Sharon (2004) have concluded that instant messages applications (e.g. instant messaging applications) joined with privacy management tools, are not suitable for mobile phones due to the small screen display and, many times, difficult to use keypad that does not encourage fast text entry. Bearing in mind the usability definition described in section *Introduction* (ISO, 1998), and the usability issues discussed by Jakob Nielsen (1999) well-designed interfaces must possess user ease of navigation, well integration of functions, friendliness, learnability, consistency, and a minimalistic design. Another important aspect related to usability, is undoubtedly the *Universal Design*, which is also known as *Design for All*, and focuses on user interfaces design without barriers to some disabled users. Therefore it is necessary that the user interface support the use of alternative interaction devices appropriate to the physical capabilities of each user, including a variety of feedback forms, such as: olfactory, gustative, tactile, auditive, and visual of course (UD, 2008).

In this way, Sanchez et al. (2005) proposes a platform for automating the generation of interfaces that comply with usability guidelines, and suitable for rendering on mobile devices with display and processing limitations. Their proposal called "EditMOS", allows to specify user interfaces by means of XML, and to generate interfaces for mobile devices (in XHTML or WML) with equivalent functionality. Prototypical results show that "EditMOS" makes easier the adaptation of regular interfaces to interfaces for mobile devices. A similar approach is presented by Georgieva & Georgiev (2007), the authors specify a methodology to recognize the characteristics of mobile devices, and develop or adapt adequate applications according to its screen resolution, screen mode, supported languages (e.g. markup language, script language, etc.), and supported multimedia files among others.

According to (Su & Yee, 2007) instant messaging applications depend on text as the sole communicative element lacks in the ability to convey non-verbal cues presented in FtF communication. Several research works have conducted to enrich the user experience by integrating behavioural expressiveness such as angry, upset, and other into avatars and emoticons in interface design. Su & Yee (2007) focus on usable interface design for mobile group chat systems considering navigation and visualization to track messages achieving minimal key-pressed and fast message retrieval. In addition the authors incorporate avatars and emoticons to facilitate both the identification between the community members, and the understanding of the message content.

Other good example of improvements for regular instant messaging applications is the research work presented by Ogura et al. (2010); they propose a new approach called *Kairos* which is equipped with three streams of time whose velocities are different. The authors found that users naturally accepted the multiple streams of time without any concrete instructions on how to use each lane.

Another related work is presented by Torsi et al. (2009). The authors propose an interdisciplinary, user-centered approach. They outline a set of design concepts directly based on HCI (Human Computer Interaction) and usability principles oriented to the design of healthcare technologies. Torsi et al. (2009) apply their proposal to the design of the interface and environment of the system "SMART 2", which emerges from several analyses of the patient experience. The "SMART 2" is aimed to take advantage of new technologies to support the different aspects of self-management, which marks a shift for the patients from a passive attitude to a more proactive role in their own care.

DESIGN-REQUIREMENTS FOR USABLE E-HEALTH COMMUNITIES IN MOBILE DEVICES

Problems, Issues, and Controversies

How can interaction with real world entities help people with special needs? Currently this is one of the most interesting questions in HCI (Human-Computer Interaction), c.f. (Hewett et al. 1996). Thus, the HCI community is creating and adapting research methodologies, tools, and infrastructure for specific challenges and opportunities, such as e-health and mobile technologies (Nakhimovsky et al., 2009).

Subsequently, a number of novel approaches oriented to provide users with the possibility of accessing and sharing information about health issues have emerged recently, e.g. e-health communities on social networks. On the other hand, the use of mobile devices to access information has become very popular. People have mobile phones, smartphones and PDAs which they take with them almost everywhere. Mobile devices have become a pervasive part of our everyday lives. According to Pabllo et al. (2008), the use of mobile computing can seriously contribute to enhance the relationships between users (public and professionals) and e-health. Nevertheless, other works (e.g. Harding et al., 2009) claim that interacting with mobile applications and services remains difficult for users because of the impact of mobility on both device capabilities and the cognitive resources of users.

Although current technology advances enhance the hardware capabilities of mobile devices, they are not adequate enough to support the most of web applications interfaces. For example, the iPhone 4 has a 640-by-960 pixel resolution at 326 ppi display (http://www.apple.com/iphone/specs.html, accessed June 22nd, 2010). According to PC Magazine, the iPhone was the most popular phone in the United States from January to October 2009 (www.pcmag.com; accessed December 17th, 2009).

Notwithstanding, in many countries the iPhone is generally a luxury too expensive for most people. In several locations, the most of the mobile phones that people uses have displays ranging from 240-by-320 pixel resolution to 360-by-640 pixel resolution (See for example sub-subsection *Shapping our Proposal*). These differences suggest special adaptations to the interfaces of traditional web applications, even after they have adapted to certain mobile devices.

Another current assumption in e-health communities (based on informal chats and blogs) is the need of having more focus on the interface between the social and the technical, that is, between users and the system (see e.g. Hesse & Shneiderman, 2007). Vronay et al., (1999) states that despite popularity the user interface of current chats consists merely of a list of chatters, a type message text-area, and the text-file history of messages, in fact no many design improvements has been from the initial and very limited, user interface design.

Alike, Suggs et al. (2006) stress the need of methodologies for the adequate design and evaluation and measure of usability aspects in e-health applications.

According to Schusteritsch et al. (2007), a number of factors should be considered when setting up an observation system for mobile devices. Different mobile usability projects will have varying requirements and constraints, and they may change as the project evolves over time. In the same way, these authors say that for most mobile usability studies, enabling natural interaction with the device can be more challenging than in a desktop-based environment because mobile phones come in a diverse range of shapes and run a variety of operating systems.

Additionally, it is necessary to establish frameworks to reduce the gap between e-health and the organizational structures for development and evaluation (Dansky et al., 2006).

Solutions and Recommendations

Shaping Our Proposal

As mentioned before, the objective of this chapter is to see how an e-health community supported by an instant message and blog based application can be improved by enhancing the usability of the user interface. In order to achieve this objective we establish a set of usability requirements oriented, but not limited, to be considered and applied during the design of mobile user interfaces. Foremost, it is very important to mention that we consider two pivotal aspects to naturalize our proposal:

1. The research works reported in the literature (García & Jacobs, 1998, Sanchez et al., 2005; Su and Yee. 2007; Toyoda & Harrison, 2002; Vronay et al., 1999).
2. And the feedback of seventy two participants on the usability of a simulated e-health community in Facebook (c.f. URL: www.facebook.com In order to attain the users' feedback, we follow the Chiasson et al. (2007; 2007) studies to conduct a simple questionnaire considering the incoming points:
    - **Participants:** We ask to one hundred undergraduate students and twenty

Alumni, from the IT and computer science career, to collaborate in this research work. We contact them by e-mail using a confidential data base from the Instituto Tecnológico de Aguascalientes. 62 undergraduate students and 10 alumni accepted our invitation to join our simulated e-health community. The participants consisted of women and men between the ages of 19 and 28 years old.

- **Apparatus:** Our e-health community was set up over the popular public social network Facebook. It is very important to highlight that we do not modify the interface style/design offered by Facebook. We required the user perception about the usability of a current very popular interface for social networks. This information allowed us to achieve a realistic user-centered proposal.
- **Tasks:** We chose "Anorexia and Bulimia" as discussion topics. Then, participants were asked to share information and personal opinions on the proposed subject for 16 days (from 2010 May 5th to May 20th). Participants were asked to access the community, from their mobile phone, at least 10 times during the specified time, regardless of the hour or day, in order to not interfere too much in their personal daily activities.
- **Questionnaire:** We structured the following Likert scale-based survey (Tulis & Albert, 2008; Brace, 2008). For this study we used 6 possible answers: strongly agree (SA), agree (A), do not know (DNK), disagree (D), strongly disagree (SD), and unable to assess (UA). We included an open question in the end to capture the participants' perception about the usability of the interface:
  - The community interface was well-suited for the mobile phone display capabilities.
  - The use and presentation of the scroll-bar was adequate.
  - The design of the interface allows an easy use and understanding of the community content.
  - Accessing the community options of the interface was agile enough.
  - The contents of the posted messages was sufficiently intelligible.
  - The posted information includes data of source and submission date.
  - The community notifies adequately about the information protection.
  - It was easier to identify other community members.
  - The community should have a section for instant messaging (chat).
  - In general terms, what is your opinion about the access, use, and navigation of the community?

We summarized below some of the most relevant observations given by the users, including spontaneous comments mentioned during an informal meeting with the participants after the application of the questionnaire.

- Most of the participants, found not suitable the regular interface of the simulated community to the capabilities of their mobile phones' displays. However, a short number of participants perceived as suitable the user interface. An important point lies in the fact that most participants used mobile phones with displays of 240-by-320 pixel resolution, being the Sony Ericsson P1i (c.f. URL: http://www.sonyericsson.com) one of the most popular mobile between the participants. A small group used mobiles with bigger displays.

- A large number of participants do not consider appropriate the way that interfaces presents the scroll-bars. Furthermore, participants expressed that some times scroll-bars were required but they did not appear. Other important concern was related to the lateral scroll use, which was identified as the most uncomfortable factor during the study.
- The vast majority of the participants found the interface design as limited and inappropriate for mobile devices. Even some of the participants, Facebook regulars, express that the Facebook platform must strengthen its user interface design for mobile devices.
- In general terms, the vast majority of the participants experienced difficulty during the use of the options available through the interface. They emphasize the need of a more agile interface to increase the popularity and use of a mobile on-line application.
- Several participants perceive the visualization of the interface elements as very limited; actually they point that some events are not visible at all, which made the navigation uncomfortable.

Previous observations provide an outline which is consistent with published approaches such as Burak & Sharon, (2004); Pabllo et al., (2008); Sanchez et al., (2005); and Su & Yee, (2007).

In addition, the data given by the survey allow us to observe that the mobile version of the generic interface offered by public platform, as Facebook (URL www.facebook.com), present certain shortcomings in important areas to be covered according to the usability design criteria (e.g. Nielsen, 1999; Sanchez et al., 2005; Su & Yee, 2007). These gaps lead the user to perceive the interface design as limited and poor.

Our Proposed Design Requirements for Usable E-Health Communities

Bearing in mind the knowledge described in the preceding sub-subsection, we establish a set of design requirements specifically oriented to construct usable interfaces for Computer-Based Communication Systems accessed through mobile devices (See Table 1).

The successful implementation of all the previous requirements should lead to a well-designed usable interface. This is important because whether a person is to use a system to its full potential, be it a web application or a traditional computer system, it is essential for them to perceive the system as easy to use and understand as possible, see e.g. (Sanchez et al., 2005; Johnston et al., 2003; Nielsen, 2005). Thus an interface easy to use and interpret could be perceived as that which allows a proper use of the system even for those inexperienced users. In addition, the interface must provide users a sense of control over the system, and to encourage a trustworthy environment between the user and the system.

Considering this, the interface of an e-health community application plays a crucial role in fostering an adequate environment (trustworthy, secure, friendly, and comfortable) between the system and users/members. One way in which this can be done is by specifying the proposed set of usability requirements into design patterns to be methodologically applied into the common stages of the development life cycle; analysis,

Table 1. Proposed usability requirements for e-health communities in mobile devices

Usability Requirement	Description
Interface Dimensions	Limiting the size of the e-health community application's interface is crucial to provide easier navigation to the user. We suggest establishing two different versions for the interface. The *A* version must be oriented to fit in 400-by-700 pixel resolution. These dimensions are within the average screen-sizes of the Top 10 most popular cell phones listed by the PCWorld Magazine (http://www.pcworld.com/reviews/collection/1671/top_10_cell_phones.html; last access November 10th, 2010). Additionally, this pixel resolution may fit even on smart phones such the Blackberry Storm 2 (http://na.blackberry.com/eng/devices/black Berrystorm). Version *B* could be fited within 640-by-960 pixel resolution for novel and vanguard mobile phones such as the iPhone 4 (http://www.apple.com/iphone/specs.htm).
User Representation	Nowadays, it is very common to hear about avatars and emoticons, which refers to a virtual, himself/herself or alter ego, representation of computer users, in the form of a three-dimensional model used in computer games, a two-dimensional icon (picture), or even a one-dimensional username (e.g. Plain text usernames) used on Internet forums and other communities to identify themselves. Figure 2 depicts some avatar examples. Combining multidimensional and one-dimensional avatars to represent the presence of the users/members in the e-health community will allow enriching the user experience by integrating behavioral expressiveness such as happiness, interest, motivation, anger, etc., into avatars and emoticons into the interface design.
Number of Screens and Distribution	We suggest to conform the e-health community application into four principal screens with the following distribution: 1. *The Authentication Screen*: This screen is oriented to authenticate the users/members' identity. The interface must meet the basic design criteria of HCISEC provided in Johnston et al. (2003) which are summarized below: • **Visibility of system status**: The user interface must inform the user about the internal state of the system (e.g., using messages to indicate that a security feature is enabled). The warning or error messages must be detailed but specific including a suggested corrective action for some security problem, and links to obtain additional information or external assistance. • **Aesthetic and minimalist design**: Only relevant security information should be displayed maintaining a simple design. The user should not be saturated with information and options. The user interface must avoid the use of technical terms as much as possible. • **Satisfaction**: The security activities must be easy to realize and understand to the user. In some cases it is convenient to use humor situations, graphics, etc. to present important security concepts to the user in an entertaining manner providing users with a satisfactory and comfortable system usage. • **Convey features**: The user interface needs to convey the available security features to the user clearly and appropriately. Graphics and figures represent a good alternative to convey security features. • **Learnability**: The user interface needs to be as non-threatening and easy to learn as possible; it may be accomplished using real-world metaphors, or graphic icons, e.g. keys and padlocks. • **Trust**: It is essential for the user to trust the system. This is particularly important in a security environment. The successful application of the previous HCISEC criteria should typically result in a trusted environment. According to Johnston et al. (2003), the concept of trust can be adapted for the HCISEC criteria of trust to "*the belief, or willingness to believe, of a user in the security of a computer system.*" The degree of trust that users have in a system will determine how they use it. For example, a user that does not trust a web site will not supply their credit card details 2. *The Welcome Screen*: May contain the name and logo of the e-health community, a list of announcements or news of interest for the community members, links to the other sections, and exit options. 3. *The Blog Screen*: This screen could be divided into two principal parts, one for the blog file, and the other one to write and post comments and information. 4. *The Chat Screen*: The interface could be divided into three parts. The first part could display the chat archive, the second part, shows the list of the connected user/members, and the third part exhibits the specific message from a particular user/member of the e-health community.
Up-Down Scroll	The Up-Down Scroll must be inserted automatically in all elements of the interface as required.
Lateral Scroll use	Even though the Up-Down scroll and the lateral (Right-Left) scroll must be inserted automatically, in mobile devices it is very important to avoid the lateral scroll as possible.

continued on following page

Table 1. Continued

Usability Requirement	Description
Date-Time in Content	Every message, notice, comment, or any other posted information must include the date and time of its creation or issuance. In this way, a better control of the logbook will be achieved.
Number of Turns	According to Vronay et al. (1999), a large number of researches on computer-based communications reveal several common problems experienced by users of chats. A typical problem occurs when a line of text is typed by any participant and envoy to other members of the chat-room, these lines of text are known as *turns*. Following the research of García & Jacobs (1998), multiple conversations occur simultaneously in chat-rooms among the participants, and the number of *turns* tends to make the conversations confused and disengaged. Furthermore this aspects cause rifts related to the loss of timing-specific information because of constant repetitions and corrections to misunderstandings of previous *turns*. The prevalent problem of *turns* in chats could be mitigated by enabling automatic settings to restrict the number of participants in a chat-room, and eliminating previous *turns* from the principal view (but not from the log) maintaining visible a small number of *turns*. Additionally, the number of *turns* is directly related to an adequate implementation and configuration of the Up-Down Scroll.
Effective Message View	According to (Su et al., 2007), it is necessary to determine a threshold if the amount of the chatting users/members of the e-health community exceed the effective reading of the message. The threshold must be dynamic and dependent on the display specifications of each model of the current mobile phones. Nonetheless, it is necessary to inform new participants about the number of users/members connected in the community. Also it is necessary to provide users/members with an option to view the avatars of all the participants, e.g. by adding a scroll bar to the section of contacts in the Chat Screen.
Redundant Clicks	The click-burden must be kept as low as possible. Most of the processes must be transparent for members/users.
Displayable Menus	The use of displayable menus in mobile interfaces seems to provide users/members with the notion of fast access. A fast access to the content adds value to the usability aspect of any application which stresses on effectiveness, efficiency and users satisfaction (Su et al., 2007).
Proper Navigation	It is very important that the interface of the e-health community application adheres to the customs and common navigation styles. But it will be necessary to consider that navigation to mobile devices should be more agile than traditional navigation.

continued on following page

design implementation, and maintenance (see e.g. Somerville, 2004).

CASE STUDY

We use a case study as a proof-of-concept, which is conducted according to the testing methodologies presented in Chiasson et al. (2007). The goal of this exercise was to obtain the users' feedback on the usability of an E-Health Community Interface-Prototype which reflects our suggested design proposal.

For this study we use an interface prototype as apparatus, created using the Adobe Dreamweaver CS5 (http://www.adobe.com/products/dreamweaver/). This prototype was entirely endowed from the knowledge offered by our proposal and was fitted into a 400-by-700 pixel resolution (See *Interface Dimensions* at Table 1). Figure 3 shows the appearance of the principal screens of our suggested E-Health Community Interface-Prototype as follows:

1. The Welcome Screen (See Figure 3A).
2. The Chat Screen (See Figure 3B).
3. The blog screen (See Figure 3C).

In this case, we design the interface's elements using an iPhone-style (http://www.apple.com/iph one) to add a modern look and to make the interface more attractive to the user view.

Table 1. Continued

Usability Requirement	Description
Aesthetic and Minimalist Design	From a computer science perspective, Human-Computer Interaction (HCI) deals with the interaction between one or more users and one or more computers using the user interface of a program (Hewett et al. 1996). Moreover, a pattern represents a proven solution for a recurrent problem within a certain environment, e.g. Design problems of security feedback (Schumacher et al., 2006). A good alternative to generating a well designed user interface consists of combining design patterns with the HCI/Usability principles. In this way, the HCI principles provide *what to do* and the design patterns indicate *how to do it* (see e.g. Muñoz et al. 2009). Applying this strategy, it is possible to achieve a comprehensible interface easy to use and interpret, which is very important for any system but imperative and critical if the adequate use and effectiveness of the e-health community depend on it. The elements of the interface must be interpreted by users/community-members as consistent, predictable, and controllable. Sanchez et al. (2005), highlights the following aspects to consider into the design of mobile interfaces: 1. Use contrasting colors. 2. Make headers look different from regular text. 3. Use at most two different font faces per screen. 4. Avoid blank lines. 5. Limit links to one line. All the html links (Traditionally showed in web pages as an underlined text in blue colour) should not exceed one line, keeping it as short as possible. 6. Limit table width. 7. Provide thumbnails for images. An adequate interface, easy to use, interpret, and manipulate, significantly contributes to reduce the operation-time of the applications. Joining both, the strategy described above and issues such as those established by Sanchez et al. (2005), it is possible to specify each issue as a design pattern. Then easily reify this knowledge into interface's elements through simple programming.
Content Complexity	Due to the nature of the e-health communities it is fairly common to find medical terms into the information managed by the users/members. Although many medical terms will be familiar to the users/members (e.g. names of medications or treatments, disease acronyms, etc.) it is highly recommended to maintain the usage of medical/technical terms as low as possible. Only essential medical information should be displayed through the interface.
Adaptability	It is very important that any e-health community counts with an interface under a barrier-free design (c.f. The Center of Universal Design, North Carolina State University (UD, 2008). The interface must allow the use of alternative interaction-devices adequate to the physic capabilities of the users.
Security	The interface must provide users with an adequate feedback related to the privacy and reliability of the information managed by the e-health community members. Similarly, the identity and the authenticity of the identity, of all the involved parties, must be guaranteed as much as possible.

Figure 2. In order of appearance: (A) An example of One-Dimensional Avatar, (B) An example of Two-Dimensional Avatar, and (C) An example of Three-Dimensional Avatar

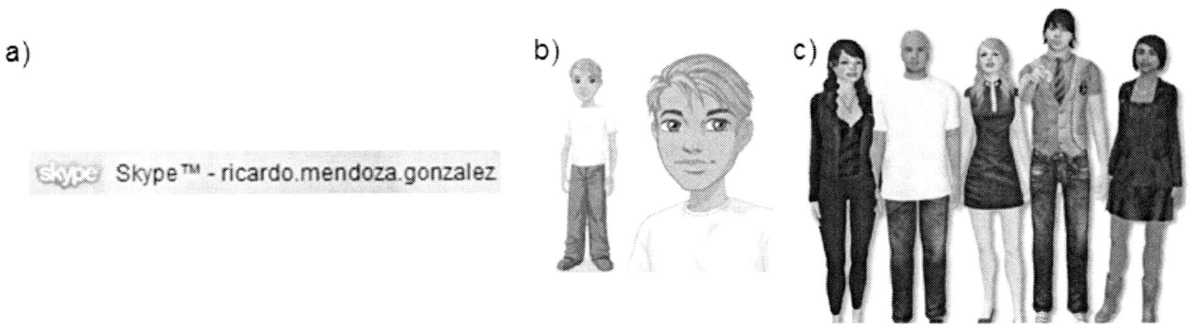

•Courtesy of Skype:
http:// www.skype.com

•Courtesy of Yahoo:
http:// www.yahoo.com

•Courtesy of Facebook:
http:// www.facebook.com

Figure 3. Principal screens of our suggested prototype

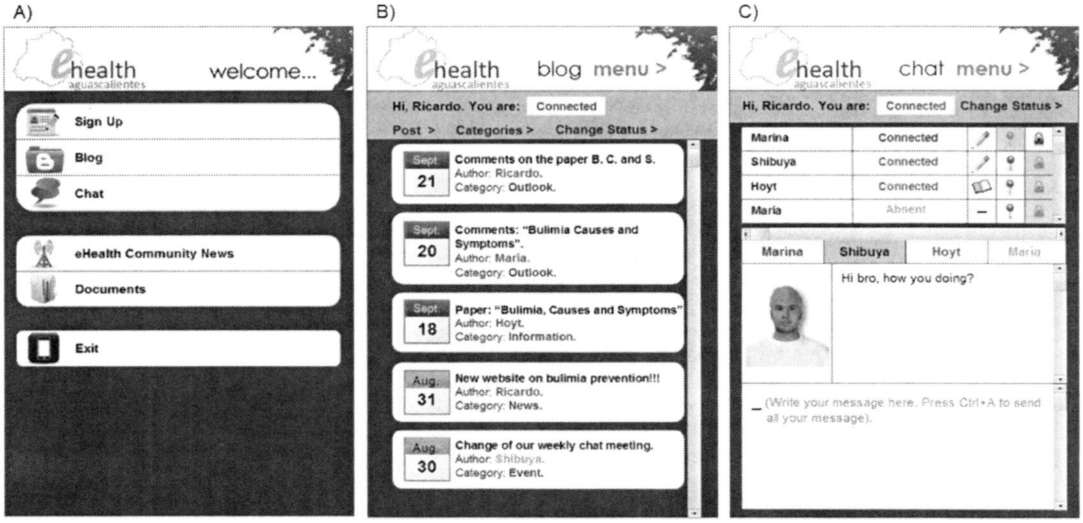

Figure 4. Elements of our suggested chat interface for mobile e-health communities

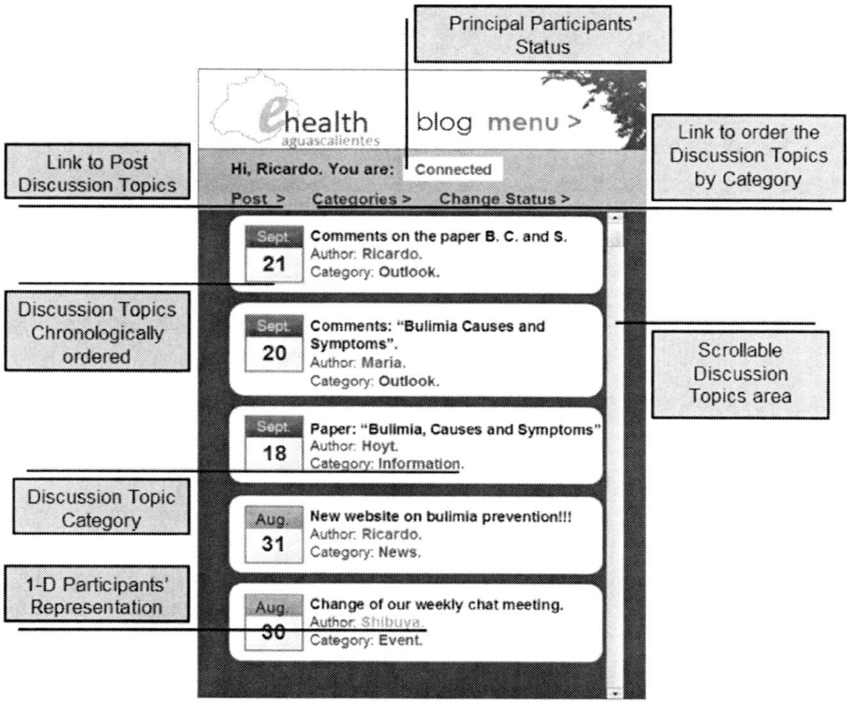

Besides style, the interface was thought to fit in the most common screen-sizes of current mobile phones. We design the interface in order to allow the participants experience the authentication process once, meaning that whether a participant is signed on the chat do not have to be signed again to use the blog.

The following sub-subsections will respectably describe in more detail the chat and blog interfaces.

Chat Interface

To design the chat interface we relied on the proposals of Su & Yee, (2007) and Vronay et al. (1999). We divide the interface in two principal sections as follows (see also Figure 4):

Section A: Display the list of participants represented by means of a one-dimensional avatar (see Figure 2). Also present the current general status of each participant, which is associated to a specific colour: Connected-Green, Absent-Yellow, and Disconnected/Blocked-Red. The section includes an informative icon to depict the current chat-activity of each participant: Pencil Icon- Writing, Open-Book Icon-Reading, and a Dash "–" - Non activity. As well as these elements, Section A presents the options "Block" depicted by the Lock icon, and "Open" depicted by the Key icon. It allows that participants literally block/unblock other particular participants. This action does not affect the general status of the participants, it means a participant may be blocked by a particular user but they stay connected to the chat/blog applications. Finally Section A present a simple greeting to the principal participant and they current status, which may be changed with the option change status, maintaining the binomial Status-Colour mentioned before. Another trait is the addition of a keyboard shortcut instead of using a button to send a collective message. This is suggested to the participant by means of text line embedded in the writing area.

Section B: This section includes the Writing and Reading messages areas. For these areas we configured both the *turns* (see *Number of Turns*, in Table 1) and the Up-Down scrollbars to show seven text-lines at the time. This *turns* configurations is wider than others available (see e.g. Su & Yee, 2007). Section B also includes a "*Tabbed Pane*" element to visualize the participants. This element allows a comfortable navigation reducing the number of redundant clicks (see *Redundant Clicks* in Table 1). The Tabbed Pane is allied to a Lateral Scroll bar (see *Lateral Scroll Use* in Table 1) configured to show four participants at the time thus minimizing the click-burden. The participants are represented by means of a One-Dimensional avatar located at the corresponding section of the Tabbed Pane maintaining their current status represented by the binomial Status-Colour mentioned before and highlighting the participant with whom they are talking. We complement the identification of the participants by including a Three-Dimensional avatar (see Figure 2).

Blog Interface

This interface is less complex than chat interface previously described and is based on the blog interface of the University of Calgary Campus mobile blog (http://www.ucalgary.ca/). See Figure 5. In this case we incorporate a simple greeting to the principal participant and their current status, which may be changed with the option change status, maintaining the binomial Status-Colour mentioned before (see sub-subsection *Chat Interface*). The "*Post*" permits to start a discussion topic and is presented like a simple text link in order to save space. Additionally, we include the option "*Category*" that allow to present the discussion topics ordered by category. In order to facilitate the identification of the discussion categories each category is associated to a particular colour as follows: Outlook-Purple (Personal points of view, opinions, etc.), Information-Pink (Announcements of interest papers, links to websites related to the community topic, among others), and Event-Brown (Meetings for the community members, announcements of social events related to the community's interest). The discussion topics are showed chronologically by default, the description of each topic was thought to be as simple as possible but trying to avoid ambiguity. We include the title of the Discussion Topic, the Author (Represented by a One-Dimensional avatar which maintain the binomial Status-Colour described before), and the category with the above mentioned format.

Data Analysis

In order to analyze our prototype, we invited 50 participants consisting of women and men between the ages of 18 and 30. All the participants were graduates of different areas.

The prototype was evaluated through the same 10 items questionnaire presented in the Section *Shaping our Proposal.*

Figure 6 depicts the participants' perception on the usability of our prototype considering just the Likert-Scale items (i.e., questions 1 to 9 only, not 10). We observe a certain consistency in the responses given by the participants, obtaining very good scores for the highest value in the Likert-Scale used (Strongly agree, *SA*).

In general terms the prototype was widely accepted by the participants. Most of them found that screens could be well adapted to their mobile phones. Furthermore, participants perceive that scrollable areas could be easy to use, and even may contribute to establishing an easier and agile navigation. Also the vast majority of the participants highly accepted the way to represent users, as the combination of One and Three Dimensional avatars greatly facilitate the identification of the participants. Additionally, they described the entire design of the prototype as "pretty cool". It is possible to observe some discrepancies on the feedback obtained by items 5 and 6; this was expected, as there was no much information and blog-content available.

It seems that the proposed set of usability requirements provide a reliable starting point to conform well designed interfaces, at least in the usability field. However, further experimentation and full usability studies will allow us to provide a more detailed analysis.

FUTURE RESEARCH DIRECTIONS

It is well known that the advances in technology increase every day. What is not possible today undoubtedly will be possible tomorrow. Bearing in mind this idea is very likely that the physical capabilities of mobile devices will be improved soon in order to support more sophisticated applications, as e-health communities applications, e-health applications to provide medical assistance to people who live in rural communities (Kulkarni, S., & Agrawal, 2008), or even e-health application for supporting self-management of chronic or mental illnesses (e.g. Torsi et al., 2009; Chang et al. 2008). We think that the approach described in this chapter is directly related with the previous idea, and represents a good alternative for future research, even a starting point for emerging trends.

In order to present a wide view about the viability of the proposed paradigm we briefly describe a soon to come research work. We have initialized an interdisciplinary project with researchers in computer science, medicine, public e-health, and psychology. This is a long term project aimed to compare directly the impact of a FtF support group against an e-health community. To achieve this objective we have structured an activity plan, some of these activities are as follows:

- We are designing our e-health community platform in collaboration with graduate students of the Instituto Tecnológico de Aguascalientes (ITA), and the Universidad Autónoma de Aguascalientes (UAA).
- Researchers in medicine and psychology of the Universidad Autónoma de

Figure 5. Elements of our suggested blog interface for mobile e-health communities

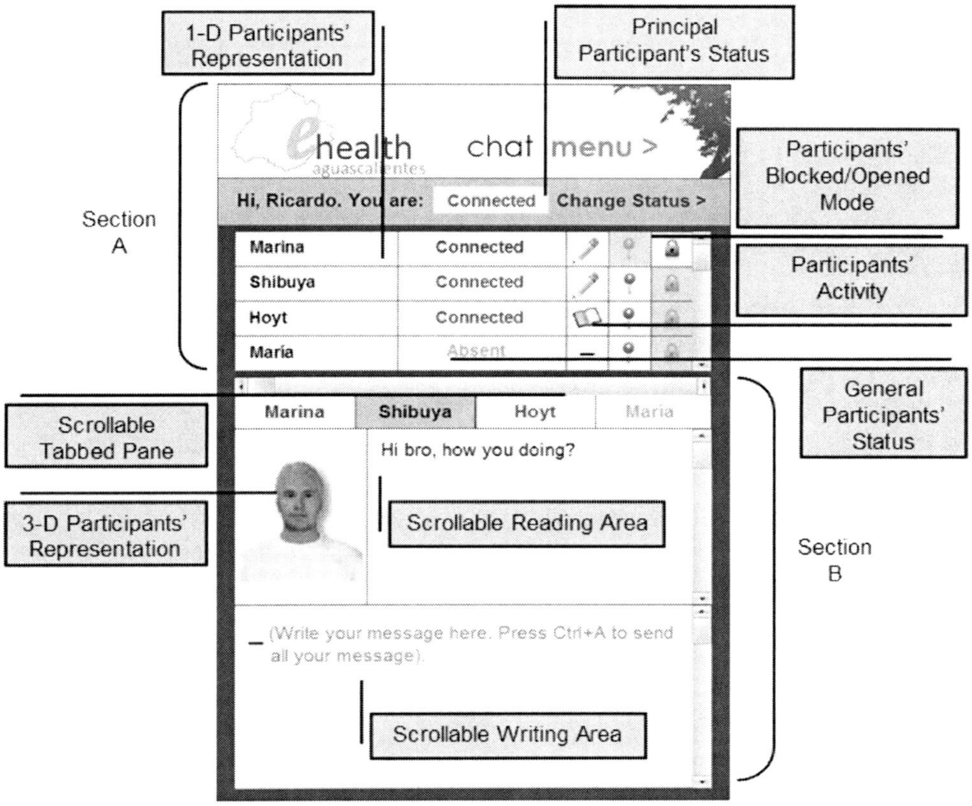

Figure 6. The perception of the participants on our mobile e-health community interface

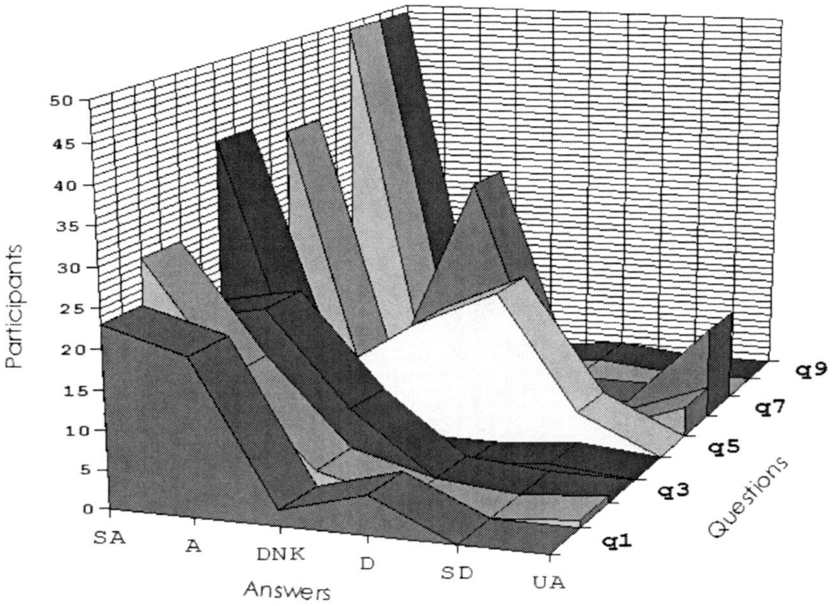

Aguascalientes invited to 340 patients with diagnosed depression to use our e-health community. These patients are currently under a depression treatment in a FtF Support Group.

- The patients will use our e-health community platform over 7 months from November 2010 to June 2011.
- We will evaluate the network quality, and the interactions quality between the community members. These measures will be obtained by means of a highly proved, but non-published, instrument property of researchers of the Universidad Autónoma de Mexico (UNAM). This instrument is regularly used by researches in the Universidad Autónoma de Aguascalientes to analyze FtF support groups. We will adapt this instrument, in conjunction with psychology and medicine researches, in order to properly measure a virtual community.
- Then we will to compare the data obtained by measuring FtF Support Group and the E-Health Community.

It is important to mention that this project is oriented to create an e-health community for traditional web, but we are discussing the adaptation of the interface to mobile devices and apply the proposal described in this chapter. As mentioned before, our project is a long term one and is open to several possibilities and contributions.

In line with the objective of this book, we believe that the emerging unique challenges from e-health, such as the well-designed e-health communities, are vast and involve a wide range of disciplines and approaches. This represents great opportunities for research and scientific collaboration that must face a particular emphasis on methodological issues.

CONCLUSION

In this chapter we summarized a non exhaustive fifteen items list of usability requirements specifically oriented to contribute to bridge the gap between usability and mobile interfaces specifically for e-health communities supported by a chat and blog-based applications.

Although the proposed requirements are specifically oriented to mobile interfaces for instant messaging-blog-based e-health communities, our findings could be applied to a variety of mobile scenarios.

We perform a usability study to structure and support our proposal taking into account the survey-obtained feedback from 72 participants who used their mobile devices to access a simulated e-health community.

Considering other studies performed in previous research (e.g. Welbourne et al., 2009), we note that most of the semi-public current available e-health communities or virtual support groups (mainly created by patients) are set up over commercial social networks platforms, as Facebook (c.f. URL: www.facebook.com), or Twitter (c.f. URL www.twitter.com), being Facebook the most popular. For this reason we select this platform to set up our simulated e-health community (see sub-subsection Case study). The obtained feedback led us to establish a preliminary set of basic yet reliable usability requirements for mobile interfaces, some of which confirm other usability aspects for mobile interfaces reported in the literature (e.g. Sanchez et al., 2005; Su et al. 2007).

We construct an interface-prototype applying our proposed usability requirements, which was analyzed and evaluated by fifty users obtaining a very good acceptance between the participants. They perceive the interface as easy to understand with elements that permit an agile and comfortable navigation. The study also reflects that the prototype provides a very well visualization of the information, specially the instant messages from the chat. In this way, we design the writing and the reading areas of the chat screen to maintain visible seven text lines (*turns*) at the time without scarifying space and design for other essential interface's elements. This configuration also permits an easier tracing of chat's conversations. This could be considered as an interesting point because the *turns* visualization represents a common problem in chat applications. Many authors consider that a good control of *turns* in mobile computer-based communications is provided by the visualization of four to eight text lines, scarifying too much space at the layout when designers choose to configure *turns* to eight text lines (See e.g. Su & Yee, 2007). It is important to note that the suggested configuration of the up and down and lateral scrollbars allows a proper visualization and control of the entire interface and content trying to harness the available space. To complement this idea we include keyboard shortcuts in the writing area of the chat screen in order to save space and use it to enhance other critical aspects, e.g. increasing the *turns* configuration.

ACKNOWLEDGMENT

We would like to acknowledge the valuable contribution of Dr. Francisco J. Álvarez-Rodríguez, and Dr. Jaime Muñoz-Arteaga in early and preliminary stages of this work.

REFERENCES

Ahern, D. K. (2007). Challenges and opportunities of ehealth research. [Elsvier]. *American Journal of Preventive Medicine*, *32*(5S), 75–82. doi:10.1016/j.amepre.2007.01.016

Arunachalan, B., & Light, J. (2007). Middleware architecture for patient care data transmission using wireless networks. In *IWCMC'07* (pp. 182–185). Honolulu, Hawaii, USA: ACM Press.

Brace, I. (2008). *Questionnaire design: How to plan, structure, and write survey material for effective market research* (2nd ed.). United Kingdom/ United States: Kogan Page Publishers.

Burak, A., & Sharon, T. (2004). Usage patterns of FriendZone—Mobile location-based community services. In *MUM'04* (pp. 93–100). Maryland, USA: ACM Press.

Calero, C., Moraha, M. A., & Piattini, M. (2008). *Handbook of research on Web Information Systems quality*. Hershey, PA: Idea Group Inc (IGI).

Chang, Y. J., Liu, H. H., Peng, S. M., & Wang, T. Y. (2008). Potential of mobile social networks as assistive technology: A case study in supported employment for people with severe mental illness. In *ASSETS '08* (pp. 239–240). Halifax, Nova Scotia, Canada: ACM Press.

Chiasson, S., Biddle, R., & van Oorschot, P. C. (2007). *A second look at the usability of click-based graphical passwords*. Best Paper Award, In Symposium on Usable Privacy and Security (pp. 1-12). Pittsburgh, Pennsylvania, ACM Press.

Chiasson, S., van Oorschot, P. C., & Biddle, R. (2007). Graphical password authentication using cued click points. In J. Biskup & J. López (Eds.), *12th European Symposium On Research In Computer Security* (pp. 359-374). Dresden, Germany. Lecture Notes in Computer Science, Springer.

Dansky, H. K., Thompson, D., & Sanner, T. (2006). A framework for evaluating ehealth research. [Elsevier.]. *Evaluation and Program Planning*, *29*(4), 397–404. doi:10.1016/j.evalprogplan.2006.08.009

Garcia, A., & Jacobs, J. (1998). The interactional organization of computer mediated communication in the college classroom. [Springer.]. *Qualitative Sociology*, *21*(3), 299–317. doi:10.1023/A:1022146620473

Georgieva, E., & Georgiev, T. (2007). *Methodology for mobile devices characteristics recognition*. In CompSys Tech'07, (1-6) Rousse, Bulgaria, ACM Press.

Grimes, A., Landry, B. M., & Grinter, R. E. (2010). Characteristics of shared health reflections in a local community. In *CSCW 2010*. Savannah, Georgia, USA: ACM Press.

Harding, M., Storz, O., Nigel, D., & Friday, A. (2009). Planning ahead: Techniques for simplifying mobile service use. In *HotMobile'09*. Santa Cruz, CA, USA: ACM Press.

Hesse, B. W., & Shneiderman, B. (2007). eHealth research from the user's perspective. [Elsevier.]. *American Journal of Preventive Medicine*, *32*(5), 97–103. doi:10.1016/j.amepre.2007.01.019

Hewett, T. T., Baecker, R., Card, S., Carey, T., Gasen, J., & Mantei, M. … Verplank, W. (1996). *ACM SIGCHI curricula for human-computer interaction*. Retrieved October 13, 2009, from http://www.acm.org/ sigchi/cdg/ cdg2.html

Ioannidis, S., & Chaintreau, A. (2009). On the strength of weak ties in mobile social networks stratis. In *SNS'09* (pp. 19–25). Nuremberg, Germany: ACM Press.

ISO International Organization for Standardization. (1998). *International ISO standard 9241-11: Ergonomic requirements for office work with visual display terminals (VDTs) - Part 11: Guidance on usability*. First edition 1998-03-15, Switzerland.

Johnston, J., Eloff, J., & Labuschagne, L. (2003). Security and human computer interfaces. *Computers & Security*, *22*(8), 675–684. doi:10.1016/S0167-4048(03)00006-3

Kulkarni, S., & Agrawal, P. (2008). Smartphone driven healthcare system for rural communities in developing countries. In *International Workshop on Systems and Networking Support for Healthcare and Assisted Living Environments HealthNet'08*, Breckenridge, CO, USA, ACM Pres

Muñoz, J., Mendoza-González, R., Vargas Martin, M., Vanderdonckt, J., & Alvarez, F. (1999). A methodology for designing information security feedback based on user interface patterns. [Elsevier.]. *Advances in Engineering Software*, *40*(12), 1231–1241. doi:10.1016/j.advengsoft.2009.01.024

Nakhimovsky, Y., Eckle, D., & Riegelsberger, J. (2009). Mobile user experience research: Challenges, methods & tools. In Workshop on Human-Computer Interaction and Security Systems, ACM CHI 2009 (pp. 4795-4798), Boston, Massachusetts, USA, ACM Press.

Nielsen, J. (1999). *Designing Web usability: The practice of simplicity*. Indianapolis, IN: New Riders Publishing.

Ogura, K., Matsumoto, Y., Yoshiyuki, Y., & Kazushi, N. (2010). Kairos chat: A novel text-based chat system that has multiple streams of time. In *CHI'10* (pp. 3721–3726). Atlanta, Georgia: ACM Press.

Pabllo, C., Soto, R., & Campos, J. (2008). Mobile medication administration system: Application and architecture. In *EATIS'08*. Aracaju, Sergipe, Brazil: ACM Press.

Sánchez, J. A., Starostenko, O., Aguilar-Castillo, E., & González, M. (2005). Generation of usable interfaces for mobile devices. In *CLIHC'05* (p. 348). Cuernavaca, México: ACM Press.

Schumacher, M., Fernandez-Buglioni, E., Hyberston, D., Buschmann, F., & Sommerland, P. (2006). *Security patterns: Integrating security and systems engineering*. Hoboken, NJ: Wiley.

Schusteritsch, R., Wei, C. Y., & LaRosa, M. (2007). Towards the perfect infrastructure for usability testing on mobile devices. In *CHI '07* (pp. 1839–1844). San Jose, CA, USA: ACM Press. doi:10.1145/1240866.1240908

Sommerville, I. (2004). *Software engineering*, 7th ed. New Jersey, Pearson/Addison-Wesley, Su, D. K., & Yee, V. S. (2007). *Designing usable interface for navigating mobile chat messages*. In OZCHI '07, (pp. 291-294), Adelaide, Australia, ACM Press.

Suggs, S., Cowdery, J., & Carroll, J. (2006). Tailored program evaluation: Past, present, future. [Elsevier.]. *Evaluation and Program Planning*, *29*(4), 426–432. doi:10.1016/j.evalprogplan.2006.08.003

Thompson, D., Canada, A., Bhatt, R., Davis, J., Plesko, L., Baranowski, T., … Zakeri, I. (2006). eHealth recruitment challenges. *Evaluation and Program Planning, 29*(4), 433-440. Elsevier.

Torsi, S., Nasr, N., Wright, P., Mawson, S., & Mountain, G. (2009). User-centered design for supporting the self-management of chronic illnesses: An interdisciplinary approach. In *PETRA '09, Article No. 43*. Corfu, Greece: ACM Press.

Toyoda, E., & Harrison, R. (2002). Categorization of text chat communication between learners and native speakers of Japanese. *Language Learning & Technology*, *6*(1), 82–99.

Tulis, T., & Albert, B. (2008). *Measuring the user experience*. Burlington, MA: Morgan Kaufmann Publishers.

UD Center for Universal Design. (2008). *The universal design principles*. North Carolina State University. Retrieved May 15, 2009, from http:// www.design.ncsu.edu/ cud/about_ud/ udprinci ples.htm

von Niman, B., Rodríguez-Ascaso, A., Brown, S., & Sund, T. (2007). User experience design guidelines for telecare (e-health) services. [ACM Press.]. *Interaction*, *14*(5), 36–40. doi:10.1145/1288515.1288537

Vronay, D., Smith, M., & Drucker, S. (1999). Alternative interfaces for chat. UIST'99, Asheville, NC. [ACM Press.]. *CHI Letters*, *1*(1), 19–26.

Welbourne, J. L., Blanchard, A. L., & Boughton, M. D. (2009). Supportive communication, sense of virtual community and health outcomes in online infertility groups. In *C&T'09* (pp. 31–40). Pennsylvania, USA: ACM Press.

Yee, K. (2003). Secure interaction design and the principle of least authority. In *ACM CHI'2003*. Fort Lauderdale, Florida: ACM Press.

ADDITIONAL READING

Baumann, K., & Thomas, B. (2001). *User Interface Design of Electronic Appliances*. CRC Press.

Beirekdar, A., Vanderdonckt, J., & Noirhomme-Fraiture, M. (2002) A Framework and a Language for Usability Automatic Evaluation of Web Sites by Static Analysis of HTML Source Code. In Kolski, C. & Vanderdonckt, J. (Eds.), 4th International Conference on Computer-Aided Design of User Interfaces, CADUI'2002, (pp. 337-348). Dordrecht: Kluwer Academics Publisher.

Bias, R. G., & Mayhew, D. J. (1994). *Cost-Justifying Usability*. California: Morgan Kaufmann Publishers.

Bouillon, L., Limbourg, Q., Vanderdonckt, J., & Michotte, B. (2005). Reverse Engineering of Web Pages based on Derivations and Transformations. In 3rd Latin American Web Congress LA-Web'05, (pp. 3- 13). Buenos Aires, Argentina. IEEE Computer Society Press.

Chong, Lee J. & McCrickard, S. (2007). Towards Extreme(ly) Usable Software: Exploring Tensions Between Usability and Agile Software Development. In Agile 2007 Conference, (pp. 59 – 71). Washington D.C., IEEE Press

Coulson, N. (2005). Receiving Social Support Online: An Analysis of a Computer-Mediated Support Group for Individuals Living with Irritable Bowel Syndrome. *Cyberpsychology & Behavior*, *8*(6), 580–584. doi:10.1089/cpb.2005.8.580

Dix, A., Finlay, J., Abowd, G., & Beale, R. (1993). *Human- Computer Interaction*. London: Prentice Hall.

Folmer, E., & Bosch, J. (2004). Architecting for Usability; a Survey. *Journal of Systems and Software*, *70*(1), 61–78. doi:10.1016/S0164-1212(02)00159-0

Jacko, J. A., & Sears, A. (2003). *The Human Computer Interaction Handbook: Fundamentals, Envolving Technologies, and Emerging Applications*. New Jersey: Lawrence Erlbaum Associates Publishers.

Lund, A. M. (1997). Another approach to justifying the cost of usability. *Interactions (New York, N.Y.)*, *4*(3), 48–56. doi:10.1145/255392.255403

Nielsen, J. (1997). Measuring the Usability of Reading on the Web. Retrieved January 10, 2009 from www.useit.com/ alertbox/ readingmetrics.html

Nielsen, J., & Landauer, T. K. (1993) A mathematical model of the finding of usability problems. In *Conference on Human Factors in Computing Systems, ACM/IFIP INTERCHI 1993* (pp. 206-213), Amsterdam, The Netherlands, ACM Press.

Preece, J., Rogers, Y., Sharp, H., Benyon, D., Holland, S., & Carey, T. (1994). *Human Computer Interaction*. Massachusetts: Addison-Wesley Publishing Company, Inc.

Rosemberg, R. S. (2004). *The social Impact of Computers*. Elsevier Academic Press.

Stephanidis, C. (2005). *Universal access in health telematics: a design code of practice, Thematic Network (Working Group) "Information Society for All*. Berlin: Springer.

KEY TERMS AND DEFINITIONS

E-Health: According to (Hesse & Shneiderman, 2007; Ahern, 2007), and in practical terms, e-health is the application of Information Technology to healthcare issues.

E-Health Community: Based on literature (Grimes et al., 2010; Welbourne et al., 2009), in general terms are oriented to contribute in the process for improving the quality of life for members of a community suffering from chronic diseases, by means of Information Technologies as the virtual social networks.

Human Computer Interaction: According to (Hewett et al., 1996), from a computer science perspective, human-computer interaction (HCI) deal with the interaction between one or more humans and one or more computers using the user interface of a program.

Mobile Devices: a.k.a. information device, handheld device, handheld computer, consumer electronic, embedded device, or small device. Represent pocket-sized computing gadgets which are small enough to be carried and used during transportation, even wirelessly. Retrieved (in Spanish) June 28, 2010, from URL: http://leo.ugr.es/J2ME/INTRO/intro_4.htm. Universidad de Granada, Granada, Spain.

Universal Design: According to (UD, 2008), universal design focuses on user interface design without barriers to disabled users.

Usability: The standard ISO 9241-11(ISO, 1998, pp. 1-2) defines usability like "Extent to which a product can be used by specified users to achieve specified goals with effectiveness, efficiency and satisfaction in a specified context of use".

User Feedback: According to (Nielsen, 1999), the term *user feedback* is often referred to as any form of communication directed from a system to the user.

Chapter 15
Australian Patient Organizations:
Using Digital Technologies to Engage Health Citizen Communities in Health Policy

Anni Dugdale
University of Canberra, Australia

ABSTRACT

Three citizen health organizations in Australia are examined for how they are consuming information and communication technologies. In particular, how they are actively domesticating and taming the internet as part of their everyday practices and how this is transforming participation, citizenship, and civil society in the health sector are explored. The organizations, Diabetes ACT, Health Care Consumers' Association of the ACT, and AIDS Action Council of the ACT are all located in Canberra in the Australian Capital Territory (ACT). The chapter focuses on how each organization imagines and configures their communities and how this leads to differences in their ways of interacting with the internet.

INTRODUCTION

The last three decades have seen a growing role for patient organizations in the production of health policies and services. These citizen health organizations are increasingly engaging with healthcare professionals and government decision-makers in the health policy arena in order to advance the interests of their constituencies. Changes in terminology from patient self-help group to health-care consumer organization to citizen health organizations abound, reflecting differences between missions, countries and also

DOI: 10.4018/978-1-60960-866-8.ch015

in the time-period during which the organization was established (Brown, Zavestoski, McCormick, Mayer, Morello-Frosch, & Altman, 2006; Callon & Rabeharisoa, 2008; Epstein, 2007). In this chapter the term citizen health organization is preferred and applied generally to describe any organization of patients, users or civil society; although it warrants attention it is beyond the scope of this chapter to take up debates about who counts as a citizen or is entitled to state funded health care (Tyler, 2010), the term citizen here is interpreted inclusively to mean residents or inhabitants. The organizations discussed here can be characterized as made up of people who are not health professionals or certified experts but ordinary people who are concerned with health care, often because of their experience with diseases and health conditions. The increase by lay people in health policy and service design has occurred simultaneously with Government Departments and Ministries of Health looking to the active participation of users of health services, and calling on them to contribute their knowledge to the better governance of health. This chapter looks at three different models for organizing citizen participation in health care adopted by patient organizations in Australia's capital city of Canberra. Of particular interest is how Information and Communication Technologies (ICT) are facilitating and enabling such engagement.

BACKGROUND

Information and communication technologies (ICT) and the internet particularly continue to be portrayed as radically transformative of civil society. The qualities of the internet, its decentralized and distributed character, and the ease and speed with which information can be distributed have been seen by many as forces to strengthen civil society and the participation of citizens in the design of government policies and services (Chadwick & Howard, 2008; Gibson, 2009; Williamson, 2009). ICT have been hailed as democratizing the relationship between health care systems and their consumers. More informed patients it is said will participate as equals in their individual treatment decision-making, and in the transformation of health policies and services (Wathen, Wyatt & Harris, 2008). It has become commonplace in science and technology studies or science, technology and society (STS), to critique such technological determinist arguments that proceed from the characteristics of a technology to social and behavioral change, assuming that the technology itself will drive change (MacKenzie & Wajcman, 1999). This chapter starts from the assumption that there are no *a priori* boundaries between the technical and the social, between technoscience on the one hand and politics on the other, providing neat categories that can be studied as a simple linear matter of the impact of a technology on society (Asdal, Brenna & Moser, 2007). These are conceptual boundaries of our making, found in our imagination, and as researchers we have as Latour suggests (Latour, 1987) followed the actors and their categories. Accordingly, this chapter sets out to show the entanglement in everyday, real-life, empirical situations of human and non-human actors, material and symbolic practices and resources, values and machines. To do otherwise is to dodge our responsibilities as researchers.

The chapter is based on research commenced at the end of 2007 and continuing with interviews through 2008 and beyond that through ongoing website observation to investigate the "consumption" of ICT in third-sector, not-for-profit citizen health organizations. This research project set out to explore how ICT are transforming participation, citizenship, civil society and democracy in the health sector. It investigated the contradictions and complexities faced by contrasting citizen health organizations in Canberra, Australia's capital city located in the Australian Capital Territory (ACT), as they grapple with increasingly ICT mediated participatory processes with governments and health service providers, at the same time utilizing ICT to build and empower their constituencies to intervene in the production of health services and health policy.

The impetus for this work comes in particular from work in STS urging attention to the study of mundane technologies and to the downstream processes of innovation. ICT designers have much to learn from a focus on end-users and their appropriations, or more accurately their re-inventions, of technologies. E-health communities are not merely adopting technologies off the shelf but are actively engaged in the designing of sociotechnical systems as they translate ICT into everyday use. This chapter explores the internet and ICT at the interface between government, health consumers living with chronic illness and three ACT health organizations. These three organizations typify three different modes of re-ordering in response to the challenges and opportunities offered to citizen health organizations by ICT. The core argument is that ICT and the politics of participation are co-productions, that new ways of being citizens, of doing politics, of technically supporting information and communication flows are co-evolving, in other words that they are fabricated in conjunction (Asdal et al., 2007).

The chapter builds on earlier work in STS that looks at how ICT designers imagine users and how consumers matter. It has been inspired by work such as Jeanette Hoffman's, 'Writers, texts and writing acts: gendered user images in word processing software' (1999) that explores how users of early word processing software were imagined differently by different software developers and how this shaped their different constructions of word processing. Ruth Schwartz Cowan's pioneering work on the "consumption junction" drew attention to the active processes involved in the consumption of technologies and called on historians and other scholars to pay close attention to how consumption shapes and reshapes technologies (Cowan, 1987), a tradition that continues to inform more recent work such as Oudtshoorn and Pinch's 2003 edited collection, *How users matter*. Steve Woolgar (1992) coined the widely adopted phrase "configuring the user" to draw attention to the ways in which technology design is constitutive of users. Paralleling these trends in STS, ICT scholars built their own tradition around the concept of "domestication" showing how information and communication technologies from television to the telephone, and from mobile phones to home computers are actively worked together with the routines of everyday life, becoming tamed through specific processes that adapt them to the various practices in different residential and organizational contexts, altering users and their contexts during such adoption processes (Lie and Sørensen, 1996; Silverstone, 1992).

The cases reported here are drawn from a study that utilized a multiple case-study design. The organizations were selected purposively to cover a mix of newer and older and differently sized self-help and advocacy organizations formed to represent people with various health conditions. Three interviews of about 1 hour each were conducted in every organization, one with the CEO and two with other workers or volunteers. Semi-structured interviews were conducted with topics covered including how networked digital ICT had become embedded in the activities of the organization, barriers and facilitators to the adoption of ICT, and the co-evolution of ICT and the activities & goals of the organization. In addition, websites were explored and analyzed along with other relevant documents such as reports and newsletters. This chapter compares three of the seven case study organizations that participated in the study, chosen because they represent different ways of domesticating ICT and the internet into organizational practices, and different ways of imagining and configuring e-health communities.

THE MAKING OF E-HEALTH COMMUNITIES IN CITIZEN HEALTH ORGANIZATIONS

Diabetes ACT is one of the older organizations. It was established in 1967 by mothers of diabetic children as a self-help group to support families living with type-I diabetes and to provide cheaper access to products, later the organization expanded to cover the ever growing number of people living with type-II diabetes. Health Care Consumers Association of ACT (HCCA) was established in 1978 to give a political voice to consumers of health care services and to undertake advocacy by and for consumers in the shaping of health care policies and services. AIDS Action Council (AAC) of the ACT was established in 1985 after a group of gay men living in the ACT met to respond to the AIDS crisis. Their immediate aim was to engage the government in the response to the looming AIDS crisis. Comparing the consumption of the internet in these three organizations can provide insights that might encourage future design practice that better articulates with users and leads to better systems of health citizenship and health activism.

Diabetes ACT

Diabetes ACT has evolved from being a relatively small self-help organization in its early days to seeing itself as potentially a very large association of members organizing to meet the needs of all people diagnosed with diabetes and everybody at risk of developing diabetes living in the ACT. With predictions that this could reach 1 in 4 people in the Australian population this is a large disease based group indeed. Diabetes ACT had about 3000 members at the time of our interview and we found ourselves squeezed between the desk of one of our interviewees and piles of glossy magazines that were about to be posted out to all 3000 of its members. Membership matters to Diabetes ACT and they have successfully negotiated with governments to be able to provide free membership to children diagnosed with diabetes and for the 1st twelve months to anyone newly diagnosed with diabetes who joins the National Diabetes Service Scheme, the scheme through which a government subsidy is provided on certain equipment purchases made regularly by people with diabetes. In fact Diabetes ACT has contracted with the Commonwealth Department of Health and Aging to conduct the National Diabetes Services Scheme (NDSS) on its behalf in the Canberra area. In the ACT which has a population of about 350,000, thirteen thousand people were registered with the NDSS for subsidized syringes, testing agents & equipment. These are supplied and receipts processed through the Diabetes ACT small suite of offices in a decommissioned old high school in the Canberra suburbs that houses a number of community organizations. Diabetes ACT does run a small shop, but the people wanting NDSS products visit one of a network of over 40 pharmacies spread across the region that work with Diabetes ACT as points of supply.

Diabetes ACT provides some health services, employing diabetes educators to run groups and see individuals. Fundraising is a big part of Diabetes ACT's business and there are a number of high profile fundraising events over the year, a gala ball, car raffle and fashion show amongst others which receive considerable support from local celebrities and media. Funds are distributed between its diabetes education, health promotion and prevention programs, with some funds donated for diabetes research. Diabetes ACT is a social enterprise, a not-for-profit company registered under the Commonwealth Corporations Act and complying with the ISO 9000 quality management system standards of the International Organization for Standardization, no mean feat for a social enterprise organization of its size. This brings Diabetes ACT under the regulatory control of ASIC, the Australian Securities and Investment Commission responsible for corporate, market and financial regulation in Australia. Diabetes ACT has a Board of Directors that includes a medical specialist, and people with expertise in management, public relations and health promotion; when we visited Diabetes ACT to conduct interviews there was a staff of about eight employed workers.

Diabetes ACT may have begun as a group that drew on its members' experience to help each other's families learn to live a good life with a child with type 1 diabetes. But this story whilst still a living part of the organization marks its past and differentiates this from the present. This feminized past, a story of mothers and children, care and daily life, emotional and social support where the medical and technical aspects of diabetes treatment are left to the medical professionals, has been transformed. Diabetes ACT now presents itself as a dynamic, hard-edged business, a key player in a war on the "tsunami" of chronic diseases that are threatening to overwhelm our health systems (Interview with CEO). Diabetes ACT pursues patients as members and enters partnerships with the government and with health professionals and researchers based on its membership data. It is seeking empowerment for its members politically by turning the knowledge, desires and experience of its members into effective policy campaigns and the kind of feedback that can be used to improve service provision. This is not so much about individual empowerment, it is primarily the staff that become active in lobbying governments and negotiating with services. What we see here is a well resourced, professional organization that can speak on behalf of a large membership joining together with the health system to wage war on their disease. This is what Brown (2004) called an embodied health movement. In the words of the CEO,

... we need to be looking at how we approach government in terms of our advocacy role to look at public policy. We've got to look at how we can work with government to create more healthy public policy, so that people can basically make the healthy choice the easy choice.

Diabetes ACT, with sister organizations in each of Australia's states and territories, is actively organizing to challenge knowledge and practice concerning the disease, particularly its prevention. It contributed to a submission calling for the banning of junk food advertising on children's television from Diabetes Australia to a Senate Enquiry, lobbies the Australian Government to fund insulin pumps for children with type I diabetes, pressures the health system to improve standards of care for people with diabetes, and presses for the direction of much greater resourcing to diabetes detection, prevention and support for people with diabetes to live healthy lives. Brown used the new terminology of the embodied health movement to distinguish a new kind of civil society health movement aimed at more than health services access, and going beyond traditional constituency based health movements focused on inequalities and the specific interests of a particular categorical group such as women, workers, older people or residents of a particular geographical area. Embodied health movements tend to be more critical of health systems, sometimes critiquing the dominant science and sometimes working with scientists and health professionals to overcome disproportionate responses or oversights in the system. Their mode of organizing is grounded in their personal awareness and the lived experience of their disease.

When entering the online site of Diabetes ACT moving balloons appear and float over a picture of a child running through grass trailing a string of balloons. This was and still is the most sophisticated site visually of the seven citizen health organizations explored in this research project. Moving balloons create an identity for Diabetes ACT and its members about the size of the diabetes community and its relative neglect. " 3.2 million Australians have diabetes or prediabetes", "a third of adults with diabetes are unaware they have the condition", "diabetes is Australia's fastest growing chronic disease" announce a series of pop-up balloons that float onto the site

(Diabetes ACT, 2010). The site itself uses a more standard static format and presents information rather than inviting comment and contribution. The information is a mix of health information and health promotion, news of events, and information about services. Nevertheless, the look and feel of the website maintained by Diabetes ACT is highly professional. It presents as an organization in partnership with health professionals and researchers. Indeed Diabetes Australia, its parent body, includes health professional organizations and research organizations in its membership alongside the state and territory based groups like Diabetes ACT.

Diabetes ACT has a strong focus on being up to date and efficient in ICT adoption, seeing this as essential to a modern, professional organization. It sees this as being driven from three directions, its partnerships with government, the competitive fund raising environment and member expectations, all of which shape the information that is being generated. The emphasis in the organization on membership and fundraising has led to the development of transaction software that visitors to its website can use to join, pay membership fees, or make a donation.

The focus on information on the website and in events and services is on the transmission of up to date information from science and medicine to people diagnosed with diabetes or to the wider community to prevent diabetes. Diabetes ACT is an organization that works within the existing system and biomedical model. Biomedical knowledge has a privileged place in assisting people living with the disease to develop strategies to craft new identities and learn new ways of life. The coping with diabetes page of the website, for example, recognizes that living with diabetes presents more than physical challenges but jumps to a medicalized model offering appointments with psychologists and depression education sessions. Whilst there are support groups where peer to peer interactions are more prominent, these are relatively recent additions to the program and the number of meeting per year is not large.

The co-evolution of ICT and health citizenship at Diabetes ACT has been focused on its role as an active government partner in service provision. Whilst continuing to lobby for a more appropriate and bigger response to the importance of diabetes in Australian society, Diabetes ACT has been able to expand the number of participating pharmacies by using the at-a-distance capabilities of the internet, to take one example. For its members this means an improved service with delivery of NDSS subsidized products occurring closer-to-home and at more convenient locations. The Subagent Connectivity software was developed at the national level but Diabetes ACT played a key role in its implementation nationally and put its participating pharmacies onto the system locally. Instead of patients filling in forms that were mailed to Diabetes ACT by the participating pharmacy, information about supply and the health consumer's unique NDSS identifying number are submitted electronically online. Data is entered directly into a central database with highly secure operating procedures, fulfilling the terms under which the products are distributed, allowing auditing to insure against abuse of the subsidy, and enabling efficient control of stock movements. The number of participating pharmacies has increased from nine to forty and the products now available from pharmacies has expanded to include non-subsidized items like the lances used in blood glucose meters that people were previously driving out to its offices to receive (NDSS manager interview). Here there is a direct link between Diabetes ACT and improvement of a health service to its members through the restructuring of its interface with pharmacies using the internet. Another example of how Diabetes ACT is engaging its membership in service design is in its health education programs. As the provider of services such as diabetes education and nutrition information some funded by government but others funded through its fundraising, Diabetes

ACT surveys its membership every two years seeking their input on issues that are important to them. Responses on the 2006 survey, for instance showed that members were concerned about feet issues so since then group education sessions about feet have been included in the monthly program (CEO interview). Diabetes ACT has co-produced new modes of organizing data and communication involving new software, new servers and significant investment in new hardware, new processes and procedures and new orientations for the organization. By entering partnerships with government and positioning themselves as a capable and effective business organization able to deliver efficiently on service contracts they have positioned themselves as a forefront organization with up-to-date knowledge on the best ways to intervene in one of Australia's biggest burdens of illness. Consultation and quality control using consumer inputs plays a role in this, but so to do the resources, particularly the large membership database with its reach into the diabetes community. We now turn to another citizen health organization where a very different domestication of ICT has occurred and a very different form of health citizenship and conglomeration of ICT strategies, and membership and organizational practices have been co-produced.

Health Care Consumers' Association of the ACT (HCCA)

Health Care Consumers' Association of the ACT is a member based organization, established 32 yrs ago. HCCA sees its main business as engaging health system consumers to participate in policy, planning, and health service decision processes. It has a membership of 70-80 individual members and 15 member organizations. But whilst it is a "membership organization" (CEO interview) it is not acting as an association seeking to represent the interest merely of its members. Rather it seeks to recruit active members who can represent health care consumers across the population, working with them to "identify and develop issues from a consumer perspective". As an HCCA member told us in our interview "we're not there to represent ourselves on committees, we're representing consumers *per se*." Members access, cultivate and mobilize consumer knowledge and feedback, ensuring that the consumer voice is an integral part of local health services monitoring, planning, and policy change. The engagement and participation of local health care users is aimed at making the health system better, at ensuring that user needs are better understood and their requirements better met, that system problems are identified and solved in a timely manner, and that the quality and delivery of health care is subject to continuous improvement. In the words of the HCCA Annual Report of 2008-2009 (HCCA, 2009, p.4):

> *Consumer participation is so important to the quality and safety of health care and this year we have continued to work with ACT Health to provide a consumer perspective on policies and programs through our very strong consumer representatives program and our research.*

HCCA is a formal organization, an incorporated association operating under the Incorporations Act. It is in receipt of Government funding and employs the equivalent of about 6 to 8 staff, some employed part-time and some contracted on specific projects. It has a CEO and is governed by a Board elected at an Annual General Meeting required under the Incorporations Act. HCCA core business is to "identify, train and support consumer representatives" who feed into the ACT health system. Nearly 50 such volunteers were placed by HCCA in the 2007-2008 financial year in positions as consumer representatives on various health committees across the ACT health system, and HCCA held regular meetings and several forums for its consumer representatives to meet together and discuss matters of common concern. Other mechanisms for building a culture of active health citizenship include holding forums on issues of interest to health care consumers. In the year we conducted our interviews for instance, such forums were held on e-health and on Nurse Practitioners who the Government is funding to join General Practice Clinics where they will complement the role of doctors and take on some tasks that would previously have been performed by doctors. Another strategy for representing the consumer perspective in the policy process is to participate in major government planning agendas, making policy submissions that draw on the expertise of members or draw together such expertise from consumers through special forums; in 2007-2008 such submissions were made for example to the chronic disease strategy, the consent to treatment policy, and to the Government's Diabetes Plan (HCCA Annual Report 2007-8).

HCCA has a well developed website that was substantially overhauled in the year we conducted our interviews. For HCCA their website has several different functions. It has a public relations function, to inform members of the public who are increasingly online of their existence, letting them know what the HCCA is doing. It provides some resources and links to empower health care consumers in their dealings with health care services - a list, "10 questions to ask your doctor", information on how to make a complaint, and a pamphlet prepared by the Australian Council for Safety and Quality in Health Care called "10 tips for safer healthcare". It is also a recruiting tool providing contact information and inviting people to get involved. People experiencing problems with health care services sometimes contact HCCA and this begins a dialogue which can results in their becoming members, even consumer representatives. But the HCCA sees the most important function of its website as the building of a community of consumer representatives and members who share information, as a "tool to provide information useful to consumer representatives" and "for our reps and members to feed information to us" (CEO interview). The newsletter produced twice per month and circulated mainly as an email attachment is a key way that HCCA manages the temporal aspects of this task. The newsletter circulates a calendar of events and provides information that is currently pertinent to consumer negotiations with the health care system.

Shortly after our interview HCCA commenced a Blog using Blogger™ primarily to build an online community for its representatives. Despite the patronage of the ACT Health Department, HCCA does not focus on raising money from its membership so its capacity to fund ICT costs are considerably constrained. It relies on external payments and a relationship with external organizations and coordinating between them to manage its web tools. At the time of the interview this was causing problems as staff were limited in being able to change the website to making changes in text. The blog was anticipated as a means of solving this problem, of putting more flexibility into the hands of staff. ICT training could also be a problem, as a small community organization, HCCA has quite a high turnover of administrative staff. With volunteers helping out too there is a constant need for training. Decisions about moving to a Blog and the decisions about how to run it were shaped by these contingencies. Equally, the enthusiasm of the CEO for Web 2.0 played a role as did the Boards willingness to experiment with new ways of moving information, seen as HCCA's core business. Moreover, the Board recognized that in a changing environment innovation is constantly needed to support its consumer representatives. As consumer representatives and members began encountering web 2.0 applications in other settings some became enthusiasts, and as the complexity and formality of government consultation and engagement of consumers, now mandatory, increased, consumer representatives began seeing themselves as needing to match the information processing capacity of the bureaucrats and health professionals they were negotiating with; ready access to digital documents became an important matter of infrastructure development for HCCA.

Posts and comments on the Blog are vetted and then posted by HCCA staff, but posts are written by staff, board members and consumer representatives, occasionally by members. From the beginning the Blog became a valuable and searchable repository of resources and information. In the first six months of 2010 the Blog was being updated regularly with 13 posts made during this time providing detailed reports and links to important resources for events and consultations relevant to health care consumers. Taking a one month period as an example, Blogs posted covered a symposium on GP super-clinics being proposed by the Federal Government, information from a forum held by HCCA where the Government reported on a Ministerial Health Study Tour of the United Kingdom and Scandinavia, a call for people interested in consumer representative training to attend a training session being run by HCCA, a comment giving HCCA's position on the building of a 3rd hospital in response to a media article in which this idea was discussed by the Chief Minister, and a call for contributions about individual's experience with personally held health records in response to a recommendation in the National Health and Hospital Reform Commission.

HCCA are imagining and configuring a community here as a community of practice where the members of the community develop the knowledge, resources, and shared perspectives and positions constitutive of a new kind of expert, health consumer experts. This is not a community of naive users; it is an activist community usually with deep and prolonged experience of the health care system brought together by their desire to translate their experience into effective interventions into health services reform and improvement. It takes training to turn a system-user into a consumer representative. As one of the representatives we interviewed said:

People get in to Health Care Consumers' Association because they've had issues with the health system, some still have issues hanging over them. That's part of the reason why we like to train reps so that when they do become consumer reps on various health committees they don't ... direct their anger, or whatever, at that committee.

HCCA imagines and constitutes a community of expert users of health care services. Users have to be turned into heath care consumer experts who can represent other users. This is achieved through face-to-face technologies like workshops but also through its internet site and blog. The blog looks professional and is moderated by paid staff who ensure that posts written by consumer representatives are not in breach of the confidentiality provisions under which the health policy and services committees operate. HCCA is reaching out to a broad constituency, after all most people use health care services at some time in their lives. The internet and blog present HCCA as a professional organization, and at the same time are constitutive of an interest bloc, health care consumers, with a perspective that can be modelled and displayed. From the size of the membership, despite its openness to new members, it is clear that the new media are not being employed here to build a large membership organization whose credibility in lobbying governments lies in the number of people choosing to belong to it. Organizations like Diabetes ACT recruit many more members but most of these join to receive product discounts and the regular magazine with its local events and national information encouraging readers to live well with diabetes; most members are happy to leave the policy interventions to the professional staff. HCCA by contrast brings together people who are passionate about health care systems and getting the most from them and makes these individuals into policy activists and policy experts. The internet, the blog and the newsletter are integrated into the socio-material mechanisms for turning experience as health care service users into expertise to act as representatives of consumer interests, expertise that is responsive to consumers on the one hand but also to the policy process and the policy makers and service managers on the other. Listen for example to Russell, a longstanding policy activist in HCCA, weave together a narrative of personal experience and expert understanding of the policy constraints of the health care arena in a 2008 blog post that preceded a forum for consumer input being held by the National Blood Authority (HCCA, 2010):

I have been a frequent user of blood and blood products in the past – at one stage receiving as many as six units a month as my enlarging spleen started to consume all the blood my bone marrow could produce. ... As a result I have followed the evolution of blood service arrangements in this country with some interest. The latest development is that private hospitals in NSW are to be charged for the blood that they use. ... This will be seen by some as exploitation of donors (including my daughters) who give blood freely to help the health system do its job. ... Blood is often used inappropriately in health care when other therapies would be more cost effective and probably would produce better outcomes for consumers. So at a time when threats to the blood supply are looming larger than ever before, it makes a lot of sense to set some price signal... (HCCA Blog)

The effectiveness of consumer representatives relies on a claim to legitimacy based not on medical expertise, nor on the numbers of individuals represented, but on skill at building a new kind of knowing, a skill of fashioning a narrative of knowing the perspective of the user, and of negotiating with and working through consensus decision-making processes with other kinds of experts to produce policies and ensure quality. The blog and other internet resources produced by HCCA model such narratives and are thus integral to the informational processes that reshape experienced users into expert consumer representatives, at the same time constituting the representatives as consumer representatives by making a spectacle of their accountability in a public forum.

AIDS Action Council of the ACT

The AIDS Action Council of the ACT (AAC) was formalized and incorporated in 1985 with the ideal of creating a 'world where no one gets newly infected with HIV and those that have HIV enjoy a good quality of life' (Tabone, 2005); today its aims are supporting the communities most impacted by HIV/AIDS (AAC, 2008), 'minimizing the social and personal impacts of the disease' and preventing transmission of the virus (AAC website, About Us). In Australia at the time of the formation of AAC the gay male community was the community most impacted by the HIV/AIDS epidemic, and many in the Gay community recognized that their biggest enemy in confronting the epidemic was discrimination, homophobia, ignorance and stigmatization. AAC was established as a grassroots community organization for a community in crisis and under siege. It quickly became a politically important organization whose partnership was recognized by Australian governments as integral to an effective response to the epidemic. With many in the gay community knowing people diagnosed with HIV/AIDS and people who had died with the disease, joining AAC became an imperative for many in the gay, lesbian, bisexual, transsexual (GLBT) and communities. As the community development team leader put it,

..if you felt part of that community you would be a member of a council like the AIDS Council ... there was a sort of civic sort of thing that you become a member

In 2006 the AAC had 128 members and support from 92 volunteers. For year ending 30 June 2007 its budget, largely sourced from government was $925,480. The AIDS Action Council is contracted by the ACT Government to run peer support, volunteer practical support, and counseling services aimed at minimizing the "social and personal impacts" of HIV/AIDS, and to develop and disseminate education and prevention programs and in particular programs aimed at behaviour change amongst communities with higher HIV transmission rates. AAC also hosts People Living with HIV/AIDS (ACT) which is constituted as a political and advocacy organization.

The AIDS Action Council of the ACT (AAC) employs about 12 fulltime equivalent staff. The organization, being a non-profit, was, like HCCA, able to choose to become an incorporated association under the Associations Incorporation Act of the ACT Government. This legislation is designed for the regulation of non-profit community organizations and is less onerous than supervision by ASIC, the Australian Securities and Investment Commission responsible for corporate, market and financial regulation in Australia. AAC is run by a Board, and being an organization that receives funds from the ACT Government is required to regularly review and improve its governance standards. It is a well run organization with a budgetary surplus and rigorous standards of transparency and accountability. The General Manager and a staff representative sit on the Board alongside a president, secretary, treasurer and 3 ordinary members elected at the Annual General Meeting. Board members tend to be drawn from HIV/AIDS affected communities but also to bring the legal, financial and management skills well represented in those communities to the Board. Information and Communication Technology is highly valued in the organization, with staff ICT skill and web development investment reflecting this priority. In this way it is like the other organizations reported on in this chapter, all three organizations shared a high awareness of ICT and all three gave priority to the development of their internet infrastructure.

The communities served by AAC include people living with HIV and their families and friends, the GLBT communities, injecting drug users, and sex workers and their clients. These are the communities most impacted by HIV/AIDS and the communities at the heart of AAC continue to develop as the profile of the epidemic changes. For instance with treatments now available many people living with HIV are living longer lives and this community now includes significant numbers of women, immigrants, children, and haemophiliacs. Young men who have sex with men also constitute an important community with growing rates of new diagnoses and different behaviours and forms of identity that do not automatically link them to the AAC.

AAC imagines and configures its health community very differently from either Diabetes ACT or HCCA and these differences have shaped its strategies for the domestication of ICT and the building and support of its online communities. For the AAC, communities are tangible, living cultures where people interact on a regular basis. Communities change over time and this requires organizational strategies to engage them with the AAC and invigorate them as health activist communities. AAC employs a community development worker and sees his job as empowering communities to take control, "to actually take hold of issues and run with them themselves" (AAC employee). This is neither a community enacted as an association of members, nor a community of practice made up of health policy activists. The communities that the AAC imagines and helps configure are shaped by the particular history of Australia's Gay community as an outsider community that both celebrated its difference through activities such as Sydney's Gay and Lesbian Mardi-Gras and defined itself as a sexual minority struggling for recognition of equal human rights, whilst being vilified and stigmatized by mainstream organizations as a life-style choice that threatened the Australian nation. This outlaw status was exacerbated by the AIDS/HIV epidemic; the AIDS epidemic was used by the anti-homosexual lobby to claim that homosexuality was unnatural, un-Godly and immoral in campaigns against law reform to end discrimination against gay men. The gay community, significant health professionals and successive Australian Governments recognized the need to enter partnerships and work together to counter such prejudice for transmission prevention strategies to be successful and in order to provide effective, non-discriminatory health care. This is recognized by AAC's community development team leader when he talks of the recent re-emphasis on community development at AAC:

Until 2000 there was still a lot of priority, politically (we were) still a very important agency... we've been trying to change the focus of our health promotion work from education to community development... one of the side effects of that disengagement with the gay community and the AIDS councils is that gradual increase in infections...

The specificities of its history have oriented AAC towards community development, the strengthening of gay, lesbian, bi-sexual, transsexual, queer, injecting drug user (GLBTQI), sex-worker and other relevant communities, the enhancing of their capacity to counter such homophobic and other toxic social contexts at the individual and community levels, and the building of capable peer support networks for peer-to-peer promotion of safe sex and for care and support for people living with and impacted by HIV/AIDS.

Vibrant communities of confident, informed, and capable people are built from the ground up through information groups, 'coming out' sessions, and major annual events including a candlelight memorial, a fair day held as part of the SpringOut Festival organised by a coalition of GLBTQI organizations, World AIDS Day and the World AIDS Awareness Week. These are long term community events, part of the established local GLBTQI calendar. But AAC is also responding to community changes. Changes in the epidemic itself and in particular in the effectiveness and, in Australia, widespread and affordable access to antiretroviral therapy has meant, as several of our interviewees reported, that AIDS has been less of a priority in the gay community and that this has led to a declining membership of AAC. Young people in particular have not identified with AAC yet young gay men have emerged over the last few years as a group with comparatively higher HIV transmission rates.

In order to address this lack of identification with AAC amongst young people, the organization launched a community development project to bring young GLBT people together around the creation of a publication including short fiction, poetry, non-fiction, cartoons and artwork about being young and same sex attracted in Canberra. This enabled a group of young people to come together, form friendships and literally make a sub-community of gay and lesbian youth who were out and confidently able to speak about their sexuality and issues such as HIV/AIDS. This more active group reached out more broadly to GLBTQ young people and to groups such as Bit Bent, a GLBTI youth group started by a recreation studies student to build participation in the 2002 Gay Games, and Jellybabies, a campus based GLBT student group, strengthening the links between GLBTQ individuals, youth oriented community groups and AAC. As the community development team leader reflected:

We launched In Our Own Write ... a community development project where the entire project was driven by young people, it got young people involved in all sorts of different ways. ... Before we did that project there were very few links that we had with ... some of the youth groups, we didn't really have very strong links with those groups,... young people that hadn't been involved in the community before now had some contacts and links and so on. So there's a book with their name in it but there was a whole lot of other outcomes from that project more than just the book.

Community here is being restored as a place of inclusion, of face-to-face encounters, a place where people are drawn together in processes of mutual support and solidarity. Community development projects for AAC nurture belonging and a sense of identification with a real community, and are fed by the social justice rhetoric of the social movements of the 1970s and 80s that shaped AAC's early years. In the words of Stephanie Buckle, retiring as AAC's counsellor after twenty years (AAC, 2010):

It was inspiring to me in the early days to see the ways in which the community came together to support gay men who had HIV, and to stand together to fight discrimination and prejudice. For all the horror and sadness that HIV brought, and the devastation to the gay community, it cannot be denied that it also provided a context in which the community claimed the right to be out and visible, and found strength from mutual support (Buckle, 2010).

The community that arose organically in the face of the early HIV/AIDS maelstrom is to be treasured and has to be continuously reinvented, cultivated and recreated in the new millennium of the hyper-individuated and fragmented society. This is the refurbishment of community as a realm of non-formal, person-to-person, give-and-take relationships that can provide the social glue that makes mutual support and advocacy possible, and hence hopefully lead to a decline in the higher rates of HIV/AIDS transmission experienced by young gay men.

The internet is often associated with community decline, with the breakdown of the processes that draw people into what are assumed to be the more substantial, embodied interactions that occur in the flesh with other family members, neighbours and the local community. This discourse of community decline argues for a restoration of community values, juxtaposing them to individual libertarian values that espouse the liberalising of heterosexual and gender normativity, the white picket fenced household where marriage is "between a man and a woman" and children are wholesomely raised, boys to become real men and women to be their handmaids. Not surprisingly the AAC does not posit community in opposition either to individual freedoms or to the online world. Rather, the networked online world is a part of its community space and it is actively engaged in community development with online communities. The internet has replaced bars and nightclubs as "the number one way of finding a sexual partner for gay men" (AAC community development team leader), indeed the ACT was the first place in Australia where this occurred, hence AAC has followed its community online:

we have campaigns on Gaydar, the Gaydar website which is one of the most common I think in Canberra for meeting sexual partners but also for... I think men are also using it to get involved in the community and that sort of thing. We use that and that works actually fairly well for attracting people into our programs (AAC community development team leader),

The website of the AIDS Action Council of the ACT reflects and engages directly with this building of a tangible 'our community', bringing the diverse groups affected by HIV/AIDS together into a single online space. The website reaches out to bring people together in the face of messy divisions. For this community is not homogenous and has often been wedged apart by bitter public policy entanglements fought against a background of extreme and sometimes unexpected adversity.

In the centre panel of its website AAC calls up its community, as I write this wishing 'our community' Merry Christmas 2010 to celebrate its 25th year. This is closely followed by the coloured buttons for different visitors to the website familiar from many portals – 'people living with HIV/AIDS', 'gay lesbian bi trans', 'students and teachers', 'health care workers', 'journalists and media' to name a few. The first of the above to take one example is linked to the home page of People Living with HIV/AIDS (PLWHA) which identifies as part of a *world wide movement to empower and support people living with HIV/AIDS and their partners, friends and families to live full, creative and meaningful lives free from fear, ignorance and prejudiceinformation (AAC website)*

From here you can link to community services provided by AAC including peer networks, counselling, complimentary health services, and home assistance; take part in the 'experiences of HIV seroconversion study', a government funded study being conducted by three universities in conjunction with state based AIDS Action Councils; participate in the Tracking Changes Survey, a survey of HIV treatments being run by the Australian Research Centre in Sex, Health and Society; find out about the Positive Support groups next meeting; learn about the latest information on treatments or the best chat groups online; get practical support from the Trevor Daley fund to help with bills and treatment costs; or link to the National Association of People Living With HIV/AIDS (NAPWA) "Treataware" online program which

aims to support people living with HIV make informed decisions about their treatments, and support their partnerships with doctors and clinicians (AAC website – Treataware).

This community of people living with HIV/AIDS is online, is accessing health and other services over the internet, and is being reached out to over the internet by researchers, support services, and government funded information and service providers with online programs. The 'gay lesbian bi trans' provides a pathway to link to the events, groups and activities of the wider sexuality identified communities in a city with a relatively high population turnover and a steady stream of new arrivals coming for government jobs, to attend university, and with Defense Force rotations, these being the city's main industries. There is an online community blog hosted by AAC for queer youth with bulletin boards such as 'meeting people', 'Wat U look for in a guy', 'law reform', and 'music, books, movies', with over 200 regular contributors and many more logging in anonymously as 'guests'. You can find out about the bush dance, the springout fair day, the Gay and Lesbian Qwire, Pink Tennis Club and so forth. And you can link to other online communities such as personals sites, and the email list ACT Queer. This is a more diffuse community than that imagined and configured by HCCA and constitutes a distinctive involvement in community-building around connections that foreground identity politics unlike the approach of Diabetes ACT. Here a space for belonging is being performed into existence, AAC is engaged in fabricating and crafting an inclusive community where there are no apologies or special pleading for equality, but in the words of a 1990s Act Up (AIDS Coalition to Unleash Power) Australia slogan 'we're here, we're queer, get used to it', and that means online as well as offline.

FUTURE RESEARCH DIRECTIONS

What is the community being imagined and instantiated through the practices of citizen health organizations and how are communities being made-over as online activities increasingly become worked into those practices? More research is needed into how communities are 'being done', how they are being brought into existence in the increasingly technoscience spaces that citizen health organizations are becoming. Helen Verran talked about technoscience and its absent imaginaries in her 2001 book *Science and an African Logic*. The book begins with an account of teaching children to measure length and of how everyday practices of doing number in Yoruba culture could not be accommodated in western imaginaries of measurement. Verran was opening a space for critical discussion of the specificity of Western technoscience imaginaries, using the term imaginary to indicate a particular domain to be opened up for investigation. The domain of the imaginary is not be conflated with the real world technoscience seeks to represent, nor with the symbolic realm of the representations of that reality technoscience produces. An imaginary is not a mental conceptual map of something that somehow pre-exists it; it emerges through and in practices that clot together human actors, natural materials, technical devices, and ways of talking, representing and symbolising (Verran, 2001, pp. 1-47). The relationship between the internet, citizens, and citizen (patient) organizations needs to be seen in this way, as an arena for investigation where citizens and indeed the very meaning of citizenship are being made. How communities are imagined and fabricated through the ICT practices of citizen health organizations is not simply a technical matter of bringing about the most effective and efficient mode of engagement with 'the community'. Rather, the design of ICT for and with citizen health organizations will shape what comes to count as community, as citizenship and as democracy. The intersection between imagined communities and the technoscientific imaginaries of ICT is calling out for ongoing investigation. Here it is worth keeping in mind that democracy is not a noun – something a nation is or is not, but a verb – a constant becoming of openness and exchange through which governments become open to the influence of citizens and citizens have the capacity to exert such influence (Rancière, 1999). More research is needed into the imaginaries of community and how they are being done in and with ICT and citizen health and other civil society organizations. In addition, something that has been beyond the scope of this chapter, research is needed to trace the impacts and realignments between the performative power of sustaining e-health communities and the state. As is often claimed there may be a potential here to reinvigorate democracy, but its realization is an empirical matter requiring case by case research.

CONCLUSION

In conclusion, this chapter has attempted to do four things. First it has reported on a detailed empirical investigation into how the new information and communication technologies and in particular the internet are becoming part of the everyday practices of citizen health organizations, sometimes called consumer health or patient organizations, at three field sites in Australia. Second, it aimed to put forward the argument that an understanding of socio-technical change requires detailed investigation of the downstream social and material processes through which new technologies become part of the everyday life of organizations, and that relatively mundane and possibly unnoticeable distinctive values and features of organizations come to be performed and re-performed through new socio-technical forms. Third, the chapter has sustained a focus on how each organization imagines and configures its community through its unique domestication of the internet. Finally, it has sought to contribute to conceptualisations of citizenship and society, politics and policy that foreground the *making* of citizenship not as something that we are, or that we have, or that is conferred legally by the nation state, but that is the complex outcome of material-semiotic-socio-technical dynamics.

ACKNOWLEDGMENT

Many thanks to Catherine Settle for her diligence as a research assistant, the many interviewees, the University of Canberra for a small grant, and science studies at Lancaster University for all kinds of support during the development of the chapter.

REFERENCES

AAC. (2008). *AIDS Action Council Annual Report 2007 – 2008*. Retrieved April 2011, from http://www.aidsaction.org.au/ content/publications/annual_reports/

AAC. (2010). *AIDS Action Council of the ACT website*. Retrieved December 2010, from http://www.aidsaction.org.au

Asdal, K., Brenna, B., & Moser, I. (2007). The politics of interventions: A history of STS. In Asdal, K., Brenna, B., & Moser, I. (Eds.), *Techno-science: The politics of interventions* (pp. 7–53). Oslo, Norway: Unipub Oslo Academic Press.

Brown, P., Zavestoski, S., McCormick, S., Mayer, B., Morello-Frosch, R., & Altman, R. G. (2004). Embodied health movements: New approaches to social movements in health. *Sociology of Health & Illness*, *26*(1), 50–80. doi:10.1111/j.1467-9566.2004.00378.x

Buckle, S. (2010). *Farewell Stephanie Buckle*. Retrieved December 2010, from http://www.aidsaction.org.au/ content/events/25_jubilee/farewell_stephanie_buckle.php

Callon, M., & Rabeharisoa, V. (2008). The growing engagement of emergent concerned groups in political and economic life: Lessons from the French Association of Neuromuscular Disease Patients. *Science, Technology & Human Values*, *33*(2), 230–261. doi:10.1177/0162243907311264

Chadwick, A., & Howard, P. N. (Eds.). (2009). *Routledge handbook of internet politics*. New York, NY: Routledge.

Cowan, R. S. (1987). The consumption junction: A proposal for research strategies in the sociology of technology. In Bijker, W., Hughes, T., & Pinch, T. (Eds.), *The social construction of technological systems*. Cambridge, MA: MIT Press.

Diabetes, A. C. T. (2010). *Diabetes ACT: Rising above diabetes website*. Retrieved September 2010 from http://www.diabetes-act.com.au

Epstein, S. (2007). Patient groups and health movements. In Hackett, E. J., Amsterdamska, O., Lynch, M., & Wajcman, J. (Eds.), *New handbook of science and technology studies*. Cambridge, MA: MIT Press.

Gibson, R. K. (2009). New media and the revitalisation of politics. *Representation*, *45*(3), 289–299. doi:10.1080/00344890903129566

HCCA. (2008). *Annual report 2007 –2008: Health Care Consumers' Association of the ACT Inc*. Retrieved November 2010, from http://www.hcca.org.au

HCCA. (2009). *Annual report 2008 –2009: Health Care Consumers' Association of the ACT Inc*. Retrieved November 2010, from http://www.hcca.org.au

HCCA. (2010). *Health Care Consumers' Association of the ACT Inc. website*. Retrieved November 2010, from http://www.hcca.org.au

HCCA. (2010). *Blogspot*. Retrieved November 2010, from http://hcca-act.blogspot.com/

Hoffman, J. (1999). Writers, texts and writing acts: gendered user images in word processing software. In MacKenzie, D., & Wajcman, J. (Eds.), *The social shaping of technology* (2nd ed.).

Latour, B. (1987). *Science in action: How to follow scientists and engineers through society*. Cambridge, MA: Harvard University Press.

Lie, M., & Sørensen, K. (Eds.). (1996). *Making technology our own? Domesticating technology into everyday life*. Oslo, Norway: Scandinavian University Press.

MacKenzie, D., & Wajcman, J. (Eds.). (1999). *The social shaping of technology* (2nd ed.). Buckingham, UK: Open University Press.

Michael, M. (2006). *Technoscience and everyday life: The complex simplicities of the mundane*. Milton Keynes, UK: Open University Press.

Rancière, J. (1999). *Disagreement: Politics and philosophy*. Minneapolis, MN: University of Minnesota Press.

Silverstone, R., & Hirsch, E. (Eds.). (1992). *Consuming technologies: Media and information in domestic spaces*. London, UK/New York, NY: Routledge. doi:10.4324/9780203401491

Tabone, J. (2005). *Joey Tabone's speech at the 22nd International AIDS Candlelight Memorial*. Retrieved April 2011, from http://www.aidsaction.org.au/ content/events/ candlelight_memorial/2005/ presidents_speech.php

Tyler, I. (2010). Designed to fail: A biopolitics of British citizenship. *Citizenship Studies*, *14*(1), 61–74. doi:10.1080/13621020903466357

Verran, H. (2001). *Science and an African logic*. Chicago, IL: University of Chicago Press.

Wathen, N., Wyatt, S., & Harris, R. N. (2008). *Mediating health information: The go-between in a changing socio-technical landscape*. Basingstoke, UK: Palgrave Macmillan.

Williamson, A. (2009). Revitalising politics from the ground up: The role of digital media in promoting citizen-led democratic renewal. *Representation*, *45*(3), 301–311. doi:10.1080/00344890903129707

Woolgar, S. (1992). Configuring the user. In Law, J. (Ed.), *A sociology of monsters: Essays on power, technology and domination*. London, UK: Routledge.

KEY TERMS AND DEFINITIONS

AIDS Action Council (AAC): The AIDS Action Council, also known as the AIDS Action Council of the ACT, is a community organization serving the people of the ACT. It was formed as a grassroots response to the HIV/AIDS crisis and is affiliated with the Australian Federation of AIDS Organisations.

Australian Capital Territory (ACT): Australia is a federation of 6 states and 2 territories. Known as the ACT, the Australian Capital Territory is home to Canberra, Australia's capital city and seat of the Federal Government of Australia. The ACT has a population of just over 350,000. It has its own elected government responsible for government services including hospitals, public health services, schools, environment and resource management, and transport and municipal services.

Diabetes ACT: Diabetes ACT is a not-for-profit organization aiming to overcome diabetes in the ACT community. It undertakes advocacy and health promotion, supports research and provides education and support services for people with diabetes, their families and those at risk.

Health Care Consumers' Association (HCCA): Health Care Consumers' Association, also known as Health Care Consumers' Association of the ACT, builds direct consumer involvement in health decision making. It works with all health services and policy makers in the ACT to ensure they are responsive, respectful, accessible and affordable to all.

Science, Technology and Society (STS): STS known either as science technology and society or science and technology studies is a community of scholars interested in understanding how science, technology and medicine develop and interact with their social contexts.

Chapter 16
European E-Health Framework: Towards More "Patient-Friendly" Healthcare Services?

Korinna Zoi Karamagkioli
Alexandra University Hospital, Greece

Evika Karamagioli
Gov2u, Greece

ABSTRACT

European health systems are under mounting pressure to respond to the challenges of population ageing, citizens' rising expectations, migration, and mobility of patients and health professionals. New technologies have the potential to revolutionize healthcare and health systems and to contribute to their future sustainability. However the organizational and regulatory environment of e-health has not progressed as rapidly as technology both in national and European level. The key issue in the European sphere is whether and to what extent it interferes with public health policy and should be treated separately from the more "traditional" healthcare. The proposed chapter will define e-health from a European perspective, present the different steps of the European policy in the field, insist on the organizational and regulatory issues that arise and discuss drives and barriers towards achieving pan European "patient-friendly" healthcare services.

INTRODUCTION

Health has a central part of the European policy agenda. Under Article 152 of the Treaty establishing the European Community (Article 152), the EU has a mandate to complement the work of national health systems. This work focuses mainly on protecting people from health threats and disease, promoting healthy lifestyles and helping national authorities to cooperate on cross-border health issues. By 2050 the number of people in the EU aged 65+ will grow by 70% and the 80+ age group will almost treble. This demographic shift could cripple national health services unless

DOI: 10.4018/978-1-60960-866-8.ch016

radical changes are made. Innovative, dynamic healthcare systems, enabled by, and in combination with, new technologies, offer solutions to these mounting pressures. "New technologies have the potential to revolutionize healthcare and health systems and to contribute to their future sustainability," the strategy states (ICT Results, June 2010).

"E-health, genomics and biotechnologies can improve prevention of illness, delivery of treatment, and support a shift from hospital care to prevention and primary care. E-health can help to provide better citizen-centred care as well as lowering costs and supporting interoperability across national boundaries, facilitating patient mobility and safety" according to the European Commission's October 2007 Communication White Paper - Together for Health: A Strategic Approach for the EU 2008–2013 (COM (2007) 630 final).

Based on a recent study (se2009.eu)100,000 adverse drug events could be avoided yearly through Computerised Physician Order Entry and Clinical Decision Support, 5 million prescription errors could be avoided yearly through the use of ePrescriptions, 11,000 diabetic deaths could be avoided every year by the use of Electronic Medical Records and Chronic Disease Management and 9 million bed-days could yearly be freed up through the use of Electronic Health Records, corresponding to a value of €3,7 billion.

At EU level, the introduction of e-health services is facilitating access to healthcare, whatever the geographical location, thanks to innovative telemedicine and personal health systems (ICT for better Healthcare in Europe, 2010). E-health is also breaking down barriers, enabling health service providers (public authorities, hospitals, etc.) from different Member States to work more closely together. If a particular treatment can be provided to a patient more effectively in another country, e-health systems make it simpler to organize and carry out treatment abroad. Suppliers of e-health tools – such as databases for patient records, mobile monitors which transmit data automatically, or handling systems for patient call centres – also benefit from the development of a European market in the sector, since it has enabled them to build a strong base from which they can tackle the global market (ibid).

It is clear that e-health is not just about technology, but about changing the everyday practice of healthcare for every healthcare professional and every patient. However the organizational and regulatory environment of e-health has not progressed as rapidly as technology both in national and European level (Legally e-health, 2008). The key issue in the European sphere is whether and to what extent it interferes with public health policy and should be treated separately from the more "traditional" healthcare.

The proposed chapter will define and discuss e-health from a European perspective; namely the chapter will present the different steps that the European policy has undertaken in the particular field. The chapter will also emphasize on the discussion of organizational and regulatory issues that arise in this specific policy area and will discuss the drives and barriers towards achieving pan European "patient-friendly" healthcare services.

DEFINING E-HEALTH FROM A EUROPEAN PERSPECTIVE

E-health covers the interaction between patients and health-service providers, institution-to-institution transmission of data, or peer-to-peer communication between patients and/or health professionals (e-health: Care for me, 2010). Examples include health information networks, electronic health records, telemedicine services, wearable and portable systems which communicate, health portals, and many other ICT-based tools assisting disease prevention, diagnosis, treatment, health monitoring and lifestyle management. The appropriate utilization of those tools and services provides a better, and a more efficient healthcare system for all.

Improvement of Information Provision for Citizens

E-health systems offer patients the opportunity to be well informed – in matters related to therapies and rehabilitation, as well as on their condition, and improved standards of living – and it makes it simpler for healthcare professionals to access and share general and patient-specific information. The use of electronic patient records permits doctors to see much more of a person's medical history than paper files do. Paper files typically include only information on treatment in a single surgery or hospitalization and the option to review past examination results and old therapeutic schemes (Wilson, Leitner & Moussalli, 2004). A patient's condition via the use of electronic patient records can be monitored remotely, and thus releasing a hospital bed which would have been mandatory with previous monitoring equipment, and without minimizing care standards of the patient. On-line tools can help patients to better understand their conditions and make it easier for them to find and chat with fellow sufferers, for example through on-line support groups which boost patients' spirits in the face of serious illness(ibid). A good example is the "The Cancer Forums", which is a website for discussions about any type of cancer (http://www.cancerforums.net/). Another example comes from the UK where the Cancer Research UK launched in 2008 an online chat forum for cancer patients to swap stories and share experiences on how to cope with such a devastating disease (http://www.cancerchat.org.uk/).

Efficient Organization of Resources and Care Provision

Limited resources – both in budgetary and staffing terms – ponder constantly on healthcare providers. e-health tools and services enable a better financial planning, a more efficient organisation of resources and care provision that leads to an increased productivity (COM/2004/0356 final,. Electronic records make it easier to schedule patient-doctor visits, keep track of follow-up exams and ensure patients' general practitioners to be informed on the results of their referrals. When it comes to preventive healthcare, e-health tools can help to accomplish a much higher coverage, for example, by ensuring that children will receive full vaccinations' programme at the right age. Additionally, thanks to the improvements that e-health tools bring, healthcare providers can tackle the increasing demand for healthcare in an improved fashion, and cover the costs of new, advanced treatments.

Development of a Patient Friendly Healthcare

A widespread implementation of e-health will facilitate in the development of a more "patient-friendly" healthcare service. This will offer healthcare providers a chance to become more adaptable and improve their ability to address the differing needs of individual patients. Patients nowadays have to go to the doctor (or the doctor comes to them), but the on-line and mobile tools are already introducing the possibility of remote diagnosis. Similar tools can also help out health professionals who travel to examine patients to provide them with more sophisticated treatments. E-health services promise to raise the quality of care in remote and rural areas, owing to modern communications infrastructure.

THE EVOLUTION OF THE EUROPEAN STRATEGY

Health has a central part of the European policy agenda. As aforementioned under Article 152 of the Treaty establishing the European Community (Article 152), the EU has a mandate to complement the work of national health systems so as to address issues like health threats and diseases, the ageing of the population as well as the cooperation on cross-border health issues. New technologies are considered as a powerful tool in this effort and their use is encouraged both in national and European level.

The First E-Health Action Plan

In 2004, the Commission adopted the first e-health action plan (COM/2004/0356 final) - which covers everything from electronic prescriptions and health cards to new information systems that reduce waiting times and errors – to facilitate a more harmonious and complementary European approach to e-health. The Plan (due for revision in 2011) states that *"e-health tools or solutions include products, systems and services that go beyond simply Internet- based applications. They include tools for health authorities and professionals as well as personalized health systems for patients and citizens*" (ibid).

The plan sets out the steps needed for a widespread adoption of e-health technologies across the EU by 2010 and calls on Member States to develop tailored national and regional e-health strategies to respond to their specific needs. Cultural differences, varying population profiles and geography, all denote that regional and national health policies have to be developed separately. The EU for the first time becomes involved in encouraging each health authority to learn from the experiences of others. On the basis of best practices identified across Europe, all Member States should adopt procedures for testing and accreditation of e-health tools and services by the end of 2007. A quicker rollout of high-speed internet access, on which so many of the tools are based, is a decisive development if MS are to completely utilize the widespread benefits of e-health. At the same time, endorsing the accessibility of e-health services, particularly to groups which are least likely to have an easy internet access, such as the elderly, disabled or unemployed, is a top priority of the action plan since those groups are most likely to be in need of health services.

The Role of the European Commission

In June 2006, the Commission's ICT for Health Unit adopted a new strategy to endorse the transformation of the European healthcare landscape. It argues that in order to face the healthcare challenges such as the ageing population and other, Europe needs a *"new healthcare delivery model, based on preventive and person-oriented health systems, which can only be realized through proper use of ICT"* (ICT for Health and i2010, 2006).

The scheme is said to build upon the e-health Action Plan and to involve forward-looking research under the EU's Seventh Framework Programme for Science and Research (FP7). The strategy is also in line with the Commission's new policy framework i2010 to endorse application of ICT to improve social inclusion, public services and quality of life (EurActiv, 2009).

A report on European countries' e-health priorities and strategies (e-health ERA report, 2007), states that Member States have made advances in implementing the EU's e-health strategy but have failed to address education and socio-economic issues that fall under their responsibility. The Commission has also published a report on best practice in EU member states.

The Commission published an Action Plan for e-health at the end of 2007 (e-health Task Force report, 2007) pledging to review the possibility of adopting a legal initiative for e-health and telemedicine. It also emphasized on the need for common standards in e-health and the importance of interoperability. Greater cooperation between EU member states was encouraged.

In 2008, the European Commission unveiled plans to make e-health one of the EU's first six Lead Market Initiatives, making it a strategic priority (COM(2007) 860 final SEC(2007) 1730). The size of the market and the capacity for innovation were cited as the principal reasons for its selection. In addition, the possibility for SMEs tapping into the various sub-sectors of e-Health was underlined.

A mid-term progress report, published in September 2009 (SEC (2009) 1198 final), said the e-health Lead Market Initiative (LMI) was still at an early phase of implementation. It said the LMI can stimulate demand-side measures in EU member states but the real impact cannot be expected for another five to ten years. The European e-health market was estimated at EUR14.269 million in 2008 and is projected to reach EUR15.619 million by 2012, with a compounded annual growth rate of 2.9%.

The report suggested better coordination between the LMI and other EU projects including the Joint Technology Initiatives (JTI) and the EU Economic Recovery Plan. Industry and civil society have been actively engaged with policy creators in arguing on how to improve the environment for innovation in e-health. Microsoft has published a White Paper urging policymakers to move away from today's fragmented system towards a connected network through which data can flow. The European Public Health Alliance (EPHA) and the European Patients Forum (EPF) have also been tracking the issue.

The Support from the European Parliament

In April 2009, the European Parliament supported a proposal on cross-border healthcare which will bring greater patient mobility in the EU (COM(2008) 414 final). Patients will be able to travel for treatment in another EU state and be reimbursed by their home country. The directive is still being debated by health ministers, some of whom have reservations about how the directive affects health service planning.

However, the directive also includes measures designed to improve cross-border cooperation on e-health. Interoperable health IT systems will be required if the proposal is to be implemented smoothly and in full. The directive is helping to add impetus to efforts at developing harmonized standards to accelerate e-health adoption in Europe. Industry groups have negotiated agreement on standardised messaging to link hospitals and other healthcare provides with insurance companies and national health IT systems.

2010 Ministerial Declaration on E-Health

European health Ministers signed a declaration on e-health at the 8th Ministerial e-health Conference in Barcelona expressing a joint vision and policy priorities on how to make e-health more accessible, interactive and customised to patients.

The Declaration (Declaration, 2010) calls for policy coordination amongst the various areas where e-health can have an impact on citizens' health in order to enhance benefits for patients, healthcare systems and society. It recognizes the need for stronger synergies with policy areas like competitiveness, research and regional development both at European and national levels.

According to the declaration the importance of e-health should be underlined in the framework of the future EU 2020 Strategy and the European Digital Agenda. ICT tools for Health should be used to scale up benefits to patients, healthcare systems and society. Large scale actions at European level to link research, innovation and deployment are therefore welcomed. The Commission should report on progress in this area (ibid).

The signatories also underline the importance of involving all stakeholders in the strategic planning, validation and implementation of e-health. *"We made the right investments over 20 years to become the world leader in e-health"* noted Neelie Kroes, Commissioner for the Digital Agenda in March 2010 (SPEECH/10/90). "The investments worked because we took them early and we took them together. She also highlighted *"Now it is time to step up another gear. Our finances demand it. Our citizens expect it. The technology is ripe. We are all rightly proud of our health systems in Europe. We have every reason to be proud to be working towards e-health for all."* (ibid).

KEY ISSUES TO CONSIDER

It is clear that e-health is not just about technology, but about changing the everyday practice of healthcare for every healthcare professional and every patient. Unfortunately the organizational and regulatory environment of e-health has not progressed as rapidly as technology both in national and European level and a key issue in the European sphere is whether and to what extent it interferes with public health policy and should be treated separately from the more "traditional" healthcare.

Interoperability

One of the most imperative practical issues regarding e-health is the interoperability of the IT systems. In some hospitals, customised software in the operating theatre is not compatible with the systems used in the emergency room or in the radiology department. Experts have highlighted interoperability as a major barrier in order to maximize the potential cost savings promised by e-health (EurActiv, 2009). Sharing electronic information within and between hospitals is a challenge, but so is the larger issue of communicating across borders. In the context of the cross-border healthcare directive, interoperable health IT infrastructure has become a key priority (e-health, Innovation, 2010).

Telemedicine

In an ageing Europe, where more and more citizens live with chronic diseases, telemedicine has proved to be an important tool. Despite the potential benefits that telemedicine can provide, its' use is still limited in most parts of the EU.

Telemedicine allows the monitoring of important health parameters (such as blood sugar levels or blood pressure) to be carried out from the patient's home, avoiding troublesome - particularly for the sick or elderly – and exhausting trips to a doctor or hospital. It can improve access to specialized treatment in remote areas where access to healthcare is difficult. It can also contribute to shortening waiting lists, for example in radiology, when reading and interpretation of medical images, such as radiographs (X-rays) or Computed Tomography (CT) scans, can be performed at a distance. It has also a key role in preventative medicine which is considered as another tool for keeping people healthier for longer (COM(2008) 689).

Furthermore, telemedicine, which is already a multi-billion global industry, can contribute substantially to the growth of the European economy. European industry, especially SMEs, can tap the financial and clinical benefits from this expanding market, provided that barriers to development such as market fragmentation and legal aspects are addressed. The actions proposed by the Commission are:

1. To increase confidence and acceptance of telemedicine services among users. In particular, by encouraging provision and dissemination of scientific evidence of its effectiveness and cost effectiveness.
2. To bring legal clarity on existing EU legislation regarding telemedicine services and encourage Member States to improve provision of telemedicine services.
3. To solve technical problems such as the lack of adequate community-wide broadband infrastructure and interoperability of telemedicine devices (COM(2008) 689).

Privacy and Security

E-health applications entail the processing of information related to an identified or identifiable "subject", the patient. This type of information is known legally as personal data and is subject to the *data protection legislation* of the European Union. In Europe, such data are protected by legal rules found in a number of legal sources such

Figure 1. Key issues of concern in e-health policy area

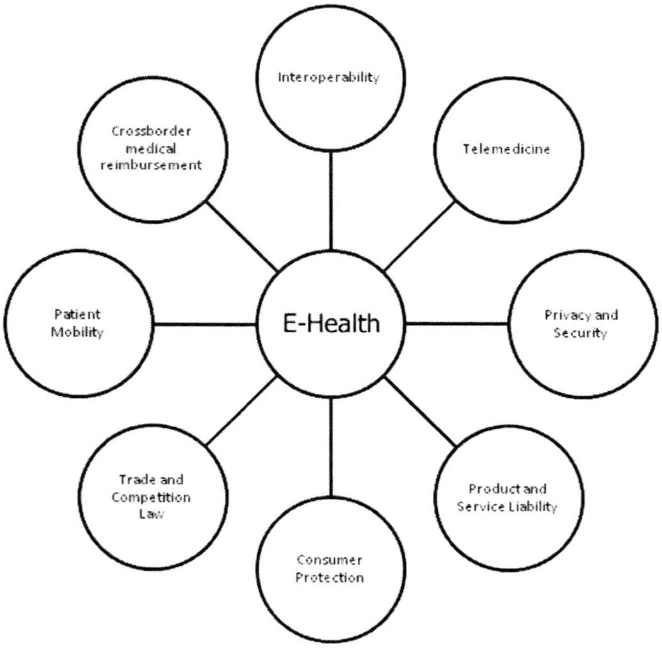

as *Article 8* of the *European Convention for the Protection of Human Rights and Fundamental Freedoms*, *Article 8* of the *EU Charter of Fundamental Rights* as well as the *Directive on Data Protection* (Dir. 95/46/EC), which has now been adopted into national data protection legislation across the EU. This Directive, however, serves an additional purpose: To allow the free movement of personal data within the European Union in the context of the internal market.

The basic principle behind this Directive in the specific content, is that if a piece of information can be linked to a person either by reasonable simple means, or with the help of a third person, then the data is considered as identifiable and, therefore, it falls into the range of the aforementioned Directive. For example the laboratory results of a blood sample test, will be covered by this legislation if the identification of the originator of the blood is possible with the use of reasonable means.

The data protection rules falls primarily into the responsibility and jurisdiction of the data controller – the person who decides the purpose and the means of the data processing and who has the legal duty to ensure that all the data are handled appropriately. In most professional cases, this will be a senior staff member who is named as the person responsible for data collection and storage by an organization. In the case of small companies or self-employed individuals (such as many General Practitioners), the data controller will be the person who has the legal and tax liability of the organization.

On the other hand, data concerning a person's health, religion, trade union activity, as well as data revealing racial or ethnic origin and judicial information, are amongst the data defined by the Directive as especially *sensitive* and, therefore, are subject to special rules. These data have the capacity, if they are exploited of infringing fundamental freedoms or privacy of the data source (patient), and thus should not be processed. This is not an absolute rule in any of the EU countries as they all accept, by principle, that medical data may be collected or processed only for certain purposes and following certain guidelines such as: (a) after the citizen's/ patient's (data subject) explicit and informed consent; (b) in the case of physical or mental incapability of the data subject in consenting for his/hers data processing, and there is a need to protect his/hers vital interest; (c) in the case of any health professional or any other subject with equivalent position which controls or processes medical data, he/she is obliged of professional secrecy concerning these data for the purposes of preventive medicine, medical diagnosis, the provision of care or treatment, or the management of healthcare services (Legally e-health, 2008).

Product and Service Liability and Consumer Protection

It is clear that the provision of e-health products, systems, and services must fulfill certain quality standards. There are various regulations that provide guarantee for any damages caused from sub-standard products or services, so as to protect the consumer. Those do not apply exclusively to e-health, but instead are applied to a general context of service provision and product delivery, whether by traditional or via electronic means.

The concept of an e-health product is sometimes difficult to understand because, in practice, most e-health products either will be software packages and interfaces (electronic health record, decision support tool, etc.) or they might be hardware devices with embedded software (radio frequency identification location trackers for locating people and objects, remotely controlled medical devices, etc.). Hence there is a broad definition of what "constitutes" an e-health product or service, so as to include anything that is sold to a medical practitioner or directly to a consumer (patient) that uses an Internet for his/ hers purchases. According to this, an e-health product might be a medical electronic record to be used by a doctor, or a monitoring device that includes a web-based interface, or even just a simple health information portal.

In order the European Commission to guarantee product liability, there are specific measures that have been implemented in the form of Directives. The *General Product Safety Directive* (Directive 2001/95/EC) has set up a general safety requirement for any product that is put on the market for consumers; including e-health products. The national legislation based on EC's *General Product Liability Directives* ensures that the buyer has the right to be compensated if the consumer goods are not fit for the purpose that they are sold. A similar concept exists also to national legislation based on Directive on the *Sale of Consumer Goods* (Directive 1999/44/EC). According to the above, when e-health products are sold as consumer goods, the provider must deliver the product in the form that is described in the sale contract.

Any e-health product which is found in the market, and is designated by its manufacturer as a medical device, will be subject to the specific additional rules regarding medical devices. The medical devices sector is covered by three directives, which cover a wide range of products. The first Directive, (90/385/EC), deals with active implantable medical devices (ex. pace-makers etc.), the second Directive, (93/42/EC), deals with medical devices in general, while the third Directive, (98/79/EC), deals with in vitro diagnostic medical devices.

National, international, and European bodies are developing standards that apply to e-health products. Examples include the *European Committee for Standardization* (CEN)[1], standard for Electronic Health Records (EHRs), the American *Health Level Seven* (HL7) standard for the Electronic Health Record (HER), or the industry standard for the Digital Imaging and Communications in Medicine (DICOM). Although these standards are not legally binding, they do provide a baseline, and thus any dispute about the quality of an e-health product, that is being covered by those standards, can be assessed and evaluated.

Directive 85/374/EC on *Defective Products* will apply to e-health products in the same way as it applies to any other product sold on the European market. This Directive intends to ensure a high level of consumer protection against damage caused to health or property by a defective product. It also aims to reduce the disparities between national liability laws, which distort competition and restrict the free movement of goods (Directive 85/374/EEC).

Additionally, there is currently no general European harmonisation of liability rules for services in which no apparent defect can be found in a device. Therefore, liability for services is governed by ordinary rules of law applicable to the Member States (Legally e-health, 2008). An exception to this may exist if a service is supplied wholly by electronic means, in which case the eCommerce Directive might apply. Therefore, any e-health service that is provided through the Internet will be subject to the national legislation derived from the eCommerce Directive of the EU, with the prerequisite that it meets the qualities of an information society service.

According to the Convention on information and legal co-operation concerning "Information Society Services" an information society service entails any service that is normally provided for remuneration, at a distance, by electronic means, and at the individual request of a recipient of the service (such as via the Internet). It covers services between enterprises or between enterprises and consumers, which are paid directly from the recipient (online transactions) or those financed by indirect means, such as advertising income or sponsoring (Council of Europe, 2010). Examples include websites of doctors promoting their activities; online selling of medicines (ePharmacy); online advice that does not require the physical examination of the patient if a fee is paid or if it is financed by advertising or sponsorship; online databases of information accessible for medical professionals or consumers if a fee is paid or if it is financed by advertising or sponsorship (even indirectly).

This principle of transparency of the site provider is included within the Commission's *Communication on Quality Criteria for Health-related Websites* (COM 2002/667). These criteria seek to increase the consistency of health-related websites and include also additional quality criteria that health-related websites should comply with, such as transparency with regards to the purpose of the website, respect of privacy, accessibility adapted to the target audience, etc. Those quality criteria may serve as a reference to the development of quality initiatives for health-related websites (COM 2002/667).

Aspects of Trade and Competition Law

The disparities that already exist, or those that are emerging in Member States' legislation and case-law in relation to healthcare, prevent the smooth functioning of the internal market, in particular by impairing the development of cross-border services and by creating distortions of competition.

Health services are, in the majority of the EU countries, funded through some form of taxation, and are organized to some degree by public bodies, thus the degree in which competition law applies to them is somewhat unclear and may be limited. To be more accurate, it is unclear just how far the rules of competition apply to all to publicly funded bodies, as well as how far the concept of Services of General Interest apply to health services, and the extent in which health services are exempted from the provisions of European competition law, on the basis of the rules on *Services of General Economic Interest* (SGEI) as supplied for in the Treaty.

Historically and socially, the provision of healthcare services has been hidden from the area of competition law. The logic behind this was not only because of its public nature, but also because healthcare generally is conceived as an intellectual service provided by professionals whose services comprise a range of skills that is not classified into separate activities subject to competition (Legally e-health, 2008). As a result, healthcare, traditionally, has not attracted the attention of competition lawyers to a significant extent. This however should not cause any problems since an e-health company is not necessarily any different from a hotel group or a car manufacturer. On the other hand the context in which e-health organisations operate might make them considerably different from other organisations, mostly because an e-health company will, in many cases, be selling its services not directly to the consumer, but to a public health services provider who, in turn, makes e-health services available to patients and citizens in the course of their usual provision of care.

For the health sector, it is important to think about the application of the rules on abuse of dominant position, and the possible exemptions of Services of General Economic Interest (SGEIs), but also about state aid, since many health service providers will be funded directly through state aid (Legally e-health, 2008). Most healthcare providers are unlikely to be legally classified as undertakers of an economic activity, since they are supplying goods and services in the execution of an exclusively social function; this denotes that this function is built on a non-profit making basis, on the principle of solidarity and thus the entitlement to services is not dependent on the amount of contributions. Their interactions with private bodies from which goods or services are purchased, for the purposes of offering healthcare, will not be subject to the rules on abuse of dominant position. A healthcare provider, however, operating outside those strict criteria, can be classified as an undertaker of economic activities and, can be therefore, subject to competition law.

Article 87 (Article 87 of the EC Treaty) states that any aid granted by a Member State, or funded by state resources, in any form what so ever, can be considered incompatible with the rules of the common market, in the situation in which it distorts or threatens to distort competition by favouring certain undertakings or the production of certain goods.

Despite the absolute character of Article 87, the European Commission has the power to decide when state aid has a social character and is granted to individual consumers (e.g. state aid to assist consumers who have suffered loss due to the collapse of a major industry) or when state aid is used to repair the damages caused by natural disasters. In the second case, such state aid may be deemed compatible with the common market. The Commission may also authorize some specific aids. In general, the Commission must be informed in advance for any project of state aid. An exception to this is aid given in the form of public service compensation that is granted to certain undertakings, and entrusted with the operation of Services of General Economic Interest (e.g., hospitals), since it is not considered as incompatible with the common market.

Patients Mobility and Cross Border Medical Reimbursement

The use of ICT in health area, has achieved significant progress but in spite of it the reimbursement for cross-border services in e-health is not regulated at the EU level (e-health Taskforce report, 2007). The mechanism used for cross-border care reimbursement in the EU, is based on Regulations, on coordination of social security systems and on the Internal Market rules concerning the free provision of services, which have been clarified by the European Court of Justice. The existing regulations provide a well-established tool that has ensured social protection for workers, tourists and patients, travelling within the EU (European Observatory, 2006). Nonetheless the system needs improvement in order to profit from the great potential for e-health applications. Every effort should therefore be made to ensure that the potential revision of legal provisions around patient mobility is fully aligned with the use of e-health goods and services, to deliver healthcare across borders.

IMPACT FACTORS, DRIVERS AND BARRIERS TO THE EUROPEAN E-HEALTH CONTEXT

Economic Factors

The major economic factors affecting indirectly e-health developments have been the rapid economic growth and income convergence. In general GDP growth, disposable incomes and resulting expenditure patterns47 are only some of the factors influencing ICT developments and spending patterns (JRC, 2008). Further explanatory variables should be incorporated when considering the special, different from the overall trend cases. These include among others ICT related public policies, institutional developments and the level of competition in the economy, the level of human capital in general and ICT skills or digital literacy in particular.

Economic growth and new investments also shape geographical disparities as regions with adequate public infrastructure supply and new private investments generally outperform those that lack such assets (ibid). The large regional disparities in GDP per capita are closely correlated with ICT penetration, poor "hard" infrastructure in the lagging regions and regions of large agricultural employment, which limits interest in the uptake of ICT skills. The income divide brings a weak presence of middle classes, which would - if they were stronger - serve the base of the demand for eServices (ibid).

Policy and Healthcare Related Factors

One important policy related factor affecting the evolution of e-health has been the low level of healthcare expenditure and under utilisation of EU funds for health. The reform of the healthcare sector has been one of the main factors affecting e-health (ibid). These reforms included the change in the financing model of healthcare services, the institutional structures providing healthcare services, the ownership of health service providers.

ICT services related to public policies can be divided to direct and indirect ones. Direct policies affect primarily the development of ICT services, such as awareness raising actions, measures supporting access to ICT infrastructure, direct government spending and programmes on ICT services. The indirect policies influence ICT developments by improving the framework conditions including such vital areas as telecom privatisation, regulation and competition policies, taxation schemes and investment promotion, R&D and education policies. While direct policies have mainly their effect on the demand side, indirect ones influence the supply side. A main health related factor has been the increase in the quality and availability of basic ICT infrastructure.

Demographic Trends

An ageing population makes the productivity challenge more urgent and Europe is caught in a demographic squeeze of declining birth rates and rising life expectancies (Creating an Innovative Europe, 2006). According to Eurostat, by 2050 the working population will decrease by 52 million, even after allowing for net migration, and there will be a sharply rising dependency ratio, with the proportion of people over 65 rising from 16.4% in 2004 to 29.9% in 2050.

Drivers and Barriers to E-Health

Within the economic, policy and health related drivers, the main ones are the growing demand from users for more efficient healthcare services, the deeper involvement of the private sector in health service provision, the access and affordability of ICT services, the foreseen shortage of healthcare professionals, the changes in the regulatory framework, the exchange of best practices and the use of EU Structural Funds.

The barriers to e-health are also divided into economic, policy and health sector related ones and include the next aspects: low level of healthcare expenditures, incomplete legislative framework, restricted healthcare structural reforms, low level of IT competence and appropriate personnel, low level of demand for eServices and efficiency versus absorption on the spending priority of Structural Funds.

FUTURE RESEARCH DIRECTIONS: TOWARDS A NEW EUROPEAN BUSINESS MODEL FOR E-HEALTH

A new study funded by the ICT for Health unit of the European Commission's DG Information Society and Media has been released in May 2010, evaluating business models for e-health in Europe. The study, coordinated by RAND Europe in partnership with Capgemini Consulting, introduces a set of policy recommendations for the European Commission and other stakeholders to improve the overall quality and efficiency of health services through e-health.

According to the study, "Business Models for e-health", senior management and staff involvement are key to make sure that business models "do not fall short of reflecting the interactions of those actors who are to use them in their day-to-day professional activities." (Valeri, Giesen, Jansen, & Klokgieters, 2010). Public policy actions need to support the development of "value-creating business models" for e-health, the study remarks. National healthcare authorities, health professional associations, healthcare delivery organisations, the industry and the research community need to share perspectives on applicable best practice and experience. The European Commission should act as the coordinating body for launching e-health pilot projects.

The set of responsibilities for the European Commission, as named by the study, includes:

- Fostering the sharing of specific best practice, for the design of value-creating and sustainable business models for e-health systems.
- Defining benchmarking parameters to ensure that individual organisations are able to monitor and compare the way that they develop and implement business models for e-health.
- Supporting the development of best practice for funding and financing individual e-health systems, via specific incentives such as tax breaks and/or different reimbursement procedures or co-funding mechanisms.
- Bringing legal clarity as to facilitate the identification and authorization of professional health staff accessing and using personal health data. The safe exchange of medical data across national borders must be ensured. The need to protect health data and the personal integrity of the patient as well as the rights of patients to give their consent to the use of their medical data, must be respected.
- Working towards the solution of technical issues and the facilitation of market developments via interoperability, common medical terminologies and technical standards as well as pre-procurement activities (ibid).

Close cooperation between Member States is a prerequisite in order to achieve the aforementioned goals. At the same time as the organization of healthcare provision depends on the social, political and economic landscape (sociopolitico-economic) of each Member State, the respect of national particularities need to be also seriously considered.

CONCLUSION

EU Health systems are under mounting pressure to respond to the challenges of population ageing, citizens' rising expectations, migration, and mobility of patients and health professionals. New technologies have the potential to revolutionize healthcare and health systems and to contribute to their future sustainability.

It is a fact that in both EU and national level, existing e-health technologies are not used to their full potential, since implementation levels often are too low. For this reason, it is clear that there is a need for political awareness and commitment, so as to ensure that the necessary organizational and regulatory changes will be realized in order to achieve sustainable and well integrated use of e-health services. Additionally, new and unfamiliar technologies can generate ethical concerns, and issues of citizen's trust and confidence must and should be addressed.

Furthermore, in order to have a successful model there is a need to identify a new modus operandi that will establish a link between politics, technology and visible benefits for patients and health professionals. This will assist in bridging the gap between experts and decision makers; better aligning ongoing e-health activities with health policies at EU and national level; strengthening the political governance of e-health; coordinating and consolidating ongoing activities at EU level; clarifying reporting mechanisms; as well as reinforcing and supporting Member States in ensuring deployment and use of existing technologies.

Finally in order to guarantee more efficient e-health services, specific legal measures need to be adopted both in EU and national level. These measures will need to: ensure that adequate protection of privacy is maintained when exchanging medical data across borders; ensure that freely given, specific and informed patient consent is guaranteed in cross-border care situations; improve legal certainty for health professionals when using medical data as input to treatment of patients from other Member States; ensure that medical data is understood and interpreted in a unified way across borders, bridge language barriers for medical records; enable the safe transfer of health data between care providers in different Regions and Member States; enable continuity of care across borders by interoperability of Electronic Health Record (EHR) systems; enable transfer of ePrescriptions, lab results and digital images in order to ensure continuity of care; enable telemedicine services and cooperation between European Reference Networks; ensure that only authorised health professionals with a treating relationship towards the patient have access to health data and last but not least ensure that the patient is identified in a secure way

REFERENCES

an Innovative Europe, C. (2006). *Report of the independent expert group on R&D and innovation appointed following the Hampton Court Summit, Jan. 2006*. Retrieved from http://www.eirma.org/ f3/ local_links.php?action=jump&id=1020&catid=55

COM. (2002). *Quality criteria for health related websites*. European Commission. Retrieved from http://eur-lex.europa.eu/ LexUriServ/ LexUriServ.do?uri=COM:2002:0667:FIN:EN:PDF

COM. (2004). *E-Health - Making healthcare better for European citizens: An action plan for a European e-Health Area*. European Commission. Retrieved from http://ec.europa.eu / information_society/doc/ qualif/health/ COM_2004_0356_F_EN_ACTE.pdf

COM. (2007). *Ageing well in the information society - An i2010 initiative action plan on information and communication technologies and ageing*. European Commission. Retrieved from http://eur-lex.europa.eu/ LexUriServ/site/ en/com/2007/ com2007_0332en01.pdf

COM. (2007). *Commission staff working document- European lead market approach: Methodology and rationale*. European Commission. Retrieved from http://eur-lex.europa.eu/ LexUriServ/ LexUriServ.do?uri=CELEX:52007SC1730:EL:NOT

COM. (2007). *White paper – Together for health: A strategic approach for the EU 2008-2013*. European Commission. Retrieved from http://ec.europa.eu/health/ ph_overview/Documents/strategy_wp_en.pdf

COM. (2008). *Proposal for a Directive of the European Parliament and the Council on the application of patients' rights in cross-border healthcare*. Retrieved from http://ec.europa.eu/health/ ph_overview/co_operation/ healthcare/docs/ COM_en.pdf

COM. (2008). *Communication from the Commission to the European Parliament, the Council, the European Economic and Social Committee and the Committee of the Regions on telemedicine for the benefit of patients, healthcare systems and society*. European Commission. Retrieved from http://ec.europa.eu/ information_society/activities/ health/docs/ policy/telemedicine/commn_telemedicine_en.pdf

Council of Europe, Human Rights and Legal Affairs. (2010). *Convention on information and legal co-operation concerning information society services*. Retrieved from http://www.coe.int/t/e/ legal_affairs/legal_co-operation/ Information_Society_Services/

Empirica. (2008). *Pilot on e-health indicators: Benchmarking ICT use among general practitioners in Europe*. Final report, European Commission, April 2008. Retrieved from http://ec.europa.eu/ information_society/ eeurope/i2010/ docs/benchmarking/ gp_survey_final_report.pdf

Euractiv. (2009). *Euroactive, e-health*. Retrieved from http://www.euractiv.com/ en/health/ e-health/ article-117474

European Commission. (2006). *ICT for Health and i2010: Transforming the European healthcare landscape-Towards a strategy for ICT for Health*. European Commission, Information Society and Media. Retrieved from http://ec.europa.eu/information_society/activities/ health/docs/publications/ ictforhealth-and-i2010-final.pdf

European Commission. (2007). *Accelerating the development of the e-health market in Europe*. European Commission, Information Society and Media. Retrieved from http://ec.europa.eu/information_society/activities/health/ docs/publications/ lmi-report-final-2007dec.pdf

European Commission. (2007). *Information society and health: Linking European policies, information society and media*. Retrieved from http://ec.europa.eu/ information_society/ activities/policy_link/brochures/ documents/health.pdf

European Commission. (2007). *Towards the establishment of a European e-health research area: E-health priorities and strategies in European countries*. European Commission, Information Society and Media. Retrieved from http://www.e-health-era.org/ documents/ 2007e-health-era-countries.pdf

European Commission. (2008). *Study on legal and regulatory aspects of e-health: Putting e-health in its European legal context*. European Commission, Information Society and Media. Retrieved from http://ec.europa.eu/ information_society/ activities/ health/docs/ studies/legally_e-health/ legally-e-health-report.pdf

European Commission. (2010). *Declaration (final) on the 8th Ministerial e-health Conference, European co-operation on e-health*. Retrieved from http:// ec.europa.eu/ information_society/ newsroom/ cf/ document.cfm?action=display&doc_id=658

European Commission. (2010). *E-health: Care for me, health – EU*. Retrieved from http://ec.europa.eu/health-eu/care_for_me/ e-health/index_en.htm

European Commission. (2010). *ICT for better healthcare in Europe, information & communication technologies for health, information society*. Retrieved from http://ec.europa.eu/ information_society/ activities/health/ index_en.htm

European Commission. (2010). *ICT research - The policy perspective: A healthy approach technology for personalized, preventative healthcare*. ISPL Publications. Retrieved from http://ec.europa.eu/ information_society/activities/health/ docs/ projects/ istresults/201006-ictresults-policy-report-health.pdf

European Commission. (2010). *ICT solutions for patients, medical services and payment institutions: Lead market initiative, enterprise and industry, policies*. Retrieved from http://ec.europa.eu/ enterprise/policies/innovation/ policy/ lead-market-initiative/e-health/index_en.htm

European Parliament. (1985). *On the approximation of the laws, regulations and administrative provisions of the Member States concerning liability for defective products*. Directive 85/374/EEC. Retrieved from http:// eur-lex.europa.eu/ LexUriServ/ LexUriServ.do?uri=CELEX:31985L0374:EN:HTML

European Parliament. (1995). *On the protection of individuals with regard to the processing of personal data and on the free movement of such data*. European Parliament, directive 95/46/EC. Retrieved from http://eurlex.europa.eu/ LexUriServ/ LexUriServ.do? uri=CELEX:31995L0046:EN:HTML

European Parliament. (1999). *On certain aspects of the sale of consumer goods and associated guarantees*. Directive 1999/44/EC. Retrieved from http://eur-lex.europa.eu/smartapi/ cgi/ sga_doc ?smartapi!celexapi!prod!CELEXnumdoc&lg=en&numdoc=31999L0044 &model=guichett

European Parliament. (2001). *On general product safety*. Directive 2001/95/EC. Retrieved from http://eur-lex.europa.eu/ LexUriServ/ LexUriServ.do?uri=CELEX:32001L0095:en:NOT

European Parliament. (2006). *European Parliament resolution of 23 May 2007 on the impact and consequences of the exclusion of health services from the Directive on services in the internal market*. European Parliament, May 2007. Retrieved from http://www.europarl.europa.eu/ sides/getDoc.do?pubRef=-//EP//TEXT+TA+P6-TA-2007-0201+0+DOC+XML+V0//EN

European Union. *(1992)*. Article 87 of the treaty establishing the European Community (nice consolidated version) part three: Community policies - Title VI: Common rules on competition, taxation and approximation of laws - Chapter 1: Rules on competition - Section 2: Aids granted by states.

European Union. (1992). *Article 152 of the treaty establishing the European Community, part three: Community policies - Title XIII: Public health*. Retrieved from http:// eur-lex.europa.eu/ LexUriServ/ LexUriServ.do?uri=CELEX:12002E152:EN:HTML

European Union. (2006). *Article 5 (subsidiarity principle) of the treaty establishing the European Commission, part one: Common provisions*. Retrieved from http://eur-lex.europa.eu/ LexUriServ/ LexUriServ.do?uri=OJ:C:2006:321E:0001:0331 :EN:PDF

European Union. (2006, June 22). Council conclusions on common values and principles in European Union health systems. *Official Journal of the European Union. L&C, 146*(1). Retrieved from http://eur-lex.europa.eu/ LexUriServ/ LexUriServ. do?uri=OJ:C:2006:146:0001:0003:EN:PDF.

Joint Research Center (JRC). (2008). *Scientific and technical reports, the development of e-health in an enlarged EU, synthesis report*. Retrieved from http://ftp.jrc.es/ EURdoc/JRC43277.pdf

Kroes, N. (2010). *A new era in e-health*. E-health Conference 2010 Barcelona, 15th March 2010. Retrieved from http://europa.eu/rapid/ pressReleasesAction.do?reference=SPEECH/10/90&format=HTML&aged=0&language=EN&guiLanguage=en

Rosenmöller, M., McKee, M., & Baeten, R. (Eds.). (2006). *European Observatory: Health systems and policies, patient mobility in the European Union: Learning from experience*. Retrieved from http://www.euro.who.int/ __data/assets/pdf_file/ 0005/98420/Patient_Mobility.pdf

SEC. (2009). *Lead market initiative for Europe, mid-term progress report*. European Commission, Retrieved from http://ec.europa.eu/ enterprise/ policies/innovation/files/ swd_lmi_midterm_ progress.pdf

Swedish Presidency for the European Union. (2009). *E-health for a healthier Europe – Opportunities for a better use of healthcare resources*. Retrieved from http://www.se2009.eu/ polopoly_fs/ 1.8427!menu/ standard/file/ EPSCO%20GH%20 -%20e-health%20for%20a%20 Healthier%20 Europe.pdf

Valeri, L., Giesen, D., Jansen, P., & Klokgieters, K. (2008). *Business models for e-health - Final report, ICT for Health unit*. DG Information Society and Media, European Commission, 28 February 2010. Retrieved from http://ec.europa. eu/ information_society/ activities/health/ docs/ studies/business_model/ business_models_e-health_report.pdf

Weerasinghe, D. (2008). *Electronic healthcare: First International Conference, e-health 2008, revised selected papers,* London, September 8-9, 2008.

Wilson, P., Leitner, Ch., & Moussalli, A. (2004). *Mapping the potential of e-health, empowering the citizen through e-health tools and services*. Maastricht, The Netherlands: European Institute of Public Administration.

ADDITIONAL READING

Database of European e-health priorities and strategies (Empirica). Available at: http://www.e-health-era.org/ database/database.html

European Observatory, Health Systems and Policies, Health Systems in Transition (HiT) country profiles. Available at: http://www.euro.who.int/en/ home/ projects/observatory/publications/ health-system-profiles-hits

KEY TERMS AND DEFINITIONS

E-Health: The term refers to the healthcare practice that is supported by electronic processes and ICT.

ePrescriptions: Defined as computer-generated prescriptions created by your healthcare provider and sent directly to your pharmacy.

European Union (EU): An economic and political union of 27 member states which are located in Europe.

Healthcare: The treatment and prevention of illness by dedicated professionals and specialized institutions.

Information and Communications Technology (ICT): It refers to the role of communications (telephone lines and wireless signals) in modern information technology. ICT consists of all technical means used to handle information and aid communication.

Patient-Friendly Healthcare Service: It refers to healthcare providers that are working in an effort to become more flexible and better able to address the differing needs of individual patients.

Telemedicine: The term is used for applications of clinical medicine where medical information is transferred through interactive audiovisual media for the purpose of consulting.

ENDNOTE

1. CEN is a major provider of European Standards and technical specifications. It is the only recognized European organization according to Directive 98/34/EC for the planning, drafting and adoption of European Standards in all areas of economic activity with the exception of electrotechnology (*CENELEC*) and telecommunication (*ETSI*).

Chapter 17
Developing Virtual Communities to Support Drug Policy Knowledge Exchange:
The Canadian Experience

Mowafa Househ
King Saud Bin Abdul Aziz University for Health Sciences, Saudi Arabia

Andre Kushniruk
University of Victoria, Canada

Malcolm Maclure
Harvard University, USA, University of Victoria, Canada & British Columbia Ministry of Health, Canada

Bruce Carleton
University of British Columbia, Canada, Children's and Women's Health Centre of BC, Canada & Child & Family Research Institute, Canada

Denise Cloutier-Fisher
University of Victoria, Canada

ABSTRACT

Within Canada, there is a growing need in the area of drug policy to develop virtual communities to facilitate knowledge exchange between academics and policy-makers. Such collaborations are regarded as a way to make research relevant by influencing the policy-making process. This chapter presents an action case study of three drug policy groups participating in various virtual knowledge exchange activities. The experiences and lessons learned by each group participating in this study are provided. Recommendations and solutions to conduct successful virtual knowledge exchange meetings based on the findings of this research are also provided.

DOI: 10.4018/978-1-60960-866-8.ch017

INTRODUCTION

A promising area of research is the development of virtual communities that support knowledge exchange using various information and communication technology tools (ICTs), such as teleconferencing, web-conferencing, and video conferencing. According to the Canadian Health Services research foundation, knowledge exchange is defined as (CHSRF, 2008):

collaborative problem-solving between researchers and decision makers [which] involves interaction between decision makers and researchers and results in mutual learning through the process of planning, disseminating, and applying existing or new research in decision making.

Much of the knowledge exchange literature focuses on how such groups engage, collaborate, and share ideas regarding research in a face-to-face setting (CHSRF, 2010). However, little is known about the impacts of knowledge exchange when it occurs within a virtual environment (Househ, Kushniruk, Maclure, Carleton, & Cloutier-fisher, 2009). The purpose of this chapter is to describe the experiences of three groups working in the field of drug policy using teleconferencing and web-conferencing technologies to support knowledge exchange activities. Each group's experience using technology to support a specific knowledge exchange tasks is provided. With this in mind, the research question posed by this project was: *what are the impacts of information and communication technologies on virtual knowledge exchange groups working in the field of drug policy?*

Here, we first provide background for the study, followed by a description of the groups, as well as the data collection and analysis methods used. A summary of our results is also provided. Finally, solutions and recommendations for conducting successful knowledge exchange are provided.

BACKGROUND

A trend in information communication technology is the emergence of various ICTs: desktop web-conferencing, videoconferencing, and collaborative technologies, including document management, application sharing, desktop sharing, white boarding, and co-browsing. These systems have been touted by proponents to have improved task performance, decision making, and collaboration in virtual groups. As healthcare groups continue to remotely communicate about and collaborate on knowledge exchange-related activities, ICTs will play a larger role in supporting such interactions.

The benefits of knowledge exchange occur when decision makers incorporate research evidence into the decision making process as a result of the knowledge exchange process. The existence of knowledge exchange networks in drug policy is not new. For example, Soumerai et al. (1997) published a paper on various factors that influence drug cost-containment policies in the United States. The authors found that one factor influencing drug policy decision making is information sharing that occurs through various stakeholders around certain Medicare policies. Similarly, a study examining drug policy knowledge exchange practices in six different countries found that knowledge exchange networks involving academics and drug policy decision makers influence various drug policies in each country (Milbank, 2001).

In Canada, there have been several examples of successful knowledge exchange in drug policy that have influenced drug policy decision makers. For example, in 1995, the British Columbia reference-based pricing (RBP) policy established a knowledge exchange group involving face-to-face interactions between academics and policy makers to produce evidence to inform drug policy decisions. The implementation of RBP led to $30 million in cost savings during the first year alone

(Maclure & Potashnik, 1997). Additionally, the Canadian Optimal Medication Prescribing and Utilization Service (COMPUS) was created to develop more effective drug policies and services to encourage the use of information in decision making among healthcare providers' and consumers' formulation for drug plans (COMPUS, 2004). One mandate of COMPUS is to facilitate knowledge exchange between clinicians, academics, and policy makers. Its purpose is to produce optimal practice information for health care providers and to improve drug prescribing and use among patients and consumers. Early indications suggest that COMPUS has been successful in influencing the use of blood glucose test strips, proton pump inhibitor therapy, and many other health-related practices.

These results demonstrate the benefits of face-to-face knowledge exchange networks between academics, clinicians, and drug policy makers. The promising results from such programs have lead to considerable interest in forging additional collaborative partnerships between various stakeholders within the drug policy domain to enhance decision making. To date however, little is known on the impacts of knowledge exchange interactions when they move from a face-to-face to a virtual setting.

METHODS

For this research study, the action case study approach was selected as an appropriate method. It uses similar data collection and analysis methods found in qualitative case studies. The major difference between action case and case studies is that the researcher is a participant within the group (Braa & Vigden, 1999). Within this project, the researcher supported the participants by providing them with technical support for either teleconferencing or web-conferencing technologies to facilitate group knowledge exchange.

Furthermore, action case is a hybrid research methodology that can be placed between action research and the case study method, as illustrated in Figure 1, adapted from Braa and Vigden (Braa & Vigden, 1999). The figure presents various methods used in information system research (Figure 1 a) and the research outcome for each method (Figure 1 b). In Figure 1 a (Methods), several methods are listed: action research, action case, soft case, hard case, field experiment, and quasi-experiment. In Figure 1 b (Research Outcome), each of these methods is mapped to a research outcome that attempts to achieve change, understanding or prediction. For example, action research is an example of a qualitative research method that studies change as a result of an intervention. Soft case studies focus on understanding what happened within a specific study. Field experiments focus on prediction and relationships between variables within the study. Hard case studies take a quantitative approach in understanding what occurred within a specific study; hard case studies fits somewhere between prediction and understanding. Quasi-experimental design focuses on understanding a change through the use of various quantitative methods; quasi-experiments fit somewhere between prediction and change. Action case focuses on understanding how an intervention took place within the study; action case fits somewhere between change and understanding.

There are a number of limitations that arise from using the action case study method. For instance, due to its similarity to case studies, one can argue that it is difficult to generalize the findings of an action case study to other times, places or settings. Another major criticism concerns researcher bias vis-à-vis participation of the researcher in the group. However, by analyzing multiple sources of data and describing the research setting, the reader of the action case study will be able to determine the similarities in the research context and determine the applicability of the research findings to his or her own setting.

Figure 1. Adapted from Braa and Vidgen (1999)

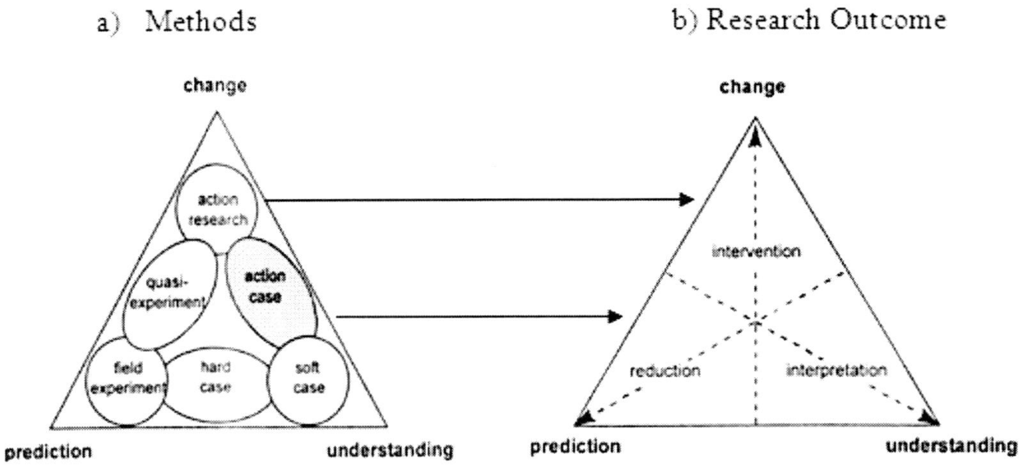

Participants

Three types of groups participated in this study: an education task group, a research task group, and a decision making task group. There were a total of 61 participants in the study.

Education Task Group

The education task group consisted of academic detailers who produce research reviews regarding new drugs for dissemination to physicians. Academic detailing involves the study of how knowledge is used, defining the objectives of knowledge, clarifying the roles that practitioners and opinion leaders have in the academic detailing process, and supporting the implementation of research knowledge (KUSP, 2003).

Of the 26 potential participants in the education task group, 20 were included in the study. The six that were excluded were observers and administrative assistants. The 20 participants included in the education task group were researchers, educators, and decision makers. This group was comprised of ten (50%) men and ten (50%) women. Of the 20, three (15%) were decision makers, three (15%) were researchers, and 14 (70%) were educators. All participants had at least a bachelor's degree. Thirteen of the educators were pharmacists by training, and one was a physician. All three researchers were experienced drug policy researchers. The educators were from five Canadian academic detailing programs located in British Columbia, Alberta, Saskatchewan, Manitoba, and Nova Scotia. A 1- to 10-year range of experience in academic detailing was noted for the different academic detailing programs. All of the researchers involved in the education task group were based in British Columbia, and each had over 10 years of drug policy research experience. The list of participants was obtained from an administrative member of the education task group. Consent to participate was obtained via e-mail. No incentives to participate in the study were offered or given to the participants. All group members had experience using e-mail, teleconferencing, and desktop computers.

Research Task Group

The research task group consisted of researchers and decision makers working together on evaluating physician education materials that focus on improving patient care. There were 17 potential participants in the group, of which 14 were included in the study. The three excluded were observers and administrative assistants. Those included were either researchers or decision makers. The research task group had nine (64%) men and five (36%) women. The group consisted of 12 (86%) researchers and two (14%) decision makers. All researchers had a level of education higher than a bachelor's degree. One of the researchers was located in the United States, and the remaining 11 were in Canada (Victoria and Vancouver, British Columbia). No incentives to participate in the study were offered to participants. The list of participants was obtained from an e-mail distribution list. Consent to participate was obtained through a consent form, which was returned via fax.

Decision Making Task Group

As part of a Health Canada-funded research program, a group of researchers met with decision makers and their staff members on a monthly basis using synchronous (live teleconferencing) and asynchronous (pre-recorded teleconferencing) communication methods to disseminate research information on the latest drug policy research trends.

There were 32 potential participants identified in the decision making task group, of which 27 were included. The five excluded were observers and administrative assistants. The 27 participants included in the decision making task group were researchers, decision makers, and staff from provincial Canadian drug plans. The decision making task group was composed of: 13 (48%) men and 14 (52%) women; and 22 (82%) decision makers/staff and five (18%) researchers. All participants had a minimum level of education, holding at least a bachelor's degree. All decision makers were senior representatives of seven major Canadian drug policy programs located in British Columbia, Alberta, Saskatchewan, Manitoba, Ontario, Quebec, and Prince Edward Island. With one exception, all researchers were university teaching professors working in the field of drug policy. No incentives to participate in the study were offered to the participants. The list of participants was obtained from an e-mail distribution list. Consent to participate was obtained via a consent form that was returned by e-mail. All group members had prior experience using e-mail and teleconferencing.

Meeting Structure

Education Task Group

With regard to teleconferencing meetings, the education task group met on the third Tuesday of every month with a rotating chair (i.e., process facilitator) to facilitate the group process. The rotating chair was selected according to location. For example, if a particular geographical area presented one month, another geographical area would present the second month and so on. The education task group members sent out an agenda several days in advance of the meeting. The meeting information and related documents were transmitted via e-mail. In the e-mail, a toll-free number and meeting code were also included so that group members could gain access to the teleconferencing meeting. Education task group members usually logged in a few minutes prior to the meeting. The group members generally opened e-mailed documents if needed during the meeting. Sample topics discussed in the education task group teleconferencing meetings included communication needs, physician education materials, relationships with funding agencies, a literature synthesis project, roles and relationships, and group identity issues.

In web-conferencing meetings, similar to teleconferencing meetings, the group met on every third Tuesday of the month with a rotating chair to facilitate the group meetings. Agenda items were sent in advance, along with a link to the web-conference meeting. Group members were asked to log in at least 20 min earlier than the designated meeting time so that any technical glitches could be addressed. The facilitator placed agenda items on the whiteboard and performed a sound check. During the sound check, the facilitator asked group members to speak into their microphones. If they heard the speaker clearly, they would signal using the voting and polling feature with a checkmark. If they did not hear the speaker clearly, they would signal with an (x). The group followed the agenda and crossed out items as they finished them. Sample agenda topics included grant proposals, physician education materials, literature, time lines and deliverables for the group evaluation project, and status reports.

Research Task Group

The research task group attempted to meet every month by web-conferencing. Approximately 1 week before the meeting, the research task group disseminated the meeting agenda with a link to the web-conferencing meeting. PowerPoint presentation slides were placed on the whiteboard for the entire group to see. A sound check was performed, in which the process facilitator ensured that all participants could be heard during the meeting. The sound check process was identical to the process followed by the education task group (above). The research task group members followed the agenda and crossed out items as they completed them. Sample group discussion topics included developing group roles, attending conferences, reviewing group methodologies, achieving project deliverables, moving to new offices, and discussing the research process. Near the end of the research project, the research task group reverted to face-to-face communication and abandoned the web-conferencing sessions.

Decision Making Task Group

The format of the live teleconferencing for the decision making task group was a 15 minutes presentation with another 5 minutes for questions. Prior to the meeting, an e-mail was sent to each participant with a number, appropriate meeting details, and PowerPoint slides. At the designated meeting time, the chair introduced the speaker and the topic. The speaker would present for 15 minutes and 5 minutes would be left for a question and answer period.

Technologies Used

The web-conferencing technology used in this study was Elluminate Live V-Class edition. This version allowed for half-duplex audio communication that permitted users to speak one at a time. Elluminate allows users to upload agendas to the whiteboard, share documents via application sharing, use instant text messaging, vote/poll participants, use emoticons, raise hands, and see participant names. These were the most relevant features used by the groups in this study.

Figure 2 shows a generic screen shot of the Elluminate Live technology. The most visible feature is the participant window (top left). In this window, the participants' names are displayed along with emoticons and the hand raising feature. Below this window is the direct text messaging feature, which allows group members to communicate using text messages. Below the direct messaging window is the half-duplex audio communication function. The group used this function to communicate using audio. The main screen is the whiteboard page. This allowed group members to share and manipulate PowerPoint slides using the whiteboard tools.

For teleconferencing, the education and decision making task groups used audio teleconferencing technology. The technology used audio-only communication in which multiple participants could speak at a time; there was no video or other media for communication. A participant simply dialed a telephone number, entered a conference code, and responded to a prompt requesting his or her name. A beep let other participants know that someone had joined the meeting. To use this technology, group members needed access to e-mail and a telephone. E-mail was necessary to inform the participants about

Figure 2. Elluminate live screen shot

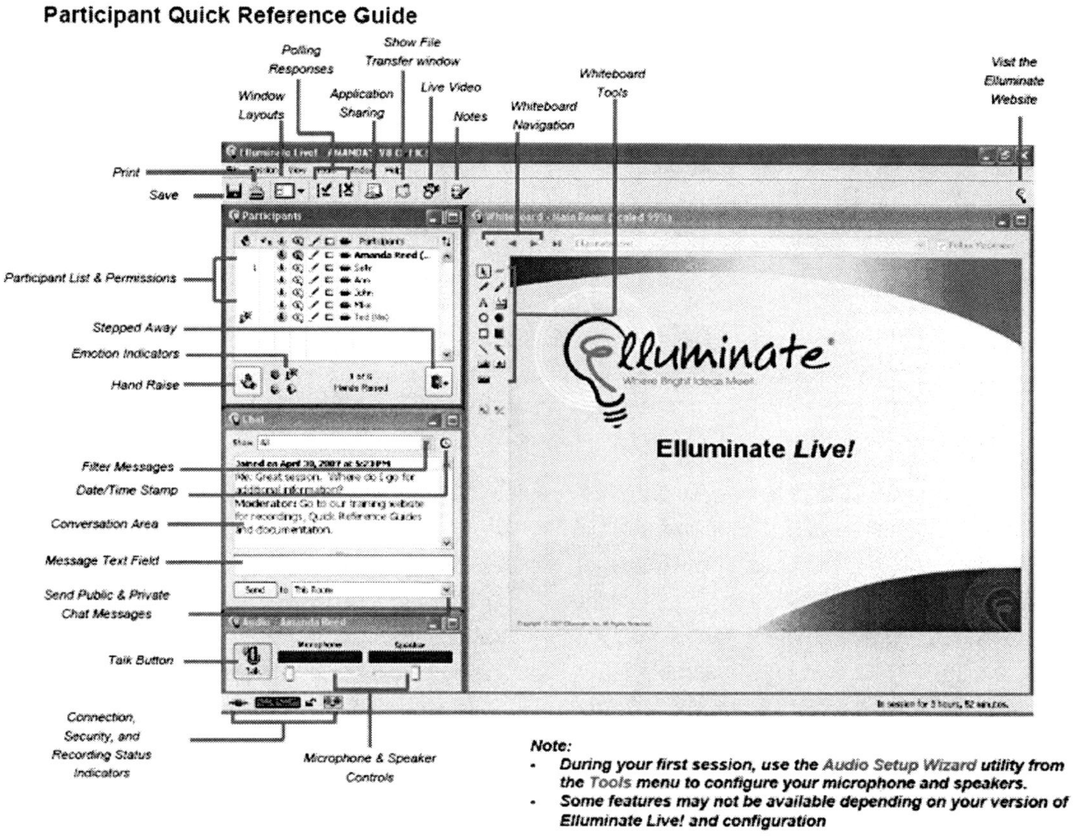

the meeting details (i.e., time, numbers to dial, and the agenda). A telephone was required to participate in the meeting.

DATA COLLECTION AND ANALYSIS

Data Collection

The data collection process took place over 3 years (April 2004 - July 2007). Different data were collected for the three drug policy groups. Phase 1 data included a compilation of baseline interviews for the researcher and educator groups and observation data for all three groups. Baseline interviews were not conducted with the decision making group. Phase 2 data included recorded meeting transcript data for the three drug policy groups. Phase 3 data included post-interview data and survey data results for the three drug policy groups. Table 1 provides a summary of the data collection phases and data types for each group.

Furthermore, the researcher transcribed all baseline interview data and hired a transcription company to transcribe the meetings and the post-interview data. The baseline interview, meetings, and post-interview data were transcribed verbatim.

Data Analysis

Content analysis was utilized to assess meeting transcripts and post-interview data. In general, content analysis is a data analysis approach that can be used to analyze qualitative data; it is a

Table 1. Types, volume, and data sources

Type	Volume	Source
Phase 1 (Baseline Interviews): Face-to-face and telephone interviews were conducted with the education and research task groups between April and July 2004.	12 education group, 9 research group, and 0 decision making task group.	Participant members. Collected by researchers.
Phase 1 (Observations): Researchers collected observational data on the three groups between 2004 and 2006.	15 pages of notes stored in Microsoft Word and Excel.	Researcher perceptions.
Phase 2 (Meeting Transcripts): Meeting transcripts were collected between March 2004 and November 2006.	Education group (6 teleconferences, 4 web-conferences); Research group (1 teleconference, 4 web-conferences); and Decision making group (7 teleconferences, one pre-recorded).	Participants. Recorded using a microphone on the telephone and Windows Media Encoder.
Phase 3 (Post-Study Interviews): Participant interviews with key stakeholders from each group. Interviews occurred between April and July 2007.	7 education group, 5 research group, and 5 decision making group.	Participant members. Collected by researchers.

systematic process of analyzing communication messages and making inferences based on the analysis (Berg, 1989) (Kondracki, Wellman, & Amundson, 2002). Content analysis involves the interpretation of textual data that has been categorized into concepts. Once concepts and categories have been identified, they are categorized into themes based on their relationships with each other (Lau & Hayward, 2000).

In this study, the analysis focused on exploring the impacts of conferencing technologies on knowledge exchange within the three drug policy groups. The analysis method used in the study was qualitative direct content analysis (Hsieh & Shannon, 2005). This method of content analysis is specific to qualitative studies. For the analysis, groups of phrases or sentences provided an appropriate level of sampling for the baseline, post-interview and meeting transcript data. A subsequent step in the analysis was to extract and compile all of the responses. In this process, responses from the education, research, and decision making task groups were separated from each other. The researcher familiarized himself with the data by reading the information for each of the groups. Sentences and phrases were selected as the basic units of analysis. Furthermore, NVIVO software was used in the qualitative data analysis process.

LESSONS LEARNED

Six key lessons were identified regarding the impact of conferencing technologies on virtual knowledge exchange groups in the field of drug policy. The basis for these lessons and how they compare with the relevant literature are discussed in this section. The lessons are summarized below in Table 2.

Finding 1: Groups Adapt to Technology

This finding applies to the education and research task groups, both of which experienced changes in social interaction norms when communicating using web-conferencing. For example, when both the education and research task groups began using web-conferencing, the technology limited their communication, allowing only one person to speak at a time. The groups implicitly started to introduce other forms for communication, such as text messaging, voting/polling, emoticons, and application sharing, to enhance the group discussions. These new discussion norms were introduced to compensate for the loss of immediacy and spontaneity in group discussion via web-conferencing interactions. This demonstrated that when encountering a highly structured approach

Table 2. Six key lessons learned on the impacts of conferencing technologies on knowledge exchange drug policy groups

Lessons Learned
Finding 1: Groups Adapt to Technology. When using new technologies, groups adapt their structure of communication around the technology's features.
Finding 2: Web-Conferencing Communication is Optimal Under Certain Conditions. Web-conferencing is an appropriate choice for knowledge exchange when there are limited budgets, large geographic dispersion, and a need for a high level of collaboration.
Finding 3: Teleconferencing is Convenient. When compared to web-conferencing, teleconferencing technology is a very simple and convenient technology to use for knowledge exchange.
Finding 4: Web-conferencing forces group interaction "within text". Web-conferencing will shift away interactions from interacting with each other to interacting via the text displayed on the whiteboard.
Finding 5: Facilitation Contributes to Successful Knowledge Exchange. When moving from a non-verbal rich medium (e.g., face-to-face) to a less non-verbal medium, such as web-conferencing, the facilitator requires strong facilitation skills to engage participants effectively.
Finding 6: Technology Impacts Information Sharing. Neither teleconferencing nor web-conferencing impacted the type of evidence that was shared between group members. However, web-conferencing and teleconferencing did impact how the information was shared between participants.

to communication, the group members resorted to other forms of communication to compensate for the lack of socio-emotional interactions found in web-conferencing. The two statements below support the above finding:

Just in the sense that if somebody was talking on and on and you wanted to interrupt them you wouldn't be able to do it vocally. You would have to do it via e-mail or a little text note or something like that [i.e., emoticons]. [Educator in the education task group]

I recall one of my problems is that I tend to interrupt when I get excited about a point. That was less possible with web-conferencing because you had to take turns more. [Educator in the education task group]

An explanation for this phenomenon may be that as the education and research task groups moved from unstructured communication environments (i.e., face-to-face or teleconferencing) to the highly structured web-conferencing, the dynamics of group communication changed. With web-conferencing, group members could only communicate vocally one person at a time using the hand raising function. The groups compensated for this loss of immediacy in communication by adapting and introducing new methods and structures for communication. Group members began using text messaging and emoticons as a way to improve group socio-emotional interactions.

This finding agrees with predictions of the theory of adaptive structuration (AST) (DeSanctis & Poole, 1994). According to AST, the use of ICTs introduces structures that influence the rules and resources that govern social interactions. Within both the education and research task groups, new forms of interaction norms were introduced to moderate the influence of technology on group social interactions.

Finding 2: Web-Conferencing Communication is Optimal under Certain Conditions

Our observations suggest that web-conferencing is an appropriate choice to facilitate knowledge exchange when groups have limited budgets, large geographic dispersion, and a need for a high level of collaboration. The education task group was able to tolerate learning the highly structured communication process required to use web-conferencing because the group had a limited budget, was geographically dispersed, and was highly collaborative. However, the research task group had a budget to support travel; its members were co-located and highly collaborative. Therefore, the research task group was not as interested in web-conferencing meetings because they had the resources to meet face-to-face.

The decision making task group had a limited budget, was geographically dispersed, and was not highly collaborative. Such a group may not have tolerated web-conferencing. In this study, it was observed that decision makers in drug policy were too busy to learn a new technology such as web-conferencing. For this group, live teleconferencing meetings were the preferred method of communication.

These results are similar to those of Orlikowski and Yates (1994) in their study of technology-enabled computer language designers collaborating on a multi-year project involving the development of various programming languages (Orlikowski & Yates, 1994). The authors found that different group inputs affected how the groups chose to communicate with each other. Over time, the group reinforced the pattern of how they communicated with each other until the technology they chose became the main method that group members used to work with each other.

From a more theoretical view, this finding can be explained by the literature on social presence. Social presence is defined as "those communication behaviors that enhance the closeness to, and non-verbal interaction with, each other" (Rourke, Anderson, Garrison, & Archer, 2001). The concept of social presence suggests that a higher degree of interaction between individuals materializes with a greater presence of non-verbal cues, body movement, and eye contact, which increase sensory stimulation (Rourke, Anderson, Garrison, & Archer, 2001). Such high-level interactions are found primarily in face-to-face interactions. According to our results, both the education and research task groups preferred meeting face-to-face due to the groups' preference for a higher degree of interaction. However, due to budget and geographical constraints, the education task group communicated via teleconferencing and web-conferencing, whereas the research task group, not affected by the same constraints, was able to meet face-to-face and later discontinued the use of web-conferencing.

Finding 3: Teleconferencing Is Convenient

Respondents noted that teleconferencing had the advantage of making the participation process easy and convenient. The teleconferencing platform provided a very simple process for enabling participation, because all participants had access to and were familiar with the technology. The participant simply called a number and entered a meeting code to participate in the meeting. It was more difficult to participate via web-conferencing than teleconferencing. In web-conferencing, the user needed a computer, a microphone, software, and skills to use the applications to participate in the meeting. As the education and research task groups noted, members needed to learn how to use the equipment before participating in the web-conference, as demonstrated in the following statements by the decision making and education task groups:

In terms of teleconferencing, it doesn't require you to get on a plane and go somewhere. It's much more convenient for regularly scheduled meetings. [Educator in the education task group]

[Teleconferencing is a] quick, easy tool that is widely available [Drug Policy Maker in the decision making task group]

Finding 4: Web-Conferencing Forces Group Interaction "Within the Text"

Education and research task group members noted that when they began using web-conferencing, their interactions changed from interacting with each other to interacting within the text. For example, when the education or research task groups met face-to-face, group members would look at each other directly and share the same space. In web-conferencing, however, the agenda would be placed on the whiteboard for all to see. All members would then interact with and talk about the agenda. The whiteboard itself represented the shared space, whereas in a face-to-face meeting, the shared space would be an office or room. Group interactions within web-conferencing were structured around the text, and the documents were shared on the whiteboard, as demonstrated by the following statements:

[Web-conferencing] allows people to engage visually in addition to being able to talk and listen, which is a key component particularly when a lot of our work was going through education materials. So [in web-conferencing], for example, everybody is looking at the same thing on a screen, and that kind of keeps the group together for one, and it also helps make sure that we're all talking about the same thing. [Educator in the education task group]

[Web-conferencing] provided the initial component to accelerate the visual aspect. For example, with the whiteboard, you can't talk it through and you need to have some visual image of the cases. [Researcher in the research task group]

Web-conferencing made us feel that we were meeting within the text. The group meets within the document or slide. It is a group space just like the difference you would feel at your home office vs. downtown in a shared space. [Researcher in the research task group]

Cramton (2002, 2001) conducted studies on the effects of text-based interactions on group communication. In studies of a performance appraisal system design firm, the author observed that due to the absence of non-verbal cues in e-mail messages, group members did not pay attention to certain messages embedded within the e-mail. The author noted that text-based interactions, especially e-mail communication, can lead to group members missing text-embedded messages. Though Cramton's (2002, 2001) studies focused on e-mail messages, it is important to note the potential ramifications of text-based interactions with regard to how information is processed by group members. The potential implication for knowledge exchange is that pieces of information may be missed or misinterpreted by decision makers or researchers.

Finding 5: Facilitation Contributes to Successful Knowledge Exchange

In the analysis, group members noted that process facilitation skills were vital to the success of knowledge exchange meetings. The group facilitators played an important role within the education and research task groups; they managed the group discussion and participation process. Without such guidance, the knowledge exchange process would likely have failed. When moving from a non-verbal rich medium (e.g., face-to-face communication) to a less non-verbal medium, such as web-conferencing, the facilitator needs to have strong facilitation skills to engage participants effectively, as demonstrated in the following statements:

I think in the face-to-face meetings, there are different kinds of cues that the facilitator can use, including visual cues, body language, etc. Whereas on the web-conferencing, you lose visual cues, but there are certain types of electronic ways to try and capture that. So on web-conferencing, the facilitator has to be a lot more conscious about the lack of cues. [Facilitator in the research task group]

The facilitator needs to be more aware of the need to check with other people. This will help make sure everybody is included. They should not move on to the next item until they checked that all discussions are finished for that item. [Facilitator in the education task group]

In a study of the effects of trained facilitators on group processes, Anson, Bostrom, and Wayne (1995) noted that process facilitation is a critical factor for improving group meetings in a technology-enabled environment. They noted that higher quality process facilitation improves the meeting process and training, and experience is important for building high quality process facilitation skills.

Finding 6: Technology Impacts Information Sharing

The data suggest that respondents in the education and research task groups believed that technology had little effect on the level of evidence shared in the group, as demonstrated by the following statements by one educator and research task group member:

We're all pretty much evidence based people, and I don't think anybody would explicitly disagree that web-conferencing affected the level of evidence. [Educator in the education task group]

No, I think the level of evidence we discussed still stayed the same. [Researcher in the research task group]

A possible explanation for this finding is that the group had arranged the documents (PowerPoint slides and PDF documents) to share before the meeting. Because they had pre-arranged the presentation of the evidence independently of the technology, the groups perceived that the technology had no real effect on the level of evidence.

Though respondents noted that technology did not affect the strength of the evidence, they acknowledged that technology did affect how the evidence was shared within the group. For example, respondents noted that web-conferencing limited the amount of information that a member could share on the whiteboard, which forced the group to summarize the information for display on the computer screen.

In general, the ICT literature on information exchange has focused on types of information (i.e., task, social, and contextual information), distribution of information, information sharing challenges, and general effects of technology on information sharing (Cramton & Orvis, 2003). Only a nominal amount of literature discusses the effects of technology on the level of evidence and how information is shared.

DISCUSSION

Our findings demonstrate that conferencing technologies had an impact on virtual knowledge exchange activities within drug policy groups. For example, respondents reported that different types of conferencing technologies (i.e., web and tele conferencing) had different effects on knowledge exchange. For the decision making task group, teleconferencing provided a simple and convenient method for participation at a distance and maintained the immediacy and spontaneity in group discussions that would be available in face-to-face meetings.

Web-conferencing was the preferred method of communication when the groups needed to collaborate, had a limited budget, and were geographically dispersed (e.g., the education task group). Groups with these traits found web-conferencing to be a more valuable medium than teleconferencing because it provided a much richer forum for interaction through its voting/polling, whiteboard, application sharing, and display of participant information functions. However, certain group respondents noted difficulties with web-conferencing, especially with the communication structure that it enforced on the group, which may have dampened social interactions.

The results of this study relate to the literature on ICTs. In general, the ICT literature tends to view social interaction norms within a group as a way to bring a form of governance to online environments. Group members learn through social interaction norms what is or is not socially acceptable within a group. Social interaction norms are crucial for the smooth operation of group meetings and interactions when technology is used to collaborate at a distance (Danis & Lee, 2005). In the education, research, and decision making task groups, our findings indicate that each group introduced various social interaction norms to facilitate group interactions in meetings. This diversity in social interaction norms can be explained by differences in group inputs, such as group characteristics, culture, and technology structure. Earlier studies on the use of collaboration technology among organizational members are found in the literature. Studying three groups within an organization for a 7-month period, Yates, Orlikowski, & Rennecker found that social interaction norms developed uniquely in the different groups. These differences were attributed to group size, task, and orientation toward the new technologies. Group members replicated similar social interaction norms within the new system and made innovations in creating new norms, including highlighting text in documents, embedding documents created in other media, and implementing faster turnaround in group-to-group discussions. (Yates, Orlikowski, & Rennecker, 1997)

Within the education, research, and decision making task groups, no explicit norms were introduced into the groups to regulate behaviors. In other studies, e.g., Ackerman et al. (1997), the groups involved in the study explicitly introduced social norms into the technology-enabled group and outlined social repercussions for not adhering to the social interaction norms. In the Ackerman et al. (1997) study, the groups used high audio quality for communication, in which users had the option to listen and speak during group discussions. The group consisted of nine members working on engineering-related projects. The group members developed social interaction norms for dealing with background noise, for knowing when someone was present and listening, and for limiting violations of personal privacy. Sanctions stopped unwanted behavior. A concerted effort was made to adhere to the social norms, and the result was improved group meetings. It is not clear why the drug policy groups did not introduce explicit social norms to influence group behavior in this study. Many of the group behaviors (i.e., expressions of social interaction norms) occurred implicitly within this study. Multiple explanations may account for why explicit rules for moderating group behavior were not expressed. Group members may have relied on the facilitator to carry out the task, may have been too busy, or may not have believed that controlling social behavior was a major issue that affected group meetings.

According to our findings, each of the three drug policy groups used a different communication media to carry out meetings. The education task group preferred web-conferencing to facilitated group communication by teleconference and face-to-face meetings. In contrast, the research task group essentially abandoned teleconferencing and web-conferencing in favor of face-to-face communication. However, the decision making task group preferred teleconferencing to facilitate group communication. This suggests that each group produced social interaction norms while using communication media, which defined how the group worked together. Over time, the three groups found the communication media that best facilitated their group interactions, becoming the norm under which group members operated. This is similar to the findings of Orlikowski and Yates (1994) in their study of technology-enabled knowledge workers and computer language designers, who collaborated on a multiyear project of developing various programming languages. The authors analyzed over 2,000 transcripts of archived e-mails, finding that when a group forms, members come to an agreement, whether implicitly or explicitly, on which communication media to use. When group members incorporate these norms into the group, they produce social interaction norms that define how the group works together. Over time, the groups studied reinforced the pattern of social interaction until it became the main method by which group members worked with each other. These social interaction norms continued to change and evolve as circumstances changed within the group.

In our findings, the drug policy groups noted the importance of having a trained process facilitator manage group interactions to improve group meetings. Similarly, Anson, Bostrom, and Wayne (1995) analyzed the consequence of group decision support systems (GDSSs) and the influence of a process facilitator on group performance and on group interaction processes. Their results demonstrate that groups that have more structure through process facilitation, but without GDSS support, demonstrated better group processes than GDSS-supported groups that lacked process facilitator support. Based on their findings, the authors observed that process facilitation is a critical factor for improving GDSSs effectiveness, higher quality process facilitation improves the meeting process, and training and experience are important for building high quality process facilitation skills. The research findings of Anson et al. (1995) were reflected in the statements of participants in the drug policy groups regarding process facilitation.

Our results showed that technology had little effect on the level of evidence in information exchange but did affect how the information was shared. In the ICT literature, many studies have focused on the use of information in problem solving tasks, such as admitting university students, general decision making, or product development (Dennis, 1996; Graetz, Boyle, Kimble, Thompson, & Garloch, 1998; Van Den Herik & Vreede Jan De, 1997). More specifically, the ICT literature on information exchange has focused on the various types of information, how they are distributed, and the challenges associated with their distribution (Cramton & Orvis, 2003). The literature discussing the effects of technology on the level of evidence and information sharing is scarce.

LIMITATIONS

There are a number of limitations in the study. First, limitations follow from using the action case study methodology. As noted in the methods section, action case study methods have been criticized for not being generalizable to other times, places, or settings. Other limitations of the study arise from the dynamic nature of drug policy groups. For example, each of the groups included in our study had a different number of participants, data types, and number of meetings. As a result, it was difficult to compare the three groups in a similar manner. Some of the interview questions had to be slightly modified to take into account group context. Furthermore, no baseline data were collected for the decision making task group. Additionally, not all of the groups used the same technologies. The decision making task group used teleconferencing, the research task group used web-conferencing and later abandoned it, and the education task group used both teleconferencing and web-conferencing. Future studies should not be limited to drug policy groups and should expand to other health and non-health related groups working on knowledge exchange activities using virtual collaboration tools.

Furthermore, this study focused on knowledge exchange, a process focused on networking and information exchange. Future studies should focus on the effects of web-conferencing, teleconferencing, and other technologies, as well as on knowledge synthesis, the contextualization of research findings, the application of research, and decision making processes.

Finally, the version of the Elluminate web-conferencing technology employed in this study allowed for half-duplex audio communication, allowing users to only speak one at a time. Future studies should examine the effects of full-duplex web-conferencing technology on knowledge exchange processes.

SOLUTIONS AND RECOMMENDATIONS

Based on our findings and experiences with the groups in this study, the following recommendations for virtual knowledge exchange groups are discussed. Five recommendations are proposed: 1) understand the group's technological needs, 2) introduce communication rules appropriate to the group, 3) take time to prepare the material shared in the meeting, 4) use a technical and process facilitator in web-conferencing meetings, and 5) include an ongoing evaluation of meetings.

Understand the Group's Technological Needs

Based on our findings, we suggest that understanding the group's technological needs based on group tasks, characteristics, context and culture will help to create successful virtual knowledge exchange groups. In the study, the education, research, and decision making task groups had different technological needs that were relevant to the specific group dynamics. Therefore, prior to introducing technologies to knowledge exchange groups, a needs assessment should be carried out to determine the types of technologies to use for the groups they will be interacting with.

The needs assessment should include three phases. In phase one, a needs assessment is carried out in the form of a questionnaire in which appropriate technologies are identified. In phase two, a review of the various technologies is carried out. In phase three, various technologies are evaluated by a group in a field setting. Figure 3 highlights the three phases.

Phase 1 and 2: Needs Phase and Technology Review

In phase 1, all or selected group members fill out a needs analysis questionnaire. The needs assessment questionnaire will help in selecting an appropriate technology for virtual knowledge exchange groups. The needs assessment can be conducted by the group coordinator or project leader. Once the interviews have been conducted, responses can be summarized outlining the needs of the group. Suggested questions, which have been adapted from Communique Conferencing, are provided in Table 3 (Communique, 2003). If it is determined that there is a need for ICTs to support virtual knowledge exchange, then a Phase 2 analysis (see Table 4), also referred to as technology review, should be conducted. A description of a scenario using the questions of Phase 1 and 2 is provided.

Phase 1 and 2 Example

The example presented below is that of the education task group that was a participant in this study. Table 5 presents the results from the needs analysis and technology review questionnaires. For this example, by interviewing key members of the group, we found that the education task group had a very limited budget (i.e., they could not afford face-to-face meetings), 10-15 participants were expected to participate monthly, the group was geographically dispersed, and there was approximately one meeting per month. Therefore, the needs analysis questionnaire determined a need for the use of ICTs to support virtual knowledge exchange within the group. For the technology review, we found that the group had a high willingness to learn new technologies and needed to share various types of content (e.g., PDF, Word, and PowerPoint files), a high level of interaction within the meetings, a hosted software solution, and both technical support and high security due to the sensitivity of the information. Based on these findings, it was found that web-conferencing would be the most viable option to support the group's virtual knowledge exchange activities.

Phase 3: Field Group Evaluation

To continue with the education task group example, because web-conferencing was determined to be the most appropriate tool for communication, a field evaluation should be conducted to determine the most appropriate technology with which the group would be comfortable, given the specifications required to support group collaboration. This process requires deploying web-conferencing software and obtaining feedback on the group's experience of using the technology while supporting a group task. Feedback from the group members determines which products are best suited for the group. The questionnaire is included in Appendix 1. The dimensions included in the survey questionnaire are overall satisfaction, technical issues, and product functionality. An online survey tool should be used to help process the results of the survey. The selection should be based on the highest survey score for a specific web-conferencing tool.

OTHER RECOMMENDATIONS

In addition to the recommendations for selecting the most appropriate technology for a virtual knowledge exchange group, other recommendations are suggested to help run successful meetings:

Introduce Communication Rules Appropriate to the Group

Experience from this research study showed that as groups use technology, each group tends to develop its own social interaction norms. For example, the education and research task groups introduced norms, such as raising a hand before speaking and carrying out a communication check

Figure 3. Needs assessment phases

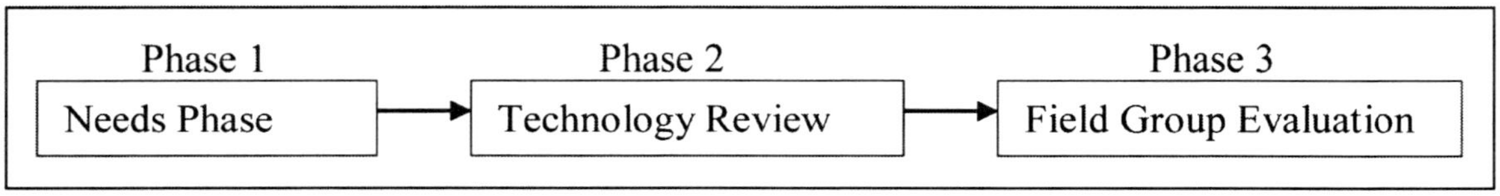

Table 3. Phase 1: Needs analysis

Does the Group Need ICT:
Q1. **Communication Budget:** What is the total monthly budget allocated to the meetings?
Q2. **Participants:** How many people are expected to participate in the group?
Q3. **Separation:** Are the individuals geographically separated from one another?
Q4. **Consistency:** Will the participants remain consistent from meeting to meeting, or will they change?
Q5. **Number of Meetings:** How many meetings will be conducted each week, month, or quarter? Will usage fluctuate depending on the time of year?

at the beginning of the meeting. The decision making task group introduced strict interaction norms on presentation times and organization of the presentation.

Such rules are important for running successful virtual knowledge exchange meetings. Group characteristics, research tasks, and cultures should be taken into account when developing rules for discussion or participation in a technology-enabled environment. For example (and based on our experience), if all of the group members know each other or if the group is small (3-5 people) in a teleconferencing session, then a discussion rule for identifying oneself is not needed because group members are likely able to identify the speaker. However, if the group is large (>5) or group members are not familiar with each other, then an explicit discussion rule of identifying oneself before speaking is needed.

In the *Houston Business Journal*, Campisi (2003) provides general etiquette for both teleconferencing and web-conferencing meetings that can be applied to virtual knowledge exchange meetings. For teleconferencing, Campisi suggests that group members should begin with introductions with each participant's name, title, and location before sharing an idea or commenting on other's ideas during the call. It is suggested that this rule

Table 4. Phase 2: Technology review

What Type of ICT would be Appropriate?
Q1. **Willingness to Learn:** Are group members willing to orient themselves with new technologies, such as web-conferencing?
Q2. **Content:** What type of content will be presented (e.g., PowerPoint slides, software applications, web-based applications, documents, and spreadsheets)?
Q3. **Interactivity:** What degree of interactivity does the group require (e.g., conversing, presenting/listening, Q&A, polling/voting, application sharing, text chatting, live video, and file sharing)?
Q4. **Software Solution:** Does the group want its own software solution or a hosted solution?
Q5. **Technical Support:** How much technical support or event management support does the group require?
Q6. **Security:** Would it matter if group discussions were heard or accessed by others?

Table 5. Phase 1 and 2 sample data

Needs Analysis: Does the Group Need ICT?
Q1. **Communication Budget:** Very limited, not more than $500 per month.
Q2. **Participants:** 10-15 participants in monthly meetings.
Q3. **Separation:** High, group members in different provinces.
Q4. **Consistency:** Range from 10-15.
Q5. **Number of Meetings:** One per month consistently throughout the year.
Technology Review: What Type of ICT would be Appropriate?
Q1. **Willingness to Learn:** Very high.
Q2. **Content:** Share PowerPoint, spreadsheets, PDF and Word documents.
Q3. **Interactivity:** Voting and polling, text chatting, application sharing, and file sharing.
Q4. **Software Solution:** Hosted.
Q5. **Technical Support:** Need dedicated facilitator to help group with technology issues.
Q6: **Security:** Sensitive information discussed; therefore, security needs are high.

be applied to large groups whose members have not yet developed a strong rapport with each other. The author also recommends that if a participant is not speaking, that person should mute his or her phone so that shuffling papers, typing on the keyboard, and side talking are not heard. If muting is not an option, group members should be reminded to minimize these potentially distracting actions. The participants in our study the study made similar comments on etiquette.

Campisi (2003) emphasizes the importance of keeping in mind that the objective of the teleconference is to streamline communications and increase productivity (Campisi, 2003). To streamline meetings, based upon experiences from this research, virtual knowledge exchange groups should encourage group members to decide on specific practices regarding sending documents for group members to review two to five business days before the meeting, scheduling monthly meetings at the same time of the month (for example, 9:30-10:00 AM, the third Tuesday of every month), keeping the agenda specific, and adhering to time limits.

For web-conferencing, Campisi (2003) suggests that members introduce only legible instant messaging texts, make legible annotations on graphs, and use clear language and font sizes. These are important factors to consider as interactions shift from a face-to-face to a text-based format. Group members should ensure that their text messaging or annotations on graphs are understandable and legible. Furthermore, Campisi emphasizes that it is important, especially in collaborative groups, that group members pay attention to the meeting and listen carefully because they may be asked to add input or to share a document. As a rule, participants should not attend to their e-mail or engage in web-browsing during the meeting.

Take Time to Prepare the Material Shared in the Meeting

Experience from this research study demonstrated that as group members move from face-to-face environments to a web-conferencing environment, the meeting shifts its focus from individuals meeting in a shared space (e.g., a room or office) to interactions that occur within the text through the computer screen. Meeting dynamics change such that the text becomes the focus of the meeting. Therefore, more extensive preparation should be made by virtual knowledge exchange groups when presenting information via web-conferencing. The information should be visually appealing to the participants, and the text should be concise and to the point. The visual aspect of the meeting via the whiteboard is what becomes important, whereas in face-to-face meetings, what the individual has to say is important. Virtual knowledge exchange groups should present materials in a way that fits the online medium. In contrast, virtual knowledge exchange groups should not be preoccupied with the effect web-conferencing will have on the level of evidence because (as respondents noted) web-conferencing has little influence on the level of evidence. Instead, the groups should focus on how to present the evidence in an appealing and credible way that is persuasive to decision makers and other stakeholders.

The Canadian Health Services Research Foundation (2000) presented a one-page document on how to give a research presentation to decision makers. The foundation suggests that in preparing the material the presenter should (CHSRF, 2000):

- Identify the specific decision that the research addresses and state it in clear, unambiguous terms;
- Understand who the decision makers in the audience will be, what they know already, and what new information they need - then tailor the presentation accordingly using plain language;

- Take into account the political, legislative, fiscal, and social factors that provide context for the issue and for the presentation; and
- Create a no-surprise environment - develop a working relationship with decision makers early on in the research process.

It is also suggested that group members distribute documents that will be shared before the presentation, even if the documents can be shared via the web-conferencing software. If any PowerPoint documents are presented, it is recommended that the content be clear and concise and that the fonts be large enough for members to read easily. When sharing documents, the process facilitator should ensure that group members can easily see the documents, easily read them, and follow along.

Use a Technical and Process Facilitator in Web-Conferencing Meetings

Bases on the experiences of this research, when introducing web-conferencing technologies to a group, it is important to plan for two distinct facilitator roles: one to facilitate the meeting process and the other to facilitate the group's use of technology. If both types of facilitators are not provided, there is a risk of overburdening the facilitation process, leading to its breakdown.

Generally, the role of the facilitator has been an active one within the group process, as the results of this research study have indicated. McFadzean, Somersall, and Coker (1999) describe three phases of group meetings in which the process facilitator plays a role in the group process. The authors noted that it is important to have group agreement on the meeting objective and on the meeting process during the pre-planning stage. The results of the authors' two field case studies indicated that groups who do not carry out these two important tasks negatively affect the meeting process (McFadzean, Somersall, & Coker, 1999). Therefore, virtual knowledge exchange groups should ensure that there are clear objectives to the meeting and that the meeting rules are clear.

According to the literature, the functions of a process facilitator include listening, clarifying and integrating information, creating an open and positive environment, directing and managing the meeting, and building a rapport with and relationships among group members (Clawson, Bostrom, & Anson, 1993). The functions of a technical facilitator include understanding the technologies and their capabilities, creating comfort with the technology, and selecting and preparing the technology for use by the group (Clawson, Bostrom, & Anson, 1993). Virtual knowledge exchange groups should ensure that both the technical and process facilitators are trained to develop such qualities.

Continuous Evaluations of Meetings Are Required

Based on our experience, it is recommended that virtual knowledge exchange groups include a meeting evaluator for technology-enabled (i.e., web- or teleconferencing) meetings. The role of the evaluator is to improve satisfaction within the meeting. The evaluator should ask the following questions at each meeting:

1. In what ways could group etiquette or the quality of person-to-person interactions be improved next time? Examples include displaying pictures of participants at the beginning of a web-conference, asking group members to introduce themselves and their work, suggesting taking 5 minutes at the beginning of the meeting for casual conversations, and reminding group members that shuffling paper can be distracting during a teleconferencing meeting.
2. In what ways could the discussion process be improved? Examples include setting

an explicit restriction on speaking time, introducing explicit directions for when to use text messaging, and emphasizing the expectation that participants do not engage in other work during the meeting.

3. In what ways could the participation process be improved? Examples include raising a hand to speak in face-to-face sessions, using the hand raising function in web-conferencing sessions, supporting the expectation that everyone must participate on every agenda item, and noting explicit directions for using the voting and polling feature.
4. Are there suggestions for how facilitation and technical assistance could be improved? For example, the process facilitator should be provided with further training, should or should not be a member of the group, needs to improve his or her credibility with the group, needs to be more engaging, and needs to do more listening and less commenting to help build group cohesiveness and rapport. With regard to the technical facilitator, he or she may require more training, should be up-to-date on newer or better technologies, should be responsive to technical issues, and should conduct a communication check at the beginning of the meeting.
5. What improvement(s) could be made to the format and content of the information exchanged? Examples include referencing statistics or academic papers when discussing evidence, using more visual presentations, providing hyperlinks to the literature, disseminating the literature or presentation before the meeting, using more graphics, using certain size fonts and colors that are visually appealing, and taking advantage of application sharing to show literature and Excel files.

Furthermore, it is important that the evaluator be encouraged to call attention to improvements within the meetings. The evaluator should document the changes and ensure that the group is following them. This will provide a continuous quality improvement process for virtual knowledge exchange and improve meeting outcomes.

FUTURE RESEARCH DIRECTIONS

Knowledge exchange activities occurring at a distance and using information and communication technologies is relatively a new field. Future research in this domain should focus on specific knowledge exchange tasks and study how conferencing technologies can impact decision maker and researcher interactions. Specifically, future studies should explore the effects of conferencing technologies on activities and processes relating to collaborative problem solving, synthesizing evidence, contextualizing evidence, applying evidence, and decision making. Future researchers should also study multiple groups in different health domains that involve researchers and decision makers employing the current technologies that were used in the study, as well as other technologies, such as videoconferencing and group decision support systems.

CONCLUSION

This study contributed to our general knowledge of understanding virtual knowledge exchange in drug policy groups. Solutions and recommendations were made on how to create successful virtual knowledge exchange meetings. The main finding of this study was that ICTs affected knowledge exchange processes in different ways. For example, drug policy groups developed different patterns for social interactions within teleconferencing and web-conferencing meetings. The recommendations proposed can be used by groups needing to communicate and collaborate on virtual knowledge exchange activities. The recommendations can be used by other groups working outside virtual knowledge exchange within drug policy domain.

In general, this study has made a significant scientific contribution to advancing our understanding of the role information and communication technologies play in shaping the knowledge exchange process within drug policy groups. The study has led to findings not previously reported. In addition, the research has important implications for the domains of knowledge exchange, ICT, and drug policy by providing lessons learned on how to conduct and improve distant knowledge exchange collaborations. In summary, the research project described in this chapter has contributed in a number of original ways to the advancement of scientific knowledge.

REFERENCES

Ackerman, M. S., Hindus, D., Mainwaring, S. D., & Starr, B. (1997). Hanging on the wire: A field study of an audio-only media space. *ACM Transactions on Human-Computer Interaction*, *4*(1), 39–66. doi:10.1145/244754.244756

Anson, R., Bostrom, R., & Wayne, B. (1995). An experiment assessing group support system and facilitator effects on meeting outcomes. *Management Science*, *41*(2), 189–208. doi:10.1287/mnsc.41.2.189

Berg, B. (1989). *Qualitative research methodology* (Bacon, A., Ed.). 3rd ed.). Boston.

Braa, K., & Vigden, R. (1999). Interpretation, intervention, and reduction in the organizational laboratory: A framework for in-context information systems research. *Accounting Management & Information Technology*, *9*(1), 25–47. doi:10.1016/S0959-8022(98)00018-6

Campisi, J. (2003, August 4). Minding manners: Conferencing technologies involve new etiquette. *Houston Business Journal*. Retrieved from http://houston.bizjournals.com/ houston/ stories/2003/08/04/ focus4.html

CHSRF. (2000). *How to give a research presentation to decision-makers*. Ottawa. Retrieved from http://www.chsrf.ca/ knowledge_transfer/ pdf/ presentation_e.pdf

CHSRF. (2010). *Knowledge exchange*. Retrieved from http://www.oise.utoronto.ca/rspe/KM_Products/Terminology/index.html

Clawson, V., Bostrom, R., & Anson, R. (1993). The role of the facilitator in computer-supported meetings. *Small Group Research*, *24*(4), 524–547. doi:10.1177/1046496493244007

Communique. (2003). *Choosing a web conferencing solution*. Retrieved from http://www.ccimeet.com/ choosingawebconferencesolution.pdf

COMPUS. (2004). *Canadian optimal medication prescribing and utilization service*. Retrieved from https://www.ccohtaccohta.ca/ compus/ compus_intro_e.cfm

Cramton, C. (2002). Finding common ground in dispersed collaboration. *Organizational Dynamics*, *30*(4), 356–367. doi:10.1016/S0090-2616(02)00063-3

Cramton, C., & Orvis, K. L. (2003). Overcoming barriers to information sharing in virtual teams. In Gibson, C., & Cohen, S. (Eds.), *Creating conditions for effective virtual teams* (pp. 214–230). San Francisco, CA: Jossey-Bass.

Cramton, C. D. (2001). The mutual knowledge problem and its consequences for dispersed collaboration. *Organization Science*, *12*(3), 346–371. doi:10.1287/orsc.12.3.346.10098

Danis, C., & Lee, A. (2005). Evolution of norms in a newly forming group. In M. F. Costabile & F. Paterno (eds.), *Proceedings of IFIP TC13 International Conference on Human-Computer Interaction — INTERACT 2005*, (pp. 522-535).

Dennis, A. R. (1996). Information exchange and use in small group decision-making. *Small Group Research*, *27*(4), 532–550. doi:10.1177/1046496496274003

DeSanctis, G., & Poole, M. (1994). Capturing the complexity in advanced technology use: Adaptive structuration theory. *Organization Science*, *5*(2), 121–147. doi:10.1287/orsc.5.2.121

Graetz, K., Boyle, E., Kimble, C., Thompson, P., & Garloch, J. (1998). Information sharing in face-to-face, teleconferencing and electronic chat groups. *Small Group Research*, *29*(6), 714–743. doi:10.1177/1046496498296003

Househ, M., Kushniruk, A., Maclure, M., Carleton, B., & Cloutier-Fisher, D. (2009). A case study examining the impacts of conferencing technologies in distributed healthcare groups. *Electronic Healthcare*, *8*(2), 10–14.

Hsieh, H. F., & Shannon, S. (2005). Three approaches to qualitative content analysis. *Qualitative Health Research*, *15*(9), 1277–1288. doi:10.1177/1049732305276687

Kondracki, N., Wellman, N., & Amundson, D. (2002). Content analysis: Review of methods and their applications in nutrition education. *Journal of Nutrition Education and Behavior*, *34*(4), 224–230. doi:10.1016/S1499-4046(06)60097-3

KUSP. (2003). *Overview of champion/opinion leader/knowledge broker*. Retrieved March 15, 2003, from http://www.nursing.ualberta.ca/ estabrooks/kusp/ DatabaseOverview.htm

Lau, F., & Hayward, R. (2000). Building a virtual network in a community health research training program. *Journal of the American Medical Informatics Association*, *7*(4), 1–3. doi:10.1136/jamia.2000.0070361

Maclure, M., & Potashnik, T. (1997). What is direct evidence-based policy-making? Experience from the drug benefits program for seniors in British Columbia. *Canadian Journal on Aging*, *1*(23), 132–146.

McFadzean, E., Somersall, L., & Coker, A. (1999). A framework for facilitating group processes. *Strategic Change*, *8*(7), 421–431. doi:10.1002/(SICI)1099-1697(199911)8:7<421::AID-JSC434>3.0.CO;2-4

Milbank. (2001). *The Cochrane collaboration: Informing judgement: Case studies of health policy and research in six countries*. Milbank Memorial Fund. New York.

Orlikowski, W. J., & Yates, J. (1994). *Genre repertoire: Norms and forms for work and interaction*. Retrieved from http://ccs.mit.edu/CCSWP166.html

Rourke, L., Anderson, T., Garrison, D. R., & Archer, W. (2001). Assessing social presence in asynchronous, text-based computer conferencing. *Journal of Distance Education*, *14*(3), 51–70.

Van Den Herik, K. W., & Vreede Jan De, G. (1997). GSS for cooperative policymaking: No trivial matter. *Proceedings of the International ACM SIGGROUP Conference on Supporting Group Work: The Integration Challenge*.

Yates, J., Orlikowski, W. J., & Rennecker, J. (1997). Collaborative genres for collaboration: Genre systems in digital media. In [). Hawaii.]. *Proceedings of the Hawaii International Conference on System Sciences*, *6*, 50–69.

KEY TERMS AND DEFINITIONS

Action Case: There is no standard definition for action case, but an action case study examines a phenomenon in its natural setting with the researcher acting as a participatory agent within the research project (Braa & Vigden, 1999).

Action Research: Action research is a methodology that links "theory with practice through an iterative process of problem diagnosis, action intervention, and reflective learning" (Lau & Hayward, 2000).

Case Study: Case study research focuses on "understanding the dynamics present within single settings" (Eisenhardt, 1989). Case studies can be referred to as either soft cases (in which the primary sources of data collection are qualitative and include archives, interviews, and observations) or hard cases (in which the primary data source is quantitative and may include data collection methods such as surveys).

ICT: ICT refers to technologies that enable groups and individuals to communicate, collaborate, and interact to share information through various technological media, including e-mail, conferencing (telephone, video and web), and discussion forums. Many ICT tools, such as PowerPoint, are included in this definition.

Knowledge Exchange: Knowledge exchange refers to collaborative problem solving between researchers and decision makers that occurs through communication and information exchanges (CHSRF, 2010).

Quasi-Experiment: A quasi-experiment is defined by Cook and Campbell as a research design having many of the characteristics of an experimental design but without random assignment of the subjects. (1979, pp. 117-118).

Teleconferencing: In this study, teleconferencing refers to the use of audio conferencing involving telephones. This technology provides an audio-only communication medium where multiple participants can speak at the same time. To use the technology, the participants dial a telephone number and enter a conference code. They are prompted to say their name, and a beep sounds to let other participants know that a new participant has joined the meeting.

Web-Conferencing: Web-conferencing describes live meetings over the Internet. During the meeting, group members use computers to synchronously communicate with other participants. To attend a web-conference, group members log onto a website using their name. To access the technology, participants typically download an application to their local computer. This type of technology allows users to upload agendas, utilize whiteboards, send instant text messages, record votes and polling results from participants, express emoticons, raise hands to indicate a wish to speak, and see participant names.

APPENDIX 1: SURVEY EVALUATING WEB-CONFERENCING TECHNOLOGY

Satisfaction – Questions Relating to Overall Satisfaction

1. How do you feel about the group's discussion? [--below--]
   [1. Very Satisfied, 2. Satisfied, 3. Neutral, 4. Dissatisfied, 5. Very Dissatisfied] -- > Select one.
2. How do you feel about the group's usage of the technology to support group tasks?
   [1. Very Satisfied, 2. Satisfied, 3. Neutral, 4. Dissatisfied, 5. Very Dissatisfied] -- > Select one.
3. To what extent did you enjoy participating in the meeting? [--below--]
   [1. Very Much, 2. Much, 3. Neutral, 4. Not Much, 5. Not At All] -- > Select one.
4. All in all, how do you feel? [--below--]
   [1. Very Satisfied, 2. Satisfied, 3. Neutral, 4. Dissatisfied, 5. Very Dissatisfied] -- > Select one.
5. What concerns/issues do you have regarding the use of web-conferencing technologies?
   Put comments here ->

Technical – Questions Relating to the Technical Aspects of the Product

1. Did you find it technically difficult to setup your computer before the meeting? [-- below --]
   [Yes, No] --> Select one please.
2. Can you list the top three technical difficulties you experienced during the meeting?
   Place list here -> 1.______________ 2. ______________ 3. ______________
3. Are there other technologies/media that you would suggest using in web conferencing meetings?
   Put comments here ->

Functionality – Questions Relating to the Functionality of the Product

1. To what extent did you find the web conferencing product to be user friendly? [-- below --]
   [1. Very Much, 2. Much, 3. Neutral, 4. Not Much, 5. Not At All]--> Select one please.
2. Did you find it easy to customize the web conferencing product to suit your visual needs?
   [1. Very Much, 2. Much, 3. Neutral, 4. Not Much, 5. Not At All] --> Select one please.

About the Contributors

Åsa Smedberg is a Senior Lecturer, Researcher and Director of PhD studies at the Department of Computer and Systems Sciences (DSV), Stockholm University, Sweden. She holds a PhD degree in Computer and Systems Sciences. Her research interests include Web-based communities and the use of ICT for continuous learning, with a focus on practical applications in the health area. She runs research in the field of web-based health communities for self-help groups. Over the years, in-depth studies have been carried out of online conversations in e-health communities. She is the author of a series of international publications, member of editorial review board of international journals and committee member of e-health conferences.

* * *

Mariano Alcañiz is Full Professor of Graphics Engineering at Universidad Politécnica de Valencia (Spain) since 2002, and he is the Director of the Human Centered Technology Lab (LabHuman). His research interests are focused in how technology can augment human ability, studying technology-augmented human cognition and action in disciplines like psychology, surgery, and education among others. Mariano Alcañiz has been principal investigator in more than 90 research projects, funded by national and European institutions. He has published over 56 articles in national and international journals, as well as several books and book chapters. He has also presented over 200 works at national and international conferences.

Rosa M. Baños is a Full Professor in Psychopathology at the University of Valencia, Spain. Her research interests include psychopathology, the treatment of psychological disorders, and the application of Information and Communication Technologies to Psychology. Dr. Banos is the director of the Master's program, "Interventions for Eating Disorders and Personality Disorders" at University of Valencia. She is a member of several scientific associations; she is in the editorial board of several journals, and expert review of several European and Spanish institutions and organizations. At this moment she is collaborating with the Spanish Ministry of Science and Innovation, as Research Manager for Psychology.

Marina Umaschi Bers is an Associate Professor at the Eliot-Pearson Department of Child Development and an Adjunct Professor in the Computer Science Department at Tufts University. She is also a scientific Research Associate at Boston Children's Hospital. Her research involves the design and study of innovative learning technologies to promote children's positive development. At Tufts, Prof. Bers heads the interdisciplinary Developmental Technologies Research Group and collaborates with Tufts' Center for Educational Engineering Outreach (CEEO).

Cristina Botella is Full Professor of Clinical Psychology at Jaume I University (Spain) since 1992. Her main line of research is the design and testing of clinical applications based on information and communication technologies (ICTs) for the treatment of emotional disorders. She has been principal investigator in more than 30 research projects. She has published over 100 papers in national and international journals, as well as 20 books and over 30 book chapters. She is the Director of the Emotional Disorders Clinic at Jaume I University that offers psychological treatments to the community and training for clinical psychologists. She is also Director of Master in Psychopathology, Health and Neuropsychology.

Kathryn A. Cantrell is a certified child life specialist and received her Master's from Eliot-Pearson Department of Child Development at Tufts University where she was a researcher with the Developmental Technologies Research Group. Her research involves the design and facilitation of virtual communities for youth with chronic illnesses to promote adjustment, adherence, and hopefulness. Kathryn is pursuing a career in pediatric psychology where she can continue designing and evaluating interventions to promote adjustment in youth with chronic illnesses.

Bruce Carleton has a lifelong goal to make medication use more effective and safer for all patients, particularly children. His research focus is on the impact of drug therapy on human health and quality of life. He is particularly interested in developing better ways to evaluate the effectiveness of drugs, medication-use models designed to improve patient health, as well as practical surveillance systems to improve the safe use of medication. Dr. Carleton has particular clinical interests in asthma, the clinical use of drugs in children, as well as the epidemiology, pharmacogenomics, and clinical management of adverse drug events.

Diana Castilla-López got her Degree in Psychology from the University of Valencia. From 2001, her main field of work is focused on the study of the Interaction Human-Machine, specifically on Usability and User-Centered Design. In 2005 she leaves her post in the private sector to join the research group LabPsiTec, directed by Dr. Cristina Botella, where she starts working as a researcher. She has taken part in the design, development and usability evaluation of different technologies in many research projects, both at a hardware and at a software level: Web, Virtual Reality, Augmented Reality, mobile devices, tactile devices, PC Architecture, rumblepads, accelerometer, and even gestural language through semantic recognition. At the present moment she is doing her PhD in the field of Usability.

Ausiàs Cebolla is a researcher at the University Jaume I of Castelló, Spain. His research interests include clinical applications based on information and communication technologies (ICTs) in the treatment of childhood obesity and promotion of physical activity. He is also interested in research on efficacy of psychotherapy and mindfulness interventions. He is a member of several scientific associations.

Stein Conradsen (born 1965) is a higher executive officer, adviser and researcher in the Patient Education Resource Center in Sunnmøre Hospital Trust, Norway. He holds a degree in education from the University of Oslo. In his academic career he has taken interest in the fields of religious education, patient education, and self-help. He gives lessons in didactical and teaching methodological aspects of patient education. He is also engaged in a program for user involvement in patient education for psychiatric care.

Anni Dugdale is a Senior Lecturer in the Government Discipline at University of Canberra where she teaches Sociology and Social Policy and Research Methodology. Her research is inspired by Science and Technology Studies (STS) and most recently investigates e-health, e-democracy, and digital governance. Anni enjoys working collaboratively with multidisciplinary teams and has worked closely with colleagues from Information Systems. Anni was a consumer representative in the 1990s although not for any of the organizations discussed here. She lives in Canberra with her partner Suzanne, a cat, and many chickens.

Gjermund Eikli is the Manager of the division for in-service training and further education at the Norwegian Net School, a non-profit company owned by 6 municipalities that offers e-learning solutions from pre-school to adult education. After 20 years as a primary school teacher, Eikli turned his focus to e-learning in 1995. Currently he guides companies and organizations that go online with their teaching and is in charge of the development of PedIT, the e-learning platform chosen by the Norwegian Study Organization for the Disabled. In partnership with Volda University College he developed a model for the in-service training of teachers that about 10% of Norwegian teachers participated in. His latest project focuses on the role of the Social Web in supporting collaborative learning processes.

Ernestina Etchemendy has a degree in Psychology from the University of Buenos Aires (Argentina). In 2007 she left Argentina to join the research group Labpsitec, directed by PhD Cristina Botella, and to start a Master in Psychopatology, Health and Neuropsychology. Currently she is studying for her Doctorate at the University of Castellon (UJI). Her research is focused on the use of information and communication technologies (ICTs) applied in the elderly population and promotion of wellbeing.

Denise Cloutier-Fisher completed her PhD at the University of Guelph in 2000 and joined the University of Victoria in July 2001 with a joint appointment that allows her to work half-time in each of the Department of Geography and the Centre on Aging. Prior to coming to UVic, Dr. Cloutier-Fisher worked as a research coordinator for the College of Family Physicians of Canada (1990-1994), a Data Analyst, and as a senior population health Consultant for the Central West Health Planning Information Network located in Hamilton, Ontario (1999-2001). Dr. Cloutier Fisher is a health geographer with a primary interest in 'healthy aging' in rural and small-town environments. Broadly speaking Dr. Cloutier-Fisher's research focuses on health and social service delivery systems, population health, and the social determinants of health. Dr. Cloutier Fisher's research approaches support the use of both qualitative and quantitative methods that are appropriate and consistent with the research questions being asked.

Anna Lisa Gentile is a Research Associate at the University of Sheffield. She is a member of the Organisations, Information and Knowledge (OAK) Group. Her research field concerns information extraction technologies. She has been involved in the EU projects WeKnowIt and SmartProducts and she currently works on the Rolls-Royce SILOET project. She has a number of relevant publications in some major conference venues such as Language Resources Evaluation Conference (LREC) and Conference on Empirical Methods in Natural Language Processing (EMNLP). She holds a PhD from the University of Bari (Italy) in the field of Natural Language Processing.

Lorna Gibson is a post-doctoral researcher with a background in e-Health and human-centred design. Her PhD "Understanding the User Experience of eHealth and the implications for social computing" was based both on her experiences working on e-Health projects with clinical partners and her personal experiences with healthcare information and misinformation and the impact this has on the individual. She has spent ten years working in the fields of accessibility, usability, and user-centred design.

Navreet Gill, BScN, RN, is a Clinical Research Nurse Coordinator at The Hospital for Sick Children in Toronto with a clinical background in pediatric cardiology. Currently she is facilitating the coordination of multiple clinical research studies in her role as a CRNC. She received her Bachelor's of Science in Nursing from the Lawrence S. Bloomberg Faculty of Nursing at the University of Toronto and is currently working towards her Master's of Science in Nursing at the same faculty. Her current research interests include pediatric pain and the delivery of self-management strategies for chronic illness through an online medium.

Ricardo Mendoza-González is a Researcher/Professor at the Instituto Tecnológico de Aguascalientes (Mexico). He holds a PhD in Computer Science (Universidad Autónoma de Aguascalientes, México, 2009), a Master's degree in Computer Science (Universidad Autónoma de Aguascalientes, México, 2007), and a Bachelor of Computer Science (Instituto Tecnológico de Aguascalientes, México, 2004). Dr. Mendoza-González has reported his work in journals such as *Advances in Engineering Software*, and prestigious international conferences such as IEEE-CCECE, CADUI, ICIMP, and IASTED-CNIS. He collaborates with researchers of the University of Ontario Institute of Technology (UOIT, Canada), and Universidad Autónoma de Aguascalientes (Mexico). His current research interests include several topics on: human-computer interaction, information security, usability, artificial intelligence, and software engineering.

Mowafa Househ is an Assistant Professor and Director of Research at the College of Public Health and Health Informatics. Dr. Househ is also the editor-in-chief of the Journal of Health Informatics in Developing Countries. Prior to finishing his doctoral studies, Dr. Househ worked for the Northern Health authority from 2006-2009 as a planning and research analyst. Dr. Househ also worked as an instructor at the University of Northern British Columbia School of Business prior to moving to Saudi Arabia. Dr. Househ has published on the topics of collaborative technology use in promoting research communication and collaboration in clinical practice and at the policy level. Dr. Househ is interested in the use of collaborative technologies in health informatics education, patient education, knowledge exchange, and in forming collaborative research partnerships. Dr. Househ's goals are the use of collaborative technologies to improve clinical and policy decision-making. He believes that such technologies can help foster communication and collaboration between various and disparate groups working in different parts of the world. In addition to this, he believes that using such technologies is one step closer to creating a more environmentally friendly world.

Korinna Zoi Karamagkioli is currently serving as a Resident in Nuclear Medicine at the Alexandra University hospital in Athens, Greece and is an MSc student at Kings College in London, working at Guys and St Thomas NHS hospitals. Previous working experience includes a residency post in Nuclear Medicine and Clinical Physiology in the department of Clinical Physiology in Sweden at the Central hospital of Karlstad, Sweden. She has also worked as a District doctor in an area of 5000 habitants at Korinthos, in the South Greece region. Dr. Karamagkioli was awarded from the President of the Greek Red Cross, for her voluntary services as a first-aid seminars trainer (March-April 2005). She also offers voluntary services (part in missions, training programmes) with the "Greek Medicines du Mondes". Dr. Karamagkioli is a member of the following professional associations: Athens Medical Association, Swedish National Board of Health and Welfare-Socialstyrelsen, General Medical Council (UK), Greek Medicines du Monde, European Association of Nuclear Medicine and European Association of Radiology. She has published several articles in the area of eHealth.

Evika Karamagioli is a jurist that serves since 2009 as Deputy Director at the Greek NGO, Gov2u. Prior to joining Gov2U she was a Grants & Research Coordinator in the Greek NGO access2democracy, Scientific Associate at the Centre for European Constitutional Law Themistocles and Dimitris Tsatsos Foundation, and responsible for European Project Management at the Athens Bar Association, Greece. She has extensive experience in designing and managing research projects funded in the areas of e-democracy, eParticipation, and eInclusion. She has also contributed as a researcher in the elaboration of a series of studies concerning public administration modernization and eGovernment. From 2007-2008 she was involved as an independent expert in the Ad hoc committee on eDemocracy of the Council of Europe (CAHDE). She holds a Master's in International Security and Defence from the University of Grenoble, France and a Master's in Crisis Management from Athens University, Greece. She is currently a PhD candidate at the University Paris 8, France. She has published extensively on the subjects of e-Democracy and human rights and ICT.

Helmut Krcmar is a Full Professor of Information Systems and holds the Chair for Information Systems at the Department of Computer Science, Technische Universität München, Germany, since 2002. His research interests include information and knowledge management, IT-enabled value webs, service management, computer-supported cooperative work, and information systems in health care and e-government.

Andre Kushniruk is a Professor of the School of Health Information Science at the University of Victoria. Dr. Kushniruk is also an Adjunct Associate Professor at the University of Toronto Faculty of Medicine and the Mt. Sinai School of Medicine in New York, and was previously an Associate Professor in Information Technology at York University. Dr. Kushniruk conducts research in a number of areas, including evaluation of the effects of technology, human-computer interaction in health care, and other domains, as well as cognitive science. His work is known internationally, and he has published widely in the area of health informatics. He focuses on developing new methods for the evaluation of information technology and studying human-computer interaction in health care, and he has been a key researcher on a number of national and international collaborative projects. His work includes the development of novel methods for conducting video analysis of computer users, and he is currently extending this research to remote study of e-health applications and advanced information technologies, including computerized patient record systems. Dr. Kushniruk has held academic positions at a number of Canadian universities, and he has taught courses in areas such as human-computer interaction, database management, and systems analysis and design. He holds undergraduate degrees in Psychology and Biology, as well as a M.Sc. in Computer Science and a PhD in Cognitive Psychology from McGill University.

Jan Marco Leimeister is a Full Professor of Information Systems and holds the Chair for Information Systems at Kassel University since 2008. He runs research groups on virtual communities, e-health, service engineering, and ubiquitous/mobile computing, and manages several publicly funded research projects. His teaching and research areas include IT innovation management, service science, ubiquitous and mobile computing, collaboration engineering, e-health, online communities, and IT management.

Malcolm Maclure's career has moved gradually from 'micro' to 'macro' sciences. At Oxford, he studied biochemistry. At Harvard, he studied and conducted chronic disease epidemiology. His teaching shifted to health services epidemiology during the decade he served in the BC Ministry of Health in the 1990s. His current investigations mainly concern pharmaceutical policy research and knowledge translation studies. Among epidemiologists, he is best known for inventing the case-crossover study design to study triggers of acute events. In health services and policy research, he is increasingly known for inventing camouflaged contacting (a method of using administrative databases to contact patients while preserving data privacy) and developing low-cost randomized policy trials (the use of randomized delays in implementation to enable rigorous evaluation with central administrative databases).

Miguel Vargas Martin is an Associate Professor at the University of Ontario Institute of Technology (Oshawa, Canada). Before joining UOIT, he was a post-doctoral Researcher at Carleton University and Alcatel Canada. He holds a Ph.D. in Computer Science (Carleton University), a Master's degree in Electrical Engineering (CINVESTAV, Mexico), and a Bachelor of Computer Science (Universidad Autónoma de Aguascalientes, Mexico). He has reported his work in over fifty journals, book chapters, conference papers, technical reports, and pending patents, and so far has supervised over 20 students at the graduate and undergraduate level. His current research interests include computer forensics, mitigation of denial-of-service attacks, security and human computer interaction, hidden communication channels, and web modeling and optimization.

Wendy Moncur completed her PhD in Computing Science at Aberdeen in 2010; her research produced a model for the provision of adaptive eHealth information to patients' family and friends. Wendy's research interests include socio-technical systems, social networks, personalisation, affect, and health informatics. She has carried out qualitative and quantitative research with users in such diverse settings as schools, Intensive Care Units and family homes. Wendy is actively involved in the international research community, serving as a committee member, panel chair and journal reviewer. She has also worked extensively in industry as a Database Designer for FTSE 100 companies.

Elia Oliver is a Researcher at the University of Valencia, Spain. Her research interests include clinical application based on information and communication technologies (ICTs) in the treatment of childhood obesity. She studied a Master in Psychopathology, Health and Neuropsychology and currently she is doing the Doctoral focused on the use of information and communication technologies (ICTs) for the treatment of childhood obesity.

Azucena Garcia-Palacios is Professor of Abnormal Psychology from 2002 at Universitat Jaume I in Castellon, Spain, and member of Labpsitec, research team leadered by Dr. Cristina Botella. She has participated as a researcher in a wide number of research proyects funded by national and European agencies, being principal investigator in four of those projects. The main lines of research Dr. Garcia-Palacios works on are the design and evaluation of cognitive-behavioral programs for the treatment of several mental disorders and the study of the use of information and communication tecnologies (ICTs) for the improvement of interventions in the field of Clinical and Health Psychology. Professor Garcia-Placios is an author of twenty book chapters and of more than 40 papers published in prestigious national and international scientific journals.

Jacob Palme was appointed to the position of tenured Professor in Computer and Systems Science at Stockholm University, Sweden, in 1998. He is now Professor Emeritus. He has authored four textbooks in the computer science area, published numerous papers in international peer-reviewed scientific journals, conferences and scientific books, and he has been invited speaker at many international scientific conferences. Jacob Palme is development manager of the very successful informational web site in the area of psychology and psychiatry, http://web4health.info/. It has about 900 informational texts, most of them translated to multiple languages, and more than one million page downloads by visitors each month. The web site has received multiple commendations, including selection as a finalist for the eEurope price 2004. Jacob Palme has also been editor in the MHTML working group that produced a standard for sending HTML-formatted documents in e-mail, which was published in March 1997 as RFC 2110/2557.

Laura C. Rodríguez-Martínez is a Full-time Professor-Researcher in Software Engineering at the Instituto Tecnológico de Aguascalientes in Aguascalientes, Mexico. She holds a PhD (2009) and a MS (2006) degrees in Computer Sciences with Software Engineering specialty from Universidad Autónoma de Aguascalientes located in Aguascalientes, Mexico. Her BS is in Computer Systems Engineering with Programming specialty from the Instituto Tecnológico de la Laguna, Torreon, Mexico (1991). She has worked as a Software Engineering in Mexican private enterprises from 1998. Her current research interest is in service-oriented software engineering, artificial intelligence and human-computer interfaces, design of software-system development life cycle, and processes of business processes modeling for software-intensive and information systems.

Shelly Rodgers is an Associate Professor of Strategic Communication at the Missouri School of Journalism. Dr. Rodgers is nationally ranked as one of the top five Internet researchers in the U.S., and is among the top 10 most cited Internet scholars in the U.S. Research areas include strategic communication, advertising, Internet advertising, interactive media, new technology, and health communication. She has been funded by state and national agencies for more than $7 million in grants. Her research has been published by many of the leading academic health communication and advertising journals including the *Journal of Advertising*, *Journal of Communication*, *Journal of Advertising Research*, *Journal of Interactive Advertising*, *Marketing Research*, *Social Marketing Research,* and *Journal of Health Communication*. She is the elected 2010 President of the American Academy of Advertising.

Hélène Sandmark is Associate Professor in Public Health Sciences at Mälardalen University, Sweden. She received her PhD in Occupational Medicine at Karolinska Institutet in 1999. For six years she has been the Director of a research program on working women's health and psychosocial stressors, as well as on studying sustainable work ability. She joined a new research program using social media in health promoting measures in collaboration with ICT researchers. Her earlier research activities focused on identifying risk factors for severe knee osteoarthrosis in work life in men and women. She has primarily used epidemiological research methodology. She teaches on all levels in the public health science program at Mälardalen University.

Karin Janina Schweizer is working with Microsoft Deutschland GmbH. She graduated from Hohenheim University in Communication Sciences in 2006. Her research interests include virtual communities, healthcare, social media, and computer-mediated communication.

David Sloan is an inclusive design Researcher with over 10 years experience researching into methods for enhancing accessibility and usability of information and communication technology to excluded groups, particularly disabled and older people. He has particular interests in web accessibility, inclusive e–learning, and educating digital content creators in inclusive design approaches; his PhD research focused on the impact of web accessibility audits on organizational approaches to inclusive design. He also leads the Digital Media Access Group, an in-house web accessibility and inclusive design consultancy group, and has advised many organizations in industry and the public sector on inclusive technology design and use.

Jennifer N. Stinson, RN, PhD, CPNP, is an Assistant Professor in the Lawrence S. Bloomberg Faculty of Nursing, at the University of Toronto. She is a Clinician Scientist in Child Health Evaluative Sciences and an Advanced Practice Nurse in the Chronic Pain Program at the Hospital for Sick Children in Toronto. Her major clinical research interests are in the area of pain and symptom management and the use of e-health technologies to improve the assessment and management of pain and other symptoms in children with chronic illnesses. She recently received a Career Scientist Award from the Ontario Ministry of Health and Long Term Care for her research on using e-health to promote chronic disease self-management in youth with chronic health conditions. She has made over 50 presentations about the broad area of chronic pain and has 35 publications to her credit.

Roar Stokken is a researcher at the Patient Education Resource Centre at Sunnmøre Hospital Trust in Norway. In its activities the resource centre collaborates with units at this hospital, with municipalities, users' organizations, academic institutions, and with other hospitals. His main research interest concerns human interaction and learning in the context of health care. Topics investigated span from self-help, via patient education and user involvement to the role of knowledge in the interaction between patient and health professional. His research is mainly qualitative, participatory and theoretically founded, drawing upon and contributing to research fields such as ICT in health care, health management, and medical sociology.

Cecilia Strand has a Master's degree in Media and Communication from Lund University, Sweden, and a Bachelor degree in Psychology from Stockholm University, Sweden. She is enrolled as a PhD candidate at the Department of Informatics and Media at Uppsala University, and plans to complete her PhD in media and communication in late 2011 with a thesis subject: Print media in Namibia, Lesotho and Uganda and their coverage of the HIV epidemic. Between 2003- 2009, Strand worked as a communication officer at UNDP Lesotho, and communication officer at Afrikagrupperna in Namibia and finally as program officer at the Swedish Embassy in Namibia.

Ye Wang is an assistant professor of journalism at the University of Missouri - Kansas City. Her research areas include online health communication, interactive advertising, and strategic communication for non-profit organizations. She has an article in *International Journal of Advertising*, a book chapter about electronic word-of-mouth, and has presented conference papers at the American Academy of Advertising and the Association for Education in Journalism and Mass Communication.

Erin Willis is an assistant professor of journalism at the University of Memphis. Her research areas include online health communities, chronic disease self-management, health communication, and health literacy. She has presented at the American Academy of Advertising, Health Communication Annual Research Conference, Kentucky Health Communication conference, and the Association for Education in Journalism and Mass Communication conference.

Jennifer Yeager is a Lecturer of Psychology and is currently engaged in research on the online social support needs of rape and sexual abuse survivors. Her research has employed a netnographic methodology to examine the support implications of survivors utilizing support groups for survivors of sexual violence. Jennifer suggests that collecting sensitive data via the internet is a viable option for social research but needs to work within strict ethical and practical boundaries in order to gain the best results. In general, Jennifer's completed and current studies aim to develop knowledge, ideas, and theories that will be of use to various professionals working with survivors of sexual abuse. This research will inform new ideas, theories, and policy for working with survivors.

Index

A

Action Case 279, 281, 292, 301
action research 180-181, 281, 301
Active Ageing 71
activist community 253
adaptive structuration (AST) 287, 300
Adherence treatment 35
adult health care system 39
advocate 19
AIDS Action Council (AAC) 245, 248, 254-258, 260-261
AIDS crisis 248, 261
American Society of Gerontology 58
anorexia nervosa 122-124, 128
anti-retroviral treatment 107, 117
application sharing 280, 284, 286, 291, 298
Assessment level 66
Association of People Living With HIV/AIDS (NAPWA) 258
Australian Capital Territory (ACT) 6, 94, 107-108, 117, 140, 165, 184, 216, 218, 245-255, 257-258, 260-261, 273

B

Basic 4, 10, 12, 22-23, 48, 104, 112, 139, 151, 196-197, 209-213, 215, 217-218, 225, 227, 240, 268, 272, 286
behavioural interventions 42
binge eating disorder 122, 126
biomedical model 250
bloggers 106, 109, 111-115, 117, 120
blogging 106-111, 113, 116-118, 120, 228
Body Mass Index (BMI) 26, 34, 123-124, 132-133, 214, 216
Books of Life 62, 64-66
bulimia nervosa 122-123, 125-126, 128
bulletin board systems (BBS) 155

C

Canadian Health Services Research Foundation (CHSRF) 280, 296, 299, 301
Canadian Optimal Medication Prescribing and Utilization Service (COMPUS) 281, 299
Cancer Patient 72-73, 77, 79
Center for Epidemiologic Studies Depression Scale (CES-D) 183
Center for Health Workforce Studies 58, 69
Centers for Disease Control and Prevention (CDC) 152, 209, 212-214, 220
chatrooms 180, 185
Childhood obesity 24-26, 32-33, 35
Chi-square tests 78
choice of conduct 6, 13, 17
chronic childhood illnesses 42
chronic disease 36, 38, 41, 50, 52, 55, 107, 161, 163, 168, 173, 210-211, 218-219, 221, 223, 249, 252, 263
chronic disease self-management 36, 38, 161, 163, 168, 173
Chronic Disease Self-Management Program (CDSMP) 161, 163, 168
chronic health conditions 36-39, 41-42, 49-50, 54, 214
citizen-centred care 263
civic literacy 212, 215-218
Clinical Support System (CSS) 24, 27-28, 31
Code of Conduct 10, 12
Cognitive-Behavioral Treatment 26
Cognitive Behavioural Therapy (CBT) 26, 42, 56, 142
collaborative technologies 280
combination phase 159, 161, 166, 168-169, 172, 176
Commonwealth Corporations Act 248
Communicative 137, 148-149, 185, 193, 212, 229
Community-building 6, 13, 17, 258

co-morbidities 195, 202
compulsive disorders 124
Computed Tomography (CT) scans 267
computer-based nutrition 26
computer-mediated communication (CMC) 5, 72, 74-76, 79-82, 84, 104, 119-120, 153-154, 210, 219, 221-222, 224, 226
constrainers 177
Constructionism 5-6, 22-23
content analysis 85, 87-88, 103-104, 106, 108, 120, 192, 208, 213, 215-217, 220-221, 285-286, 300
Content creation 6, 13-14
contingency management 49
Continuous Learning 144
controlled trial 33-35, 41-42, 47-49, 51-55
coping methods 86
critical literacy 212
cultural literacy 212, 215-217

D

data controller 268
data protection legislation 267-268
decision support tool 269
demand-control model 140
design based research 180
Design Guidelines 72, 243
desktop sharing 280
desktop web-conferencing 280
Diabetes ACT 245, 248-251, 253, 255, 258, 260-261
digital divide 61, 195, 199, 205
digital economy 194, 207
digital exclusion 195, 206
Digital Imaging and Communications in Medicine (DICOM) 269
Disease management 37, 39, 50, 55, 263
disembedding mechanisms 185
document management 280

E

eating disorders 100, 105, 121-123, 126, 128-129, 131-135, 180, 187-188, 192
eCommerce Directive 270
E-Curriculum 4, 7, 10, 23
e-health 24-27, 31-32, 35, 39, 56-57, 60-61, 68-69, 71, 119, 136, 139, 149, 152, 156, 194-197, 199-200, 203-204, 207-209, 213, 217-219, 225-234, 236, 238-240, 243-244, 247-248, 252, 259, 262-277
e-health applications 26, 57, 196, 226-227, 230, 238, 267, 271
E-health communities 136, 139, 149, 152, 195, 225-230, 232-233, 236, 238-240, 247-248, 259
e-health literacy 208-209, 213, 217-219
e-health resource 196, 199
e-health services 156, 196, 263-265, 271, 274
e-health systems 139, 152, 194-197, 199-200, 203-204, 263-264, 273
elderly population 59, 61, 67-69
Electronic Health Records (EHRs) 263, 269, 274
electronic patient records 264
Electronic Self-help Groups (ESGs) 177-178, 181-182, 186-187, 190-191, 193
emotional support 59, 72, 79, 83-86, 96-97, 100-101, 108, 182-183, 201-202, 204, 214, 224
enablers 177
environmental stressors 86
ePrescriptions 263, 274, 277
ETIOBE 24, 26-28, 30-34
European Association of Obesity (EASO) 25
European Commission 61, 106, 119, 196, 263, 265, 269, 271, 273-277
European Committee for Standardization (CEN) 269, 278
European Patients Forum (EPF) 266
European Public Health Alliance (EPHA) 266
European Reference Networks 274
European Union (EU) 25, 84, 119, 262-268, 270-278
exergaming 32, 34
existential anxiety 182
experiential knowledge 155-161, 163-164, 166, 169, 171-173, 176
externalization phase 160

F

Facebook 112, 114, 135, 185, 201, 230-232, 240
face-to-face contact 26, 201
Face to Face (FtF) 7, 9, 13, 109, 142, 226-227, 229, 238, 240
face-to-face groups 26, 155-156, 188
face-to-face self-management programs 40
face-to-face setting 164, 280
face-to-face treatments 42
Feedback Mechanisms 144
food pyramid 28-29
functional literacy 208, 212, 215, 217
fundamental literacy 212

G

gastric bypass surgery 126, 214
gay, lesbian, bisexual, transsexual (GLBT) 254-256
gay, lesbian, bisexual, transsexual, queer, injecting drug user (GLBTQI) 256
gender normativity 257

H

haemophiliacs 255
health activism 248
Health Care Consumers Association of ACT (HCCA) 248, 251-255, 258, 260-261
healthcare professional 196, 263, 267
health citizenship 248, 250-251
Health Level Seven (HL7) 269
health literacy 208-224
health portals 263
healthy habits 26, 57, 152
HIV 100, 103, 106-120, 211, 221, 254-258, 261
HIV-infection 106-108, 118
HIV-positive status 106-107
Home Support System (HSS) 24, 27-32
human-centred design 195
Human-Computer Interaction (HCI) 71, 196-197, 205-206, 229, 242, 244, 299-300

I

immediate feedback 26, 49
Information and Communication Technologies (ICTs) 26, 32, 35, 58, 60-61, 67-68, 184, 195, 198-199, 203, 205, 220, 245-247, 250-252, 255, 259, 263, 265-266, 271-273, 275-278, 280, 287, 290-293, 298-299, 301
information sharing 111-115, 137, 280, 290, 292, 299-300
Instituto Tecnológico de Aguascalientes (ITA) 225, 231, 238
interactive characters 1, 4, 10
Interactive Health Communication Applications (IHCA) 40-41, 52
interactive literacy 208, 212, 215-217
intercoder reliability 215
internalization phase 160-161
Internet based intervention 35, 40, 71
Interpersonal utility 75, 78-79
Iterative design 198

J

Joint Technology Initiatives (JTI) 266
juvenile idiopathic arthritis (JIA) 43, 47-51, 53

K

Knowledge Exchange 158, 166, 279-281, 286-287, 289-290, 292-299, 301

L

Lead Market Initiative (LMI) 266, 276-277
lecturette 166, 171

M

marital dyads 105
media literacy 213
medical history 9, 264
mega-band 200
Member States 263, 265-267, 270, 274, 276, 278
Mobile Support System (MSS) 24, 27-31
multiplayer video games 3
multi-user environment 2

N

National Center of Patient Education (NCPE) 178, 193
National Diabetes Services Scheme (NDSS) 248
Neonatal Intensive Care Unit (NICU) 201

O

Obesogenic environment 24-25, 32, 35
Online communities 22, 72-78, 80, 82-84, 110, 119, 137-139, 152-153, 174, 194-195, 207, 210-213, 216, 255, 257-258
online health communities (OHCs) 137-138, 208-214, 216-220
Online Self-Help Groups 75-76, 155-156, 171, 179-180, 195
organizational trust 177, 185-186, 188, 190-191

P

paediatric chronic illness 37
participative inquiry research methods 180
patient-friendly 262-264, 278
Patient-Friendly Healthcare Service 278
pediatric cancer patients 1, 10
peer networks 258

peer-support network 2
peer-to-peer communication 263
People Living with HIV/AIDS (PLWHA) 106, 255, 257
Personal Digital Assistant (PDA) 29-31, 33, 227
physical activity program 26
physical wellbeing 146-147
pilot testing 42
Positive Psychology 58, 69-71
Positive Technological Development (PTD) 1-2, 5-7, 10-14, 19-21, 23
Positive Youth Development (PYD) 1, 4-6, 21-23
post-transplant pediatric patients 1-2, 7
prediabetes 249
private message 93
psychiatric disorders 122
psycho-social support 106, 117
psycho-social well-being 110, 116
public health policy 262-263, 267

Q

quality of life 36-42, 48-49, 53, 58-59, 62, 68, 70-71, 95, 194, 225-227, 244, 254, 265
Quasi-Experiment 281, 301
questions and answers (Q&As) 138-139, 145

R

radiographs (X-rays) 267
reference-based pricing (RBP) 280

S

sadorexia 133
science literacy 212, 215-217
science, technology and society (STS) 246-247, 260-261
self-diagnosis 125, 132
self-help groups 73, 75-76, 103-104, 110, 113, 137-138, 155-161, 163, 170-175, 177-182, 184-187, 189-191, 193-195, 221, 245, 248
Self-help on Internet based Video Conference (SIVC) 178-181, 183, 185-186, 188-193
self-management education 37, 39-40, 52, 54
self-monitoring tools 44
self-related health (SRH) 142
Serious Games 24, 28, 31, 35
Services of General Economic Interest (SGEI) 270-271
Sexual violence 85-87, 99-101, 103
sleeping pills 129
social activity 59, 120
social climate 60
social commentary 111-114, 116
social connectedness 10-12, 67, 194, 197, 204
social exclusion 60, 194, 198, 207
social interaction 3, 73, 109-114, 158-159, 176, 286, 291-292, 294
social networking 3, 11, 67, 110, 202, 205, 226
social networks 59-60, 62, 151, 200-207, 223, 225, 227, 229, 231, 240-242, 244
social support 3, 13, 37, 40, 43-44, 59, 67, 70, 73, 75-76, 79, 83-89, 99-101, 103-105, 107-110, 113-114, 117-120, 136-137, 140, 154, 194, 196-197, 200-202, 204-207, 209, 211, 219, 221, 223-224, 243, 249
Social Support Behavior Code 85-86, 88-89, 99
sociotechnical systems 247
sound check 284
source of help 90
specified diagnosis 177, 185-186, 188, 191
stress buffering 201
stress intervention 140, 145, 147
stress management system 137-138, 142-143, 145-150
SuperETIOBE 29
Survivors Online 86, 88-89, 93, 96-97, 100-103
sustainability 262-263, 274
sympathy group 200

T

tangible assistance 88, 92-93, 100, 102-103
techno-lay people 178
technoscience 246, 258-261
Telecare 61, 68-69, 71, 243
teleconferencing 280-284, 287-288, 290-292, 295, 297-298, 300-301
telemedicine 178, 263, 265, 267, 274-275, 278
The Butler system 57-58, 61-62, 66-69
The Healthy Plate 28
The Memory Game 29
Therapeutic action level 62, 66
Therapeutic Book of Life (LVT) 62, 64-66
therapeutic management 25
therapy intelligent network (TIN) 29-30
traditional literacy 213
Twitter 112, 185, 240
type-I diabetes 248
type-II diabetes 248

U

Universal Design 198, 205, 228, 243-244
Universidad Autónoma de Aguascalientes (UAA) 238, 240
Universidad Autónoma de Mexico (UNAM) 240
user-centred design (UCD) 195, 197-200, 202-204, 207
U.S. National Institute on Aging 58

V

videoconferencing 64-66, 192, 280, 298
virtual city 1-2, 4, 6, 13, 20
Virtual Communities (VCs) 1-4, 9-10, 18, 20-22, 60-61, 65, 69, 72-73, 80, 82-85, 103, 109, 119, 153, 221, 223, 226-227, 240, 243, 279-280
virtual curriculum 2-3, 5-7, 19
virtual intervention 8, 19-20
Virtual Relationship 72, 74, 77
virtual world 1-6, 10-11, 13-14, 16-19, 21, 71, 143

W

Web 2.0 252
web-based stress management 137, 141-142, 147, 149-150
web-conferencing 280-281, 283-284, 286-298, 301-302
web-conferencing meetings 283, 288, 293, 295, 297-298
Web Content Accessibility Guidelines (WCAG) 198, 207
web forums 185
Weight loss 24, 26-27, 29-35, 42, 127-128, 130-131, 134, 138, 150, 214, 218, 223
white boarding 280
Women with Eating Disorder (WED) 180, 187-189, 192
World Health Organization (WHO) 1-3, 6-13, 16, 19, 26, 28-29, 33, 37, 41, 43, 48, 57-60, 62, 64-67, 71, 74-75, 78-79, 83, 91-92, 94-97, 103, 107, 109-110, 112, 117, 120, 123-124, 126-128, 131-134, 137-139, 142-143, 145, 147-149, 152-153, 155, 164, 168, 172, 175, 178-179, 182, 189, 194-195, 197-200, 203, 207, 210-211, 214, 219, 223-226, 238, 240, 246, 248, 251-257, 264, 268, 271, 273, 277, 282, 292, 296-297
World Wide Web Consortium (W3C) 198, 207

CPSIA information can be obtained at www.ICGtesting.com
Printed in the USA
BVOW021626241011

273893BV00008BC/1/P